PATHOLOGY OF

AIDS

A **Slide Atlas of Pathology of AIDS,** based on
the material in this book, is available. The text of
each of the chapters in this book is presented in
the slide atlas format, in separate vinyl binders,
together with 35mm color transparencies of each
figure. All figures are clearly labelled and num-
bered. Each unit also contains abbreviated slide
captions for reference when using the slides. The
complete set of slide atlas units is available in a
durable presentation slip case. The **Slide Atlas
of Pathology of AIDS** contains a total of 413
slides, some of which are composite mounts of
multiple photographs.

Unit I	Textbook of AIDS Pathology	39 slides
Unit II	Skin, Hematolympho-poietic System, and Cardiovascular System	90 slides
Unit III	Respiratory System	67 slides
Unit IV	Gastrointestinal Tract and Associated Organs	88 slides
Unit V	Urinary Tract, Genital Tract, and Endocrine System	27 slides
Unit VI	Central Nervous System	64 slides
Unit VII	Eyes	32 slides

Further information may be obtained from:

Gower Medical Publishing
101 Fifth Avenue
New York, New York 10003 USA

PATHOLOGY OF

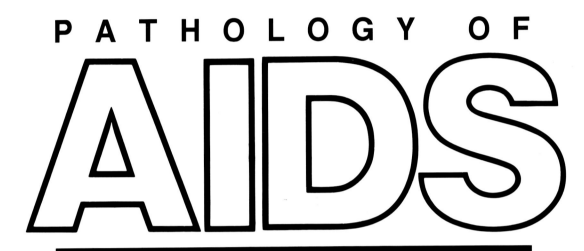

AIDS

*TEXTBOOK AND ATLAS OF DISEASES ASSOCIATED
WITH ACQUIRED IMMUNE DEFICIENCY SYNDROME*

HARRY L. IOACHIM, MD

Director, Department of Pathology
Lenox Hill Hospital
Clinical Professor of Pathology
College of Physicians and Surgeons of Columbia University
Professor of Pathology, New York Medical College

J. B. Lippincott Company • Philadelphia
Gower Medical Publishing • New York • London

Distributed in USA and Canada by:
J.B. Lippincott Company
East Washington Square, Philadelphia, PA 19105, USA

Distributed in UK and Continental Europe by:
Harper & Row Ltd
Middlesex House, 34-42 Cleveland Street, London W1P 5FB, UK

Distributed in Australia and New Zealand by:
Harper & Row (Australasia) Pty Ltd
P.O. Box 226, Artarmon, N.S.W. 2064, Australia

Distributed in Southeast Asia, Hong Kong, India and Pakistan by:
Harper & Row Publishers (Asia) Pte Ltd
37 Jalan Pemimpin 02-01, Singapore 2057

Distributed in Japan by:
Igaku Shoin Ltd
Tokyo International, P.O. Box 5063, Tokyo Japan

Distributed in Philippines/Guam, Middle East, Latin America and Africa by:
Harper & Row International
East Washington Square, Philadelphia, PA 19105, USA

ISBN 0-397-44556-3

Library of Congress Cataloging-in-Publication Data

Ioachim, Harry L., 1924–
    Pathology of AIDS.
    Includes bibliographies and index.
    1. AIDS (Disease)—Atlases.   2. AIDS (Disease)
I. Title. [DNLM: 1. Acquired immunodeficiency Syndrome—
complications—atlases.   2. Acquired Immunodeficiency
Syndrome—pathology—atlases. WD 308 I64p]
RC607.A26I65 1989   616.97'92   88-81418

ISBN 0-397-44556-3

British Library Cataloguing in Publication Data

Ioachim, Harry L.
    Pathology of AIDS
    1. Man. AIDS. Pathology
    I. Title
    616.9'792'07

ISBN 0-397-44556-3

Editor: Kristin Robie
Art Director: Jill Feltham
Cover Design, Book Design and Layout: Jacqueline Elsawaby
Illustrator: Carol Kalafatić

10 9 8 7 6 5 4 3 2 1

Printed in Singapore by Imago Productions (FE) PTE, Ltd.

TABLE OF CONTENTS

Textbook of AIDS Pathology

section ONE

Atlas of AIDS Pathology

section TWO

ACKNOWLEDGMENTS

Contributions from the following physicians, who provided photographs, tissue sections or permission to reproduce previously published material, is gratefully acknowledged:

Melvin N. Blake, DDS, Lenox Hill Hospital, New York

Jacques Diebold, MD, Faculté de Medicine, Hôtel Dieu, Paris

Alan H. Friedman, MD, Lenox Hill Hospital, New York

Deborah Greenspan, BDS, University of California, San Francisco

Herbert A. Hochman, MD, Lenox Hill Hospital, New York

Vijay V. Joshi, MD, Children's Hospital, Newark, New Jersey

Robert J. Lewis, MD, Sun Coast Hospital, Largo, Florida

Carol K. Petito, MD, New York Hospital, Cornell Medical Center, New York

Yale Rosen, MD, Brookdale Hospital Medical Center, New York

Lewis M. Rothman, MD, Lenox Hill Hospital, New York

James Sciubba, DMD, PHD, Long Island Jewish Medical Center, New York

Peter A. Seitzman, MD, Lenox Hill Hospital, New York

Gurdip S. Sidhu, MD, Veterans Administration Medical Center, New York

James A. Strauchen, MD, Mount Sinai Medical Center, New York

Harry V. Vinters, MD, University of California, Los Angeles

Also acknowledged with gratitude is the expert work of Tove Bamberger, who typed the manuscript; Kristin Robie of Gower Medical Publishing, who edited this volume, and Jacqueline Elsawaby who created and executed the book's design.

GLOSSARY

STAIN ABBREVIATIONS

STAIN	ABBREVIATION
Elastic van Gieson	EVG
Hematoxylin-Eosin	H&E
Hematoxylin-Phloxin-Saffranin	HPS
Grocott's methenamine silver	GMS
Perox-antiperox	Peroxidase-antiperoxidase
Periodic acid Schiff	PAS

In June 1981, the first report was published on the occurrence of certain opportunistic diseases in homosexual men, diseases that we have since learned to consider a characteristic part of the acquired immune deficiency syndrome (AIDS). Over the seven years that have intervened between that time and the present, the few cases initially reported have grown into a worldwide epidemic, with cases of AIDS being reported from 175 countries. By the time of the Fourth International Conference on AIDS held in June 1988 in Stockholm, Sweden, the World Health Organization had recorded more than 100,000 cases of AIDS and estimated that 5 to 10 million persons had shown seroconversion to the human immunodeficiency virus (HIV). Five hundred thousand to three million of those infected may develop AIDS by the early 1990s.[1]

In the United States, as of July 1988, 66,464 cases including 1054 children with AIDS had been reported. Of these, 37,535 have died.[2] Most of the fatalities have occurred in patients who were diagnosed during the first years of the epidemic, which indicates that the mortality rate eventually will be much higher. At present, more than 1,000,000 Americans are believed to have been infected by HIV. With so many victims to examine and so many intriguing questions to answer, interest in this new disease on the part of both the medical–scientific community and the public at large has reached unprecedented proportions. As a result, clinical data and basic research have progressed faster than ever before, and our general knowledge of AIDS has increased rapidly, as new and unsuspected aspects of the disease continue to be uncovered.

The complexity of the subject necessitates that experts in various fields collaborate with each other if any progress is to be achieved. To enable physicians and scientists to keep abreast of the large number of publications available, it is necessary from time to time to compile comprehensive reviews that update and integrate the relevant information. From the viewpoint of the clinical disciplines, AIDS has proved itself to be entirely different from any previously known diseases, in that it affects not one organ or one system of organs but practically all the tissues and organs of the human body. The background of AIDS is the deregulation of the cellular immune system caused by the HIV infection, which permits pathogenic activity on the part of a host of viruses, bacteria, parasites, and oncogenic agents. Physicians in all specialties have learned to recognize the particular manifestations of AIDS commonly seen in their fields of expertise. Dermatologists and gastroenterologists, gynecologists and pediatricians, ophthalmologists and dentists, endoscopists and neurosurgeons are presently diagnosing various forms of AIDS on a daily basis. Pathology, by its nature, encompasses the full spectrum of lesions and diseases of various organs and tissues. In patients with AIDS, pathologists making surgical pathology or autopsy diagnoses are confronted with an incomparable diversity of inflammatory, vascular, degenerative, and neoplastic changes. Since most of the etiologic agents involved are opportunistic, the pathologic changes they cause are not commonly seen in the general population, which makes their recognition even more difficult.

This atlas, *Pathology of AIDS*, was written in response to the need for help in learning to diagnose these hitherto rare infections. With the aim of assisting physicians—in particular, pathologists, who have to recognize the multiple aspects of AIDS—this volume was developed as a comprehensive, illustrated source of documentation. It is intended as a practical textbook that is easy to consult in the course of daily medical practice. It includes an illustrated inventory of histologic, macroscopic, and roentgenographic images of the lesions that are associated with AIDS. To ensure that it can be easily and rapidly consulted, the atlas is organized by organ systems. For each organ, the pathologic changes that can affect it in the course of HIV infection and its complications are illustrated. Clinical data relating to the case from which the illustrations were obtained are provided so that a proper perspective can be maintained. The presentation of pathology by organ system, while necessary for practical use, does result in a fragmentation of certain clinicopathologic entities. To restore their integrity as multiorgan or systemic diseases, the most common conditions associated with the HIV infection are described separately in the first section of this volume. The descriptions are generally succinct; no attempt is made to analyze the etiology or the pathogenesis of AIDS, which is beyond the scope of this book. Each clinicopathologic entity is, however, presented as an independent chapter containing the pertinent current information, an up-to-date list of references, and a summary table to be used as a means of quick review.

Pathology of AIDS, therefore, comprises both an integrated description and a detailed illustration of the diseases and lesions associated with AIDS. The two parts are closely coordinated and are referenced with the most pertinent publications in the medical literature up to the time of the writing of this book. The continuous increase in the proportions of the AIDS epidemic, coupled with the rapid progress of our knowledge in this field, indicates that information will continue to accumulate at a fast pace, making the need to keep current an urgent priority.

REFERENCES

1. World Health Organization Global Program AIDS —May 31, 1988— Washington, D.C.
2. AIDS Weekly Surveillance Report—US cases AIDS program—Center for Infectious Diseases, Centers for Disease Control, Atlanta, GA.

The definition of the acquired immuno-deficiency syndrome has been periodically revised to include new developments in the understanding of this new clinicopathologic entity. The latest revision was published on August 14, 1987.

REVISION OF THE CDC SURVEILLANCE CASE DEFINITION FOR ACQUIRED IMMUNODEFICIENCY SYNDROME

Reported by
Council of State and Territorial Epidemiologists;
AIDS Program, Center for Infectious Diseases,
CDC Reproduced from *Morbidity and Mortality Weekly Report*, 36:3–9, 1987.

The following revised case definition for surveillance of acquired immunodeficiency syndrome (AIDS) was developed by CDC in collaboration with public health and clinical specialists. The Council of State and Territorial Epidemiologists (CSTE) has officially recommended adoption of the revised definition for national reporting of AIDS. The objectives of the revision are a) to track more effectively the severe disabling morbidity associated with infection with human immunodeficiency virus (HIV) (including HIV-1 and HIV-2); b) to simplify reporting of AIDS cases; c) to increase the sensitivity and specificity of the definition through greater diagnostic application of laboratory evidence for HIV infection; and d) to be consistent with current diagnostic practice, which in some cases includes presumptive, i.e., without confirmatory laboratory evidence, diagnosis of AIDS-indicative diseases (e.g., *Pneumocystis carinii* pneumonia, Kaposi's sarcoma).

The definition is organized into three sections that depend on the status of laboratory evidence of HIV infection (eg, HIV antibody) (Figure 1). The major proposed changes apply to patients with laboratory evidence for HIV infection: a) inclusion of HIV encephalopathy, HIV wasting syndrome, and a broader range of specific AIDS-indicative diseases (Section II.A); b) inclusion of AIDS patients whose indicator diseases are diagnosed presumptively (Section II.B); and c) elimination of exclusions due to other causes of immunodeficiency (Section I.A).

Application of the definition for children differs from that for adults in two ways. First, multiple or recurrent serious bacterial infections and lymphoid interstitial pneumonia/pulmonary lymphoid hyperplasia are accepted as indicative of AIDS among children but not among adults. Second, for children <15 months of age whose mothers are thought to have had HIV infection during the child's perinatal period, the laboratory criteria for HIV infection are more stringent, since the presence of HIV antibody in the child is, by itself, insufficient evidence for HIV infection because of the persistence of passively acquired maternal antibodies <15 months after birth.

The new definition is effective immediately. State and local health departments are requested to apply the new definition henceforth to patients reported to them. The initiation of the actual reporting of cases that meet the new definition is targeted for September 1, 1987, when modified computer software and report forms should be in place to accommodate the changes. CSTE has recommended retrospective application of the revised definition to patients already reported to health departments. The new definition follows:

1987 REVISION OF CASE DEFINITION FOR AIDS FOR SURVEILLANCE PURPOSES

For national reporting, a case of AIDS is defined as an illness characterized by one or more of the following "indicator" diseases, depending on the status of laboratory evidence of HIV infection, as shown below.

I. Without Laboratory Evidence Regarding HIV Infection

If laboratory tests for HIV were not performed or gave inconclusive results and the patient had no other cause of immunodeficiency listed in Section I.A below, then any disease listed in Section I.B indicates AIDS if it was diagnosed by a definitive method.

A. **Causes of immunodeficiency that disqualify diseases as indicators of AIDS in the absence of laboratory evidence for HIV infection**
   1. high-dose or long-term systemic corticosteroid therapy or other immunosuppressive/cytotoxic therapy ≤3 months before the onset of the indicator disease
   2. any of the following diseases diagnosed ≤3 months after diagnosis of the indicator disease: Hodgkin's disease, non-Hodgkin's lymphoma (other than primary brain lymphoma), lymphocytic leukemia, multiple myeloma, any other cancer of lymphoreticular or histiocytic tissue, or angioimmunoblastic lymphadenopathy
   3. a genetic (congenital) immunodeficiency syndrome or an acquired immunodeficiency syndrome atypical of HIV infection, such as one involving hypogammaglobulinemia

B. **Indicator diseases diagnosed definitively**
   1. candidiasis of the esophagus, trachea, bronchi, or lungs
   2. cryptococcosis, extrapulmonary
   3. cryptosporidiosis with diarrhea persisting >1 month
   4. cytomegalovirus disease of an organ other than liver, spleen, or lymph nodes in a patient >1 month of age
   5. herpes simplex virus infection causing a mucocutaneous ulcer that persists longer than 1 month; or bronchitis, pneumonitis, or esophagitis for any duration affecting a patient >1 month of age
   6. Kaposi's sarcoma affecting a patient <60 years of age
   7. lymphoma of the brain (primary) affecting a patient < 60 years of age

8. lymphoid interstitial pneumonia and/or pulmonary lymphoid hyperplasia (LIP/PLH complex) affecting a child <13 years of age
9. *Mycobacterium avium* complex or *M. kansasii* disease, disseminated (at a site other than or in addition to lungs, skin, or cervical or hilar lymph nodes)
10. *Pneumocystis carinii* pneumonia
11. progressive multifocal leukoencephalopathy
12. toxoplasmosis of the brain affecting a patient >1 month of age

II. With Laboratory Evidence for HIV Infection

Regardless of the presence of other causes of immunodeficiency (I.A), in the presence of laboratory evidence for HIV infection, any disease listed above (I.B) or below (II.A or II.B) indicates a diagnosis of AIDS.

A. **Indicator diseases diagnosed definitively,**
   1. bacterial infections, multiple or recurrent (any combination of at least two within a 2-year period), of the following types affecting a child <13 years of age: septicemia, pneumonia, meningitis, bone or joint infection, or abscess of an internal organ or body cavity (excluding otitis media or superficial skin or mucosal abscesses), caused by *Haemophilus*, *Streptococcus* (including pneumococcus), or other pyogenic bacteria
   2. coccidioidomycosis, disseminated (at a site other than or in addition to lungs or cervical or hilar lymph nodes)
   3. HIV encephalopathy (also called "HIV dementia," "AIDS dementia," or "subacute encephalitis due to HIV")
   4. histoplasmosis, disseminated (at a site other than or in addition to lungs or cervical or hilar lymph nodes)
   5. isosporiasis with diarrhea persisting >1 month
   6. Kaposi's sarcoma at any age
   7. lymphoma of the brain (primary) at any age
   8. other non-Hodgkin's lymphoma of B-cell or unknown immunologic phenotype and the following histologic types:
      a. small noncleaved lymphoma (either Burkitt or non-Burkitt type)
      b. immunoblastic sarcoma (equivalent to any of the following, although not necessarily all in combination: immunoblastic lymphoma, large-cell lymphoma, diffuse histiocytic lymphoma, diffuse undifferentiated lymphoma, or high-grade lymphoma)
      Note: Lymphomas are not included here if they are of T-cell immunologic phenotype or their histologic type is not described or is described as "lymphocytic," "lymphoblastic," "small cleaved," or "plasmacytoid lymphocytic"
   9. any mycobacterial disease caused by mycobacteria other than *M. tuberculosis*, disseminated (at a site other than or in addition to lungs, skin, or cervical or hilar lymph nodes)
   10. disease caused by *M. tuberculosis*, extrapulmonary (involving at least one site outside the lungs, regardless of whether there is concurrent pulmonary involvement)
   11. *Salmonella* (nontyphoid) septicemia, recurrent
   12. HIV wasting syndrome (emaciation, "slim disease")

B. Indicator diseases diagnosed presumptively
    Note: Given the seriousness of diseases indicative of AIDS, it is generally important to diagnose them definitively, especially when therapy that would be used may have serious side effects or when definitive diagnosis is needed for eligibility for antiretroviral therapy. Nonetheless, in some situations, a patient's condition will not permit the performance of definitive tests. In other situations, accepted clinical practice may be to diagnose presumptively based on the presence of characteristic clinical and laboratory abnormalities.
    1. candidiasis of the esophagus
    2. cytomegalovirus retinitis with loss of vision
    3. Kaposi's sarcoma
    4. lymphoid interstitial pneumonia and/or pulmonary lymphoid hyperplasia (LIP/PLH complex) affecting a child <13 years of age
    5. mycobacterial disease (acid-fast bacilli with species not identified by culture), disseminated (involving at least one site other than or in addition to lungs, skin, or cervical or hilar lymph nodes)
    6. *Pneumocystis carinii* pneumonia
    7. toxoplasmosis of the brain affecting a patient >1 month of age

III. With Laboratory Evidence Against HIV Infection
With laboratory test results negative for HIV infection, a diagnosis of AIDS for surveillance purposes is ruled out *unless:*
    A. all the other causes of immunodeficiency listed above in Section I.A are excluded; **AND**
    B. the patient has had either:
        1. *Pneumocystis carinii* pneumonia diagnosed by a definitive method;
        2. a. any of the other diseases indicative of AIDS listed above in Section I.B diagnosed by a definitive method;
            b. a T-helper/inducer (CD4) lymphocyte count <400/mm^3.

COMMENTARY
The surveillance of severe disease associated with HIV infection remains an essential, though not the only, indicator of the course of the HIV epidemic. The number of AIDS cases and the relative distribution of cases by demographic, geographic, and behavioral risk variables are the oldest indices of the epidemic, which began in 1981 and for which data are available retrospectively back to 1978. The original surveillance case definition, based on then-available knowledge, provided useful epidemiologic data on severe HIV disease [1]. To ensure a reasonable predictive value for underlying immunodeficiency caused by what was then an unknown agent, the indicators of AIDS in the old case definition were restricted to particular opportunistic diseases diagnosed by reliable methods in patients without specific known causes of immunodeficiency. After HIV was discovered to be the cause of AIDS, however, and highly sensitive and specific HIV-antibody tests became available, the spectrum of manifestations of HIV infection became better defined, and classification systems for HIV infection were developed [2–5]. It became apparent that some progressive, seriously disabling, and even fatal conditions (e.g., encephalopathy, wasting syndrome) affecting a substantial number of

HIV-infected patients were not subject to epidemiologic surveillance, as they were not included in the AIDS case definition. For reporting purposes, the revision adds to the definition most of those severe non-infectious, non-cancerous HIV-associated conditions that are categorized in the CDC clinical classification systems for HIV infection among adults and children (4,5).

Another limitation of the old definition was that AIDS-indicative diseases are diagnosed presumptively (i.e., without confirmation by methods required by the old definition) in 10%–15% of patients diagnosed with such diseases; thus, an appreciable proportion of AIDS cases were missed for reporting purposes (6,7). This proportion may be increasing, which would compromise the old case definition's usefulness as a tool for monitoring trends. The revised case definition permits the reporting of these clinically diagnosed cases as long as there is laboratory evidence of HIV infection.

The effectiveness of the revision will depend on how extensively HIV-antibody tests are used. Approximately one third of AIDS patients in the United States have been from New York City and San Francisco, where, since 1985, <7% have been reported with HIV-antibody test results, compared with >60% in other areas. The impact of the revision on the reported numbers of AIDS cases will also depend on the proportion of AIDS patients in whom indicator diseases are diagnosed presumptively rather than definitively. The use of presumptive diagnostic criteria varies geographically, being more common in certain rural areas and in urban areas with many indigent AIDS patients.

To avoid confusion about what should be reported to health departments, the term "AIDS" should refer only to conditions meeting the surveillance definition. This definition is intended only to provide consistent statistical data for public health purposes. Clinicians will not rely on this definition alone to diagnose serious disease caused by HIV infection in individual patients because there may be additional information that would lead to a more accurate diagnosis. For example, patients who are not reportable under the definition because they have either a negative HIV-antibody test or, in the presence of HIV antibody, an opportunistic disease not listed in the definition as an indicator of AIDS nonetheless may be diagnosed as having serious HIV disease on consideration of other clinical or laboratory characteristics of HIV infection or a history of exposure to HIV.

Conversely, the AIDS surveillance definition may rarely misclassify other patients as having serious HIV disease if they have no HIV-antibody test but have an AIDS-indicative disease with a background incidence unrelated to HIV infection, such as cryptococcal meningitis.

The diagnostic criteria accepted by the AIDS surveillance case definition should not be interpreted as the standard of good medical practice. Presumptive diagnoses are accepted in the definition because not to count them would be to ignore substantial morbidity resulting from HIV infection. Likewise, the definition accepts a reactive screening test for HIV antibody without confirmation by a supplemental test because a repeatedly reactive screening test result, in combination with an indicator disease, is highly indicative of true HIV disease. For national surveillance purposes, the tiny proportion of possibly false-positive screening tests in persons with AIDS-indicative diseases is of little consequence. For the individual patient, however, a correct diagnosis is critically important. The use of supplemental tests is, therefore, strongly endorsed. An increase in the diagnostic use of HIV-antibody tests could improve both the quality of medical care and the function of the new case definition, as well as assist in providing counseling to prevent transmission of HIV.

FIGURE I. Flow diagram for revised CDC case definition of AIDS, September 1, 1987

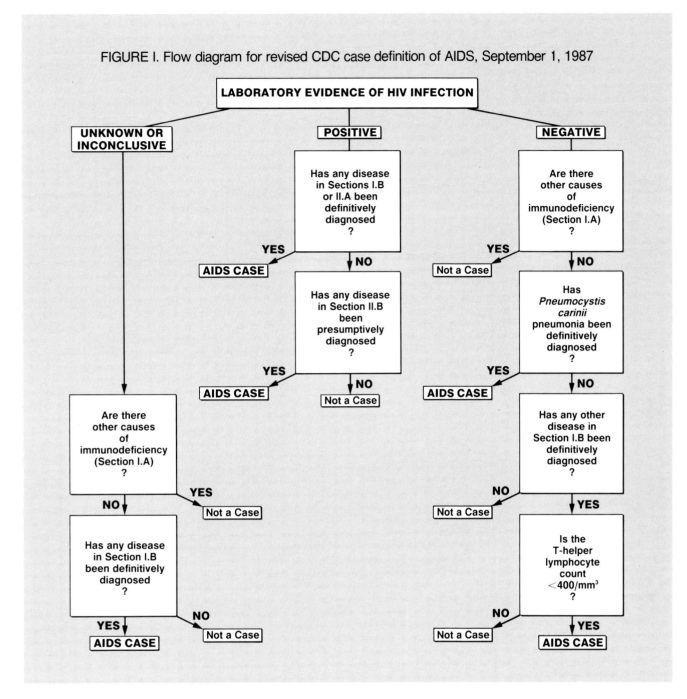

REFERENCES

1. World Health Organization. Acquired immunodeficiency syndrome (AIDS): WHO/CDC case definition for AIDS. WHO Wkly Epidemiol Rec 1986;61:69–72.

2. Haverkos HW, Gottlieb MS, Killen JY, Edelman R. Classification of HTLV-III/LAV-related diseases [Letter]. J Infect Dis 1985;152:1095.

3. Redfield RR, Wright DC, Tramont EC. The Walter Reed staging classification of HTLV-III infection. N Engl J Med 1986;314:131–2.

4. CDC. Classification system for human T-lymphotropic virus type III/lymphadenopathy-associated virus infections. MMWR 1986;35:334–9.

5. CDC. Classification system for human immunodeficiency virus (HIV) infection in children under 13 years of age. MMWR 1987;36:225–30,235.

6. Hardy AM, Starcher ET, Morgan WM, et al. Review of death certificates to assess completeness of AIDS case reporting. Pub Hlth Rep 1987;102(4):386–91.

7. Starcher ET, Biel JK, Rivera-Castano R, Day JM, Hopkins SG, Miller JW. The impact of presumptively diagnosed opportunistic infections and cancers on national reporting of AIDS [Abstract]. Washington, DC: III International Conference on AIDS, June 1–5, 1987.

Textbook of
AIDS Pathology

Clinicopathologic Entities Attributable to HIV Infection

PERSISTENT GENERALIZED LYMPHADENOPATHY (PGL)

Persistent generalized lymphadenopathy (PGL) is a frequent and important manifestation of HIV infection. It was first reported in 1981 by the Centers for Disease Control (CDC) in individuals at risk for AIDS and was described in detail by other investigators in subsequent studies.[1-7] The CDC defined PGL as a palpable lymphadenopathy of more than 1 cm in diameter that is found at two or more extrainguinal sites and has persisted for more than three months in the absence of a causative illness or infection.[8]

The patients are usually in good health before the appearance of lymphadenopathy and may present with fatigue, mild fever, night sweats, loss of appetite, and moderate weight loss.[2,3,9] The lymph nodes are indolent but may attain large proportions and persist for months or years without further complications.[6,7,9-11] More often, however, patients with PGL progress to AIDS and acquire a variety of infections and neoplastic complications.[2,3,5,6,9,12] The immunologic abnormalities induced by HIV infection that characterize AIDS are already present in patients with PGL, though to more moderate degrees. In one early study of 36 patients with PGL, the majority showed moderate decreases in total lymphocyte count and total amount of T lymphocytes. The helper/suppressor T-cell ratios were significantly decreased: the range was 0.52 to 0.81, with an average of 0.64. Though low, these values were not as low as those in patients with AIDS, in whom the range was 0.2 to 0.7 and the average 0.4.[4] Patients with PGL also show polyclonal hypergammaglobulinemia with marked elevation of at least one isotype (most commonly IgD), the presence of circulating anti-lymphocyte antibodies (specifically, anti-T helper cell antibodies), and cutaneous anergy to a variety of antigens.[2,3,10,13] Histologically, the lesions of PGL are consistent and characteristic, though none are unique or pathognomonic for the HIV infection when taken alone.[14,15] Three major microscopic patterns, probably representing pathologic stages, have been described.[2,4,11,12]

Type I (or type A) (see Figs. II.2.12–20) shows features consistent with acute lymphadenitis of viral origin.[3,4,12] These include enlarged coalescing lymphoid follicles taking serpentine or hourglass shapes (see Fig. II.2.12), with markedly hyperplastic germinal centers (see Fig. II.2.13) showing extensive cytolysis, phagocytosis of nuclear debris by tingible-body histiocytes, and cellular regeneration with numerous cells in mitosis (see Fig. II.2.14). The dendritic cell network is disrupted, and small-mantle lymphocytes may invaginate into the follicles.[6,7,16] There are multiple focal hemorrhages (see Fig. II.2.15) and aggregates of monocytoid cells located next to blood vessels (see Figs. II.2.16, 17) These large cells with clear cytoplasm and central nuclei, previously noted in *Toxoplasma* lymphadenitis, were identified by immunohistochemistry to be activated B cells (see Fig. II.2.20).[17,18] There are also clusters of polymorphonuclear neutrophils within the sinuses, which are often associated with the monocytoid cells (see Fig. II.2.17).[4,5] Finally, there are scattered multinucleated giant cells of the Warthin-Finkeldey type, commonly seen in measles, which are characterized by a grapelike cluster of nuclei (see Figs. II.2.18, 19).[4,5]

Type II (or type B) (see Figs. II.2.26, 27) is characterized by the effacement of follicles and partial or total involution of germinal centers. There is depletion of lymphocytes, accumulation of plasma cells (sometimes in prominent sheets), and excessive proliferation of blood vessels in and around the lymphoid follicles.[3-5] These features are suggestive of subacute lymphadenitis or an intermediate phase in the progression of HIV infection.

Type III (or type C) (see Figs. II.2.28–31) shows lymph nodes with atrophic, burnt-out follicles and germinal centers (see Figs. II.2.28, 30). In their place are numerous blood vessels and focal areas of hyalinization (see Figs. II.2.29, 30). Lymphocyte depletion is advanced, and plasma cells are present; however, the dominant features are the extensive proliferation of blood vessels and fibrosis (see Fig. II.2.31). The appearance is that of chronic lymphadenitis with atrophy, angiogenesis, and fibrosis.

Immunohistochemical studies using monoclonal antibodies and immunoperoxidase staining have documented in lymph-node tissues a diminished number of helper T lymphocytes and a relatively increased number of suppressor T lymphocytes, reflecting the reversed ratios of lymphocyte subsets in the peripheral blood,[19] the invasion of follicles by T lymphocytes, and the progressive loss of dendritic cells (**Fig. I.1.1**; see also Fig. II.2.23).[16,20]

The interpretation of the histologic patterns of PGL and their correlation with clinical manifestations and prognosis have been investigated in various studies.[2,7,11,12] Patients with PGL have progressed to AIDS from none to 23% over one to several years in one group.[9] In a study of 93 homosexual men with PGL, AIDS developed in 11.8% between three and 17 months of diagnosis of PGL,

with most cases occurring in those that were diagnosed earlier, indicating that the incidence of conversion from PGL to AIDS is increasing with time.[7] In our own study, clinical follow-up of 75 patients with PGL showed that after intervals of three months to eight years, 35 remained stationary and 40 progressed to AIDS. Of the 40 who progressed to AIDS, 29 died.[11] The three microscopic patterns of lymphadenitis described could be the result of more or less severe infections with HIV, or else could represent sequential stages of progression. Studies of repeated lymph-node biopsies in the same patients seem to favor the latter interpretation by showing the changes to take place in one direction, from type I to type II to type III.[11,12] Some patients may show no further clinical complications and remain with stationary PGL; in these, histologic type I may persist for long periods.[2,11] Most others, however, progress to AIDS and generally exhibit the histologic type III pattern.[2,4,5,6] Moreover, retrospective studies show that the majority of patients who had histologic type I PGL at initial lymph-node biopsy remained clinically stationary, whereas the majority of patients who initially had histologic type III progressed to AIDS and acquired fatal infections and neoplastic diseases.[11,12] It can therefore be concluded that the patterns of lymphadenitis correlate with the clinical progression and prognosis of HIV infection. Histologic types I to III appear to represent stages and progression of the disease.[11]

The etiologic agent of PGL can be detected in the involved lymph nodes. Through use of monoclonal antibodies to core proteins $P_{24/25}$ of HIV, the presence of viral antigen has been demonstrated in lymph nodes of patients with PGL (**Fig. I.1.2**; see also Fig. II.2.25).[21] This was in the form of deposits on the processes of dendritic cells in the affected follicles. Not yet known is whether the HIV-related proteins represent deposition of immunocomplexes or viral replication in the dendritic cells.[21]

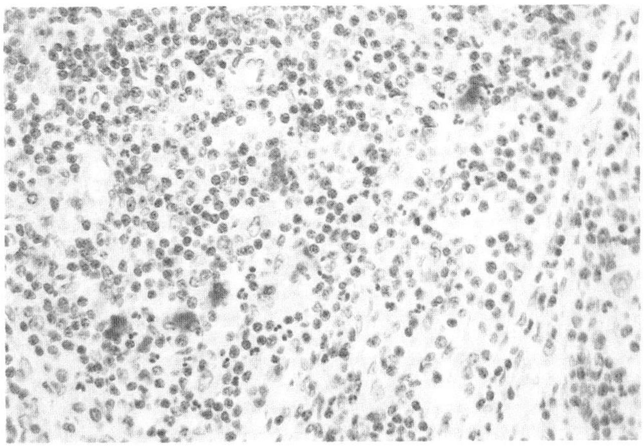

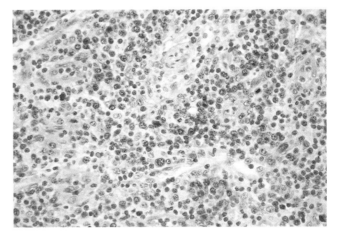

Fig. I.1.1 Few, scattered Langerhans cells stained with anti-S-100 antibody within the germinal center. (PAS, ×250)

Fig. I.1.2 Positively anti-P_{24}-stained cells include monocytoid cells, immunoblasts, and dendritic cells. (PAS, ×400)

These findings are reciprocally confirmed by electron microscopy studies that have demonstrated viral particles with the features of HIV in lymph nodes of patients with PGL or AIDS-related complex (ARC).[22-24] The viral particles described were situated exclusively in the extracellular spaces delimited by the cytoplasmic processes of follicular dendritic cells (**Fig. I.1.3;** see also Fig. II.2.24).[23] These cells linked by functional systems were usually hyperplastic and enveloped other cells within the germinal centers. The viral particles were round and 100 to 120 nm in diameter, with an electron-dense core and an electron-lucent halo. They resembled type C particles; however, budding on the cell membranes was not observed.[23] Such viral particles, though not numerous, were present in 26 of 27 lymph nodes examined in one study.[23] On the basis of their morphologic features, they were identified as HIV particles and characterized as retroviruses. Lymphocytes, endothelial cells, and dendritic cells of PGL lymph nodes may also include unusual formations that are described as tubuloreticular structures, test-tube and ring-shaped forms, and multivesicular bodies (**Figs. I.1.4** and **I.1.5;** see also Figs. II.2.21, 22).[25,26] These may be present in a majority of patients with AIDS or ARC; however, they are not specific and may occur in various viral infections and autoimmune diseases.

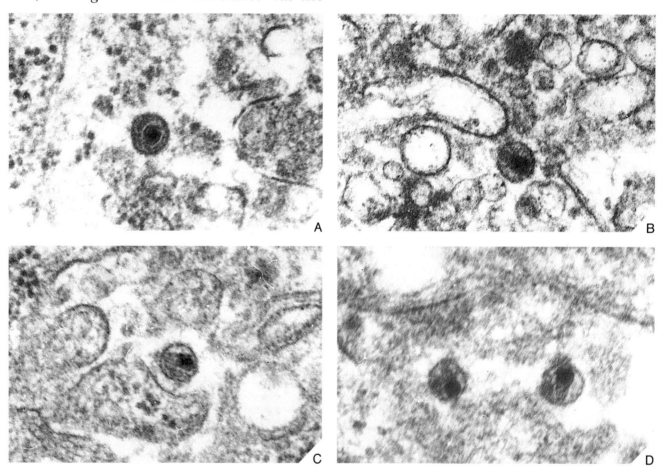

Fig. I.1.3 HIV particles with various morphologic features: **A.** Round, central nucleus. **B.** Rectangular, eccentric nucleus. **C.** Pyramidal nucleus with truncated, inconspicuous apex.

D. Conical nuclei with dark, eccentric base and truncated, inconspicuous apex. (From Le Tourneau et al, 1986.)

(×70,000)

Fig. I.1.4 Test tube or ring-shaped form next to mitochondria in cytoplasm of blood monocyte. (From Sidhu GS et al, 1985)

(×55,000)

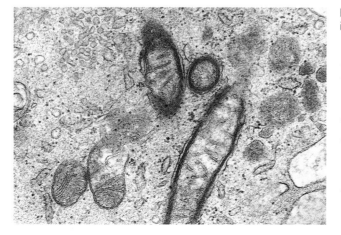

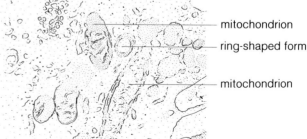

mitochondrion

ring-shaped form

mitochondrion

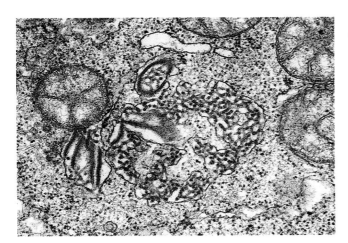

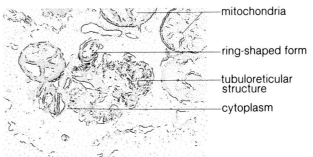

Fig. I.1.5 Tubuloreticular structures inside a test tube-shaped or ring-shaped form, or free in the cytoplasm of blood lymphocyte. (From Sidhu GS et al: *Hum Pathol* 1985;16:380.) (×55,000)

mitochondria

ring-shaped form

tubuloreticular structure

cytoplasm

PERSISTENT GENERALIZED LYMPHADENOPATHIES

Homosexual males, drug addicts, and others at risk for AIDS

Palpable lymphadenopathy, two or more sites, for 3 months

Absence of infection or apparent illness

Reversed helper/suppressor T lymphocytes ratio

Positive anti-HIV antibodies test

Acute lymphadenitis (type A pattern)

    Enlarged lymphoid follicles

    Hyperplastic germinal centers

    Cytolysis

    Tingible-body macrophages

    Hemorrhages

    Monocytoid cells

    Neutrophils

    Multinucleated giant cells

Subacute lymphadenitis (type B pattern)

    Effacement of lymphoid follicles

    Involution of germinal centers

    Partial lymphocyte depletion

    Plasma cells

    Focal angiogenesis

Chronic lymphadenitis (type C pattern)

    Absence of lymphoid follicles

    Atrophic, hyalinized germinal centers

    Lymphocyte depletion

    Extensive angiogenesis

    Plasma cells

    Fibrosis

REFERENCES

1. Centers for Disease Control: Persistent, generalized lymphadenopathy among homosexual males. *MMWR* 1982; 31:249–251.
2. Metroka CE, Cunningham-Rundles S, Pollack MS, et al: Generalized lymphadenopathy in homosexual men. *Ann Intern Med* 1983; 99:585–591.
3. Ioachim, HL, Lerner CW, Tapper ML: Lymphadenopathies in homosexual men. *JAMA* 1983; 250:1306–1309.
4. Ioachim HL, Lerner CW, Tapper ML: The lymphoid lesions associated with the acquired immunodeficiency syndrome. *Am J Surg Pathol* 1983; 7:543–553.
5. Guarda LA, Butler JJ, Mansell P, et al: Lymphadenopathy in homosexual men: Morbid anatomy with clinical and immunologic correlations. *Am J Clin Pathol* 1983; 79:559–568.
6. Brynes RK, Chan WC, Spira TJ, et al: Value of lymph node biopsy in unexplained lymphadenopathy in homosexual men. *JAMA* 1983; 250:1313–1317.
7. Burns BF, Wood GS, Dorfman RF: The varied histopathology of lymphadenopathy in the homosexual male. *Am J Surg Pathol* 1985; 9:287–297.
8. Centers for Disease Control: Classification system for human T-lymphotropic virus type III/lymphadenopathy-associated virus infections. *MMWR* 1986; 35:334–339.
9. Selwyn PA: AIDS: What is now known: III. Clinical aspects. *Hosp Pract* 1986; 21:119–153.
10. Ioachim HL: Acquired immune deficiency disease after three years: The unsolved riddle, editorial. *Lab Invest* 1984; 51:1–6.
11. Ioachim HL, Roy M, Cronin W: Histologic patterns of lymphadenopathies in AIDS: Correlations with progress of disease. Presented at the Third International Conference on Acquired Immunodeficiency Syndrome (AIDS), Washington, DC, June 1–5, 1987.
12. Ewing EP, Chandler FW, Spira TJ, et al: Primary lymph node pathology in AIDS and AIDS-related lymphadenopathy. *Arch Pathol Lab Med* 1985; 109:977–981.
13. Dorsett B, Cronin W, Chuma V, et al: Anti-lymphocyte antibodies in patients with the acquired immune deficiency syndrome. *Am J Med* 1985; 78:621–626.
14. O'Murchadha MT, Wolf BC, Neiman RS: The histologic features of hyperplastic lymphadenopathy in AIDS-related complex are nonspecific. *Am J Surg Pathol* 1987; 11:94–99.
15. Stanley MW, Frizzera G: Diagnostic specificity of histologic features in lymph node biopsy specimens from patients at risk for the acquired immunodeficiency syndrome. *Hum Pathol* 1986; 17:1231–1239.
16. Janossy G, Pinching AJ, Bofill M, et al: An immunohistological approach to persistent lymphadenopathy and its relevance to AIDS. *Clin Exp Immunol* 1985; 59:257–266.
17. Almeida de PC, Harris NL, Bhan AK: Characterization of immature sinus histiocytes (monocytoid cells) in reactive lymph nodes by use of monoclonal antibodies. *Hum Pathol* 1984; 15:330–335.
18. Sohn CC, Sheibani K, Winberg CD, et al: Monocytoid B lymphocytes: Their relation to the patterns of the acquired immunodeficiency syndrome (AIDS) and AIDS-related lymphadenopathy. *Hum Pathol* 1985; 16:979–985.
19. Modlin RI, Meyer PR, Ammann AJ, et al: Altered distribution of B and T lymphocytes in lymphnodes from homosexual men with Kaposi's sarcoma. *Lancet* 1983; 1:768.
20. Biberfeld P, Porwit-Ksiazek A, Böttiger B, et al: Immunohistopathology of lymph nodes in HTLV-III infected homosexuals with persistent adenopathy or AIDS. *Cancer Res* 1985; 45:4665s–4670s.
21. Tenner-Racz K, Racz P, Bofill M, et al: HTLV-III/LAV viral antigens in lymph nodes of homosexual men with persistent generalized lymphadenopathy and AIDS. *Am J Pathol* 1986; 123:9–15.
22. Armstrong JA, Horne R: Follicular dendritic cells and virus-like particles in AIDS-related lymphadenopathy. *Lancet* 1984; 2:370–372.
23. Le Tourneau A, Audouin J, Diebold J, et al: LAV-like viral particles in lymph node germinal centers in patients with the persistent lymphadenopathy syndrome and the acquired immunodeficiency syndrome-related complex. *Hum Pathol* 1986; 17:1047–1053.
24. Tenner-Racz K, Racz P, Dietrich M, et al: Altered follicular dendritic cells and virus-like particles in AIDS and AIDs-related lymphadenopathy. *Lancet* 1985; 1:105–106.
25. Ewing EP, Spira TJ, Chandler FW, et al: Unusual cytoplasmic body in lymphoid cells of homosexual men with unexplained lymphadenopathy. *N Engl J Med* 1983; 308:819–822.
26. Sidhu GS, Stahl RE, El-Sadr W, et al: The acquired immunodeficiency syndrome: An ultrastructural study. *Hum Pathol* 1985; 16:377–386.

LYMPHOCYTIC INTERSTITIAL PNEUMONITIS (LIP)

Pulmonary involvement is common in AIDS patients. It is caused by a variety of infectious agents and by neoplastic processes. In addition to the inflammatory pulmonary lesions in which specific etiologic agents—i.e., viruses, bacteria, fungi, and parasites—have been identified, a type of pneumonia of unknown cause has been also reported. More common in children than in adults, this variety of pneumonia may occur in population groups at risk for AIDS during early stages of the HIV infection (e.g., the AIDS-related complex [ARC], or persistent generalized lymphadenopathy) or during later stages, sometimes at the same time as another complication, such as candidiasis or Kaposi's sarcoma.[1-4] It consists of bilateral pulmonary interstitial infiltrates with lymphocytes causing the symptoms of pneumonia (see Figs. II.4.4, 5).

Lymphocytic interstitial pneumonitis (LIP) was recognized as a clinicopathologic entity before the beginning of the AIDS epidemic.[4,5] Significantly, many cases were associated with various forms of immune disorders such as dysproteinemia, Sjögren's syndrome, chronic hepatitis, chronic thyroiditis, systemic lupus erythematosus, myasthenia gravis, and autoimmune hemolytic anemia.[3-7]

The association of LIP with AIDS was first noted in children, particularly in infants of mothers at high risk for AIDS, and was included in the revised definition of AIDS issued in 1985 by the Centers for Disease Control.[8-10] Subsequently, similar cases were recognized in adults. The incidence was 2% in one series of 150 cases of AIDS, and other studies may yield higher figures.[3] Lymphoid interstitial pneumonia was reported to occur more frequently in Haitians:[4] of seven cases of LIP observed in the Miami area, six involved Haitian immigrants and their offspring. The patients present with moderate fever and weight loss, a nonproductive cough, and increasing dyspnea. Radiologic examination reveals a focal accentuation of interstitial markings initially that progresses to bilateral, diffuse reticulonodular densities.[2-4]

The diagnosis is made histologically through examination of lung tissues obtained by transbronchial biopsy or, if this fails, through open lung biopsy (see Figs. II.4.1–9).[11] The lesions appear as randomly distributed interstitial cellular infiltrates. They comprise a mixed monocellular population that is predominantly lymphocytic, with occasional plasma cells and histiocytes (see Figs. II.4.3, 9). The lymphocytes are of the small, mature type and of the polyclonal B-cell phenotype.[3] The accumulations of cells in the interstitial spaces form nodules that may be sharply demarcated or may extend along the interalveolar septae (see Figs. II.4.1–3, 6–8). In the absence of additional opportunistic infections, the prognosis for LIP is generally favorable; response to corticosteroid treatment has been noted.[3,12]

For some time, the etiology of this entity remained obscure, as all attempts to isolate and identify one of the usual pulmonary pathogens proved unsuccessful. More recently, however, both HIV and anti-HIV antibodies were isolated from bronchoalveolar lavage fluids and from the blood of patients with LIP associated with AIDS.[13,14] The ratio of HIV-specific IgG to total IgG was higher in the bronchial fluid than in the blood, which suggests a local specific humoral immunity to HIV.[13] When an in situ molecular hybridization technique was applied to sections of lung tissue from patients with AIDS-associated LIP, a significant number of cells were found to be positive for HIV RNA.[15] These studies strongly suggest that HIV is directly implicated in the development of LIP, which appears to be one of the initial manifestations of HIV infection in the population groups that are at risk for AIDS.[15]

LYMPHOCYTIC INTERSTITIAL PNEUMONITIS (LIP)

Associated with AIDS and with other immune disorders

AIDS-associated LIP is more common in children than adults

Nonproductive cough, fever, dyspnea

Bilateral, diffuse, reticulonodular pattern

Interstitial infiltrates of lymphocytes, histiocytes, plasma cells

Lymphocytes small, mature, polyclonal B-cell type

HIV and HIV-antibodies in bronchoalveolar lavage fluids

HIV RNA expressed by cells of pulmonary infiltrates

REFERENCES

1. Grieco MH, Chinoy AP: Lymphocytic interstitial pneumonia associated with the acquired immune deficiency syndrome. *Am Rev Respir Dis* 1985; 131:952–955.

2. Kradin RL, Mark EJ: Benign lymphoid disorders of the lung with a theory regarding their development. *Hum Pathol* 1983; 14:857–867.

3. Morris JC, Rosen MJ, Marchevsky A, et al: Lymphocytic interstitial pneumonia in patients at risk for the acquired immune deficiency syndrome. *Chest* 1987; 91:63–67.

4. Saldana MJ, Mones J, Buck BE: Lymphoid interstitial pneumonia in Haitian residents of Florida. *Chest* 1983; 84:347.

5. Liebow AA, Carrington CB: Diffuse pulmonary lymphoreticular infiltrations associated with dysproteinemia. *Med Clin North Am* 1973; 57:809–848.

6. Benisch B, Peison B: The association of lymphocytic interstitial pneumonia and systemic lupus erythematosus. *Mt Sinai J Med* 1979; 46:395–401.

7. Strimlan CV, Rosenow EC III, Weiland LH, et al: Lymphocytic interstitial pneumonitis: Review of 13 cases. *Ann Intern Med* 1978; 88:616–621.

8. Centers for Disease Control: Revision of the case definition of acquired immunodeficiency syndrome for national reporting: United States. *Ann Intern Med* 1985; 103:402–403.

9. Oleske J, Minnefor A, Cooper R, et al: Immune deficiency syndrome in children. *JAMA* 1983; 249:2345–2349.

10. Scott GB, Buck BE, Leterman JG, et al: Acquired immunodeficiency syndrome in infants. *N Engl J Med* 1984; 310:76–81.

11. Marchevsky A, Rosen MJ, Chrystal G, et al: Pulmonary complications of the acquired immunodeficiency syndrome: A clinicopathologic study of 70 cases. *Hum Pathol* 1985; 16:659–670.

12. Stover DE, White DA, Romano PA, et al: Spectrum of pulmonary diseases associated with the acquired immune deficiency syndrome. *Am J Med* 1985; 78:429–437.

13. Resnick L, Pitchenik AE, Fisher E, et al: Detection of HTLV-III/LAV specific IgG and antigen in bronchoalveolar lavage fluid from two patients with lymphocytic interstitial pneumonitis associated with AIDS-related complex. *Am J Med* 1987; 82:553–556.

14. Ziza JM, Brun-Vezinet F, Venet A, et al: Lymphadenopathy-associated virus isolated from broncho-alveolar lavage fluid in AIDS-related complex with lymphoid interstitial pneumonitis (letter). *N Engl J Med* 1985; 313:183.

15. Chayt KJ, Harper ME, Marselle LM, et al: Detection of HTLV-III RNA in lungs of patients with AIDS and pulmonary involvement. *JAMA* 1986; 256:2356–2359.

SUBACUTE ENCEPHALITIS

Neurologic involvement in AIDS was largely underestimated in the early years of the epidemic. More recently, studies have shown that the central nervous system is a major target of HIV infection and its complications. Large series of cases revealed unexpectedly high incidences, severe clinical symptoms, and devastating pathologic lesions. In several of these series, more than 40% of patients with AIDS had neurologic symptoms and signs.[1–3] Moreover, it has been determined that about 10% of all AIDS patients have neurologic problems at initial presentation.[1] Even these high figures, however, fail to indicate the real extent of CNS involvement. According to histopathologic studies, as many as 74% of AIDS patients have neurologic lesions at autopsy.[1,4]

About 30% of the neurologic complications of AIDS are focal processes produced by opportunistic infections and tumors, such as cerebral toxoplasmosis, cryptococcal meningitis, progressive multifocal leukoencephalopathy, and lymphoma.[5] The most common neurologic syndrome in patients with AIDS and ARC, however, is a particular form of subacute encephalitis that leads to cerebral atrophy and progressive dementia. About 60% of AIDS patients with neurologic symptoms have encephalitis; in one series reported on in 1985, 43% of all AIDS patients had this disease.[1,2] It is estimated that as many as 60% of AIDS patients may eventually suffer from dementia. In the early stages of the disease, many AIDS patients complain of loss of ability to concentrate, forgetfulness, and mild confusion.[1,5] A few months later, these patients may become very confused and unable to speak or function. Accompanying these cognitive changes are focal motor symptoms and signs, such as leg weakness, unsteady gait, and poor condition. Cases of hemianopsia, myoclonus, and seizures have been reported.[3] Some patients are unaware of their status, whereas others become apathetic, withdrawn, mute, agitated, or depressed.[1,5] The clinical course of subacute encephalitis is slowly progressive over the course of several months; profound dementia develops gradually.[1,5] Of the AIDS patients who exhibit neurologic symptoms, about 10% show these symptoms before any other manifestations occur, about 40% show them during the ARC phase, and 50% show them after they have already had other complications of AIDS.[5]

The methods available for diagnosing subacute encephalitis are not very efficient. Cerebrospinal fluid analysis yields abnormal results in about 75% of cases, but the findings are somewhat nonspecific—mild protein elevation (50 to 100 mg/dL), mild hypoglycorrhachia, and mild monocellular pleiocytosis.[1,3] Electroencephalography shows diffuse, nonspecific slowing in some cases.[1] A CT scan generally reveals progressive, generalized cortical atrophy with a proportionate enlargement of the ventricles and cortical sulci (see Figs. II.9.1, 5).[1,5]

Histopathologic studies of brains with subacute encephalitis show haphazardly scattered, sparse collections of multinucleated giant cells, accompanied by macrophages and lymphocytes, which involve the white matter of the cortex, midbrain, brainstem, and spinal cord, as well as the gray matter deep in the thalamus and basal ganglia.[2,6] These poorly defined collections of cells are located in areas of demyelination, frequently around blood vessels. (**Fig. I.1.6**; see Figs. II.9.2, 3, 6, 8). In more advanced cases, mineralization of blood vessels, in the form of iron and calcium deposition in vessel walls, can be seen (**Fig. I.1.7**; see Fig. II.9.7).[2,4] The multinucleated giant cells (**Fig. I.1.6**; see Figs. II.9.2, 3, 4, 8) are small, with the cytoplasm obscured by three to five overlapping oval, dark nuclei; they are very similar to the giant cells seen in the lymphadenopathies of ARC and AIDS patients and in tissue cultures infected with HIV.[2,7–9] Other studies of encephalitis asso-

ciated with AIDS, mostly in children, have described an additional type of giant cell—one that is larger, with abundant, irregularly shaped eosinophilic cytoplasm and peripherally arranged nuclei resembling those of Langhans cells—and suggested that the two types of giant cells represent different stages of development.[10] The origin of these giant cells, as demonstrated by histochemical staining, appears to be in the circulating monocytes that are attracted to the brain and fuse there into multinucleated cells under the influence of HIV.[2,7,8] With them may be a few mononucleated macrophages, lymphocytes, microglial cells, and atypical astrocytes.

Electron microscopic examination of brain tissues shows typical retroviral particles budding from and associated with the plasma membranes of infected cells.[3,4,7] These are identified as mononucleated or multinucleated macrophages by the presence of lipid vacuoles and of lysosomes containing myelinlike material.[8,10] The free virus particles are 90 to 140 nm in diameter, with a central zone surrounded by a double electron-dense membrane. Whereas the immature particles have a clear central zone, the mature particles have eccentric, roughly spherical, electron-dense cores measuring about 40 nm in diameter that appear as solid cones or bars, depending on the plane of section.[7,8,10] Retroviral particles have not been observed to bud from oligodendroglial cells, astrocytes, lymphocytes, or endothelial cells.[8] HIV was isolated and identified by in situ hybridization and Southern blot analysis in the brain tissue and cerebrospinal fluid of patients with AIDS encephalitis.[11–13] Tissue sections from the cortices of patients with subacute encephalitis examined by

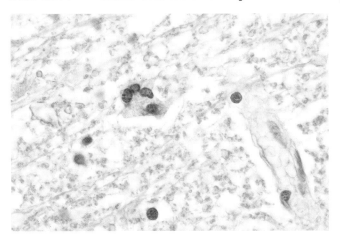

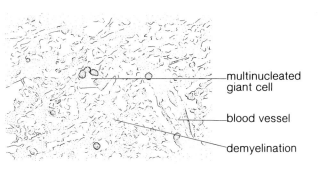

Fig. I.1.6 Subacute encephalitis in HIV infection. Demyelination of cortical white matter and multinucleated giant cell near blood vessel.   (HPS stain, ×1,000)

multinucleated giant cell

blood vessel

demyelination

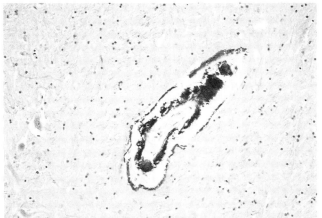

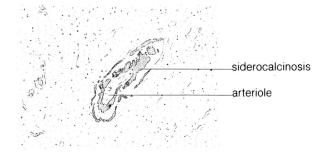

Fig. I.1.7 Subacute encephalitis in HIV infection with siderocalcinosis of cerebral arteriole.   (HPS stain, ×200)

siderocalcinosis

arteriole

in situ hybridization show that 15% to 70% of multinucleated giant cells contain HIV RNA.[8] Besides the giant cells, only a few mononuclear cells in areas of demyelination also contained viral RNA. It appears, therefore, that macrophages, mononucleated and multinucleated, are the cells that actively synthesize HIV, produce mature viral particles, and are the main reservoir for the virus.[8]

In HIV infection, the virus is also known to infect and multiply in T_4 lymphocytes, as demonstrated by in vitro studies.[9] The finding of HIV replication in macrophages, however, calls to mind the CNS disease of sheep in which Visna virus, a lentivirus related to HIV, infects monocytes in the peripheral blood, from which location it is transported along with the cells to the brain, possibly through the cerebrospinal fluid. In subacute encephalitis, it is not clear how brain damage is produced by HIV, that is, whether the damage results from direct action on neural cells through specific recognition of cross-reacting antigens or from the action of factors released by the infected macrophages, which may cause tissue injury and impair neural transmission.[8]

SUBACUTE ENCEPHALITIS

Neurologic symptoms in one third, CNS lesions in two thirds of AIDS patients

Subacute encephalitis, most common neurologic disease in AIDS patients

Slow, progressive, relentless course

Cognitive changes, focal motor symptoms, gradually increasing dementia

Cerebral atrophy, enlargement of sulci and ventricles on CT scan

Focal areas of demyelination; scattered, small cellular infiltrates

Multinucleated giant cells, macrophages, lymphocytes, glial cells

Retroviral particles replicating in mononucleated and multinucleated macrophages

Virions with electron-dense cores surrounded by double membranes

HIV isolated from CSF and brain tissues

HIV RNA in mononucleated and multinucleated macrophages

REFERENCES

1. Levy RM, Bredesen DE, Rosenblum ML: Neurological manifestations of the acquired immunodeficiency syndrome (AIDS): Experience at UCSF and review of the literature. *J Neurosurg* 1985; 62:475–495.
2. Petito CK, Cho E-S, Lemann W, et al: Neuropathology of acquired immunodeficiency syndrome (AIDS): An autopsy review. *J Neuropathol Exp Neurol* 1986; 45:635–646.
3. Snider WD, Simpson DM, Nielsen S, et al: Neurological complications of acquired immune deficiency syndrome: Analysis of 50 patients. *Ann Neurol* 1983; 14:403–419.
4. Anders KH, Guerra WF, Tomiyasu U, et al: The neuropathology of AIDS: UCLA experience and reviews. *Am J Pathol* 1986; 124:537–558.
5. Navia BA, Jordan BD, Price RW: The AIDS dementia complex: I. Clinical features. *Ann Neurol* 1986; 19:517–524.
6. Navia BA, Cho E-S, Petito CK, et al: The AIDS dementia complex: II. Neuropathology. *Ann Neurol* 1986; 19:525–535.
7. Epstein LG, Sharer LR, Cho E-S, et al: HTLV-III/LAV-like retrovirus particles in the brains of patients with AIDS encephalopathy. *AIDS Research* 1984/85; 1:447–454.
8. Koenig S, Gendelman HE, Orenstein JM, et al: Detection of AIDS virus in macrophages in brain tissue from AIDS patients with encephalopathy. *Science* 1986; 233:1089–1093.
9. Popovic M, Sarngadharan MG, Read E, et al: Detection, isolation, and continuous production of cytopathic retroviruses (HTLV-III) from patients with AIDS and pre-AIDS. *Science* 1984; 224:497–500.
10. Sharer LR, Epstein LG, Cho E-S: Pathologic features of AIDS encephalopathy in children: Evidence for LAV/HTLV-III infection of brain. *Hum Pathol* 1986; 17:271–284.
11. Ho DD, Rota JR, Schooley RT, et al: Isolation of HTLV-III from cerebrospinal fluid and neural tissues of patients with neurologic syndromes related to the acquired immunodeficiency syndrome. *N Engl J Med* 1985; 313:1493–1497.
12. Levy JA, Shimabukuro J, Hollander H, et al: Isolation of AIDS-associated retrovirus from cerebrospinal fluid and brain of patients with neurological symptoms. *Lancet* 1985; 2:586–588.
13. Shaw GM, Harper ME, Hahn BH, et al: HTLV-III infection in brains of children and adults with AIDS encephalopathy. *Science* 1985; 227:177–182.

VACUOLAR MYELOPATHY

The spinal cord, in patients with AIDS, may show various forms of degenerative lesions particularly bilateral degenerations of the long tracts. The most common of these is vacuolar myelopathy, which in three large series of autopsies on AIDS patients was found in 13% to 29.6% of cases.[1-4] Its lower incidence in other series and the relatively few studies in the literature probably reflect the fact that the spinal cord is not routinely removed at autopsies of patients with AIDS.[2]

The morphologic changes characteristic of vacuolar myelopathy resemble those found in subacute combined degeneration of the spinal cord; however, AIDS patients have normal levels of vitamin B_1 and folic acid.[3] The prime clinical symptom is spastic ataxic paralysis, often accompanied by urinary and fecal incontinence.[2,3] The myelopathy involves the dorsal columns and the lateral corticospinal tracts and is more severe at the cervical and thoracic levels.[2,4] It consists of symmetric vacuolation (see Fig.II.9.61,9.62), caused by edema within the myelin lamellae, and areas of liquefaction necrosis showing microcavitation and accumulations of lipid-laden macrophages. There are also spongiform alterations with myelin loss, in which the tissue elements seem to be separated.[4] In cases of severe involvement, there is secondary axonal degeneration with varicose axons and axonal spheroids, as shown by silver stainings; however, myelin loss significantly exceeds axon loss.[4] In some cases, similar changes—myelin degeneration and spongiform alteration with collections of macrophages and multinucleated giant cells—are seen to affect the long tracts in the internal capsule as well as in the spinal cord (see Fig.II.9.61).[4] In cases of focal necrosis in the internal capsule, wallerian degeneration has been observed to occur in the corticospinal tracts in the brainstem and sometimes to continue into the spinal cord.[4]

The vacuolar myelopathy observed in AIDS patients, with lesions resembling those of subacute combined degeneration, appears to be another effect of HIV infection. It is not clear at present whether it is the result of degenerative and necrotic lesions in the internal capsule or whether it may occur independently, since in one reported series approximately 60% of AIDS patients with vacuolar myelopathy did not have a multinucleated cell subacute encephalitis.[2,4]

VACUOLAR MYELOPATHY

Bilateral, symmetrical degenerations of the long tracts

Dorsal and lateral columns involved

Lesions of internal capsule often associated

Severe wallerian degeneration of corticospinal tracts

Edema

Spongiform change

Vacuolation

Microcavitation of myelin

Axonal disruption and degeneration

Spastic-ataxic paralysis and incontinence

HIV probable etiologic agent

REFERENCES

1. Anders KH, Guerra WE, Tomiyasu U, et al: The neuropathology of AIDS: UCLA experience and review. *Am J Pathol* 1986; 124:537–558.
2. Petito CK, Cho E-S, Lemann W, et al: Neuropathology of acquired immunodeficiency syndrome (AIDS): An autopsy review. *J Neuropathol Exp Neurol* 1986; 45:635–646.
3. Petito CK, Navia BA, Cho E-S, et al: Vacuolar myelopathy pathologically resembling subacute combined degeneration in patients with the acquired immunodeficiency syndrome. *N Engl J Med* 1985; 312:874–879.
4. Rhodes RH: Histopathology of the central nervous system in the acquired immunodeficiency syndrome. *Hum Pathol* 1987; 18:636–643.

PERIPHERAL NEUROPATHIES

Inflammatory demyelinating peripheral neuropathies associated with AIDS have been described in patients in the late phases of AIDS, when the various opportunistic complications develop, as well as in patients in the early phases of the HIV infection, when few or no other simultaneous symptoms are present.[1,2] In the late phases, patients have painful sensory neuropathies, and electrodiagnostic studies indicate substantial axonal loss.[1] In the earlier phases, patients with peripheral neuropathies also present with fever, night sweats, and lymphadenopathies, or are otherwise symptomless.[1,3]

In a series of nine patients (eight men and one woman) with documented HIV infection, six had chronic inflammatory demyelinating polyneuropathies, and three had the acute form of inflammatory demyelinating polyneuropathy also known as the Guillain-Barré syndrome.[1] In a series of 12 homosexual males, sensory symptoms predominated, though regional weaknesses, headaches, and cranial nerve dysfunctions were also noted.[3] Cerebrospinal fluid was abnormal in all cases; most patients showed increased protein levels (mean, 193 mg/dL) and pleocytosis (mean, 23 cells/μL).[1,3] No abnormalities were noted on CT scans of the brain.[3] The T_4/T_8 ratios were reversed, and HIV antibody tests yielded positive results. The findings from nerve conduction studies were characteristic of demyelination.[1]

Peripheral nerve biopsies in three studies showed similar histologic changes:[1,3,4] demyelination, present in 78% of 20 patients in one study; axonopathy, present in 31%; and mononuclear cell infiltration, present in 40%.[4] The demyelination was patchy and sometimes accompanied by macrophage-mediated myelin stripping and wal-lerian-like degeneration.[1,3,5] One study noted a significant loss of myelinated fibers, with a disproportionately greater loss of the large fibers (see Figs.II.9.63,64).[5] Axons showed attenuation, fragmentation, and sometimes axonal spheroid formation.[1,4,5] There was subperineurial edema and perivascular cuffing by lymphocytes, without involvement of the vascular walls. Endoneurial fibrosis was occasionally observed.[4] Identification of the inflammatory cells by immunohistochemical staining showed the cellular infiltrates to be composed of T cells, predominantly of the T_8 subset, and macrophages without B cells.[4]

The etiology of peripheral neuropathies still is not clearly understood although in recent years the strong neurotropism of HIV and its direct role in the development of subacute encephalitis have been demonstrated. In addition, HIV has been isolated from a sural nerve of a patient with inflammatory demyelinating peripheral neuropathy.[6] Nonetheless, the neural lesions are probably not the result of direct viral action; it is more likely that they reflect viral-induced autoantibody- or macrophage-mediated tissue destruction.[1,4] The profound immune alterations associated with HIV infection may initiate autoimmune reactions directed against myelin and Schwann cells.[1] This process is not unique in HIV infection, which is known to have induced the production of autoantibodies against platelets and lymphocytes. The favorable therapeutical results obtained with corticosteroids and plasmapheresis tend to support this explanation.[1,3]

In contrast to most other manifestations of AIDS, peripheral neuropathies in patients with no other complications may remit spontaneously in as many as 50% of cases.[3]

PERIPHERAL NEUROPATHIES

Early and late phases of HIV infection

Chronic and acute inflammatory, demyelinating polyneuropathies

Painful sensory symptoms

Regional weaknesses

Cranial nerve dysfunctions

CSF abnormal, with increased protein and cellular content

Demyelination

Axonal fragmentation

Monocellular infiltrates

Autoimmune reactions against myelin and Schwann cells

Occasional spontaneous remission

Favorable results with corticosteroids

REFERENCES

1. Cornblath DR, McArthur JC, Kennedy PGE, et al: Inflammatory demyelinating peripheral neuropathies associated with human T-cell lymphotropic virus type III infection. *Ann Neurol* 1987; 21:32–40.
2. Snider WD, Simpson DM, Nielson G, et al: Neurological complications of acquired immune deficiency syndrome: Analysis of 50 patients. *Ann Neurol* 1983; 14:403–418.
3. Lipkin WI, Parry G, Kiprov D, et al: Inflammatory neuropathy in homosexual men with lymphadenopathy. *Neurology* 1985; 35:1479–1483.
4. De la Monte SM, Gabuzda DH, Ho DD, et al: The immunopathology of peripheral nerve disease in AIDS, abstract. Presented at the Third International Conference on AIDS, Washington, DC, June 1–5, 1987.
5. Mah V, Vartavarian L, Akers MA, Vinters HV: Abnormalities of peripheral nerve in patients with acquired immune deficiency syndrome (AIDS). *J Neuropathol Exp Neurol* 1987; 46:380.
6. Ho DD, Rota MA, Schooley RT, et al: Isolation of HTLV-III from cerebrospinal fluid and neural tissues of patients with neurological syndromes related to acquired immunodefiency syndrome. *N Engl J Med* 1985; 313:1493–1497.

THYMIC DYSPLASIA

Normally, the thymus undergoes progressive involution with age, a process that is occasionally accelerated by stress and disease. This involution is characterized by a reduction in thymocytes and the persistence of Hassall's corpuscles and epithelial clusters.[1] The function of Hassall's corpuscles has not been clearly determined, though it is believed that they synthesize thymosin and thymopoetin, hormones that affect T-cell differentiation.[2]

Thymic dysplasia is known to occur in some of the genetic immune deficiencies, such as the severe combined immunodeficiency syndrome, and in graft-versus-host reactions in which Hassall's corpuscles and the thymic medullary epithelium are injured.[3] In AIDS patients, morphologic changes characteristic of thymic dysplasia have been described in adults and children.[1,4,5] In two Haitian women with AIDS and fatal complications of CMV and *Pneumocystis* infections, the thymuses were depleted of thymocytes. There was no distinction between cortex and medulla, there were small infiltrates of plasma cells, and, most important, there were no Hassall's corpuscles and epithelial clusters—the characteristic picture of thymic dysplasia (see Figs. II.2.10, 11). The thymuses of age-matched controls, by contrast, contained numerous epithelial clusters and prominent Hassal's corpuscles.[1] In four children, aged 22 months to 10 years, who died of AIDS, the thymuses were markedly reduced in size and weight, were severely depleted of lymphocytes, exhibited obscured corticomedullary differentiation, and were almost entirely devoid of Hassall's corpuscles.[5] Only by step-serial sections could remnants of Hassall's corpuscles, in the form of calcified cell clusters or microcysts, be found. Profound lymphocytic depletion involving both T and B cells also affected the Peyer's patches of the ileum, the appendix, the lymph nodes, and the spleen.[5]

It is noteworthy that whereas the thymic epithelium is severely damaged in the late phases of AIDS, consistently elevated serum levels of thymosin α_1 have been recorded in the early phases of HIV infection. In one study of eight healthy homosexual males and two patients with Kaposi's sarcoma who had inverted helper/suppressor T-cell ratios, serum levels of thymosin α_1 were markedly increased.[6] The sequence of morphologic changes in the affected thymus and their relationships with its function are not yet well understood. In thymic dysplasia associated with AIDS, these changes are similar to those previously described in other types of immune deficiencies, both congenital and acquired.

THYMIC DYSPLASIA

Adults and children with AIDS

Marked reduction in size and weight of thymus

Severe depletion of thymocytes

Effacement of corticomedullary differentiation

Degeneration and absence of Hassall's corpuscles and epithelial clusters

Lymphocyte depletion of all extrathymic lymphoid tissues

Elevated serum levels of thymosin α_1

hvmic dysplasia in AIDS similar to that in congenital and acquired immune deficiencies

REFERENCES

1. Elie R, Laroche AC, Arnoux E, et al: Thymic dysplasia in acquired immunodeficiency syndrome. *N Engl J Med* 1983; 308:841–842.
2. Trainin N, Pecht M, Handzel ZT: Thymic hormones: Inducers and regulators of the T-cell system. *Immunol Today* 1983; 4:16–21.
3. Borzy MS, Schulte-Wisserman H, Gilbert E, et al: Thymic morphology in immunodeficiency disease: Results of thymic biopsies. *Clin Immunol Immunopathol* 1979; 12:31–51.
4. Grody WW, Naeim F: Histopathology of thymus in acquired immune deficiency syndrome. *Lab Invest* 1984; 50:23A.
5. Joshi VV, Oleske JM: Pathologic appraisal of the thymus gland in acquired immunodeficiency syndrome in children. *Arch Pathol Lab Med* 1985; 109:142–146.
6. Hersh EM, Reuben JM, Rios A, et al: Elevated serum thymosin α_1 levels associated with evidence of immune dysregulation in male homosexuals with a history of infectious diseases or Kaposi's sarcoma. *N Engl J Med* 1983; 308:45–46.

BONE MARROW AND PERIPHERAL BLOOD ABNORMALITIES

Individuals infected by HIV may present as asymptomatic carriers, as patients with AIDS-related complex (ARC) that is, fever of unknown origin, chronic diarrhea and weight loss, as patients with lymphadenopathies—or as patients with the characteristic infections and neoplasias of AIDS. In all these phases of the HIV infection, patients may have anemia, granulocytopenia, and thrombocytopenia in various associations and degrees, according to the severity of the underlying clinical disease. To evaluate these commonly occurring forms of pancytopenia in persons at high risk for AIDS, bone-marrow aspirations and biopsies are frequently performed. Consequently, large series of cases are available for investigation, which makes detailed hematologic studies possible.

In some cases, particularly in AIDS patients, the systemic disease may involve the bone marrow, which then shows the local manifestations of the general infection or neoplasia. Granulomas, with or without necrosis, may be present in the bone marrow in the course of mycobacterial or fungal infections (see Figs. II.2.4, 5).[1,2] Acid-fast or silver stains usually reveal the presence of *Mycobacterium tuberculosis*, the *Mycobacterium avium-intracellulare* (MAI) complex, *Histoplasma capsulatum*, or other organisms. (see Figs. II.2.6, 7). Not infrequently, however, the immunodeficient patient is unable to form granulomas, and MAI is cultured from the peripheral blood or bone marrow, while the tissue sections show no characteristic changes. In one study of 55 bone marrow biopsies, granulomas were not found in six cases with positive MAI cultures.[1] In another eight cases from the same study, granulomas were present, but acid-fast organisms could be demonstrated in only four. In general, bone marrow granulomas in AIDS-associated cases are ill-formed, frequently consisting of a loose aggregate of epithelioid cells without giant cells or necrosis. Overall, culture of bone-marrow aspirates appears to be a more sensitive method than acid-fast staining of tissues for demonstration of MAI infection.[1] Hodgkin's and non-Hodgkin's lymphomas may involve the bone marrow in AIDS patients; occasionally, probably more often in AIDS patients than in non-AIDS patients, they represent the primary location of the neoplastic process (see Figs. II.2.8, 9).[3] Kaposi's sarcoma has not been reported to involve the bone marrow, even when it is widely disseminated.[1]

More difficult to interpret are those bone-marrow biopsies of patients with AIDS or ARC that do not show granulomas or other morphologic changes identified with specific diseases. These actually make up the majority of bone-marrow biopsies in patients with the HIV infection, whether the infection is complicated by other AIDS-associated diseases or not. The bone-marrow changes, although nonspecific, constitute a characteristic pattern that, with minor variations, has been described by all the authors of bone-marrow studies in AIDS patients.[1,2,4-11] Study of the peripheral blood reveals anemia in as many as 83% of all patients with AIDS, leukopenia in as many as 66%, and thrombocytopenia in as many as 100%.[7,10] Pancytopenia that is severe enough to necessitate a bone marrow biopsy has been recorded in more than 60% of cases of AIDS and ARC.[9] In contrast with the decrease in the cellular amount of one or all hematologic series in the peripheral blood, the hematopoietic bone marrow almost invariably appears hypercellular.[1,2,5,8-11] Except in the late stages of AIDS, when the exhausted bone marrow finally becomes hypocellular, there is marked hematopoietic hyperplasia (see Figs. II.2.1-3). The hematopoietic bone marrow is evenly expanded, separating without effacing the adipose tissue.[5,8] The myeloid/erythroid ratio is increased, because the cellular hyperplasia affects the white blood cell series more than the red. There is also a marked increase in the total amount of megakaryocytes, which are usually present in clusters, a tendency often associated with myeloproliferative disorders (see Figs.

II.2.1-3).[8,9] The occurrence of peripheral pancytopenia in conjunction with bone-marrow hypercellularity is an indication of ineffective hematopoiesis or of peripheral cellular destruction.

In addition to the quantitative changes, morphologic cellular abnormalities are usually noted. In the myeloid series, immature, blast-like cells with high nuclear/cytoplasmic ratios and unusual irregular, folded nuclei have occasionally been described; they are considered to represent cellular dysplasia.[9] More striking are the morphologic changes found in the megakaryocytic series, in which abnormal, dysplastic megakaryocytopoiesis is expressed by the presence of immature and atypical forms (see Figs. II.2.2, 3).[8,9] There are numerous megakaryocytes with hyperchromatic, poorly lobulated, apparently pyknotic nuclei surrounded by a small amount of cytoplasm; there are megakaryocytes with large, bizarre nuclei that resemble megakaryoblasts or leukemic cells; and there are bare nuclei, devoid of cytoplasm, that are scattered throughout the hemopoetic bone marrow cells.[8,9] Lymphocytic nodules and mixed collections of small and large lymphocytes, usually not in a paratrabecular position, are common.[1,2,4,10,11] Increased numbers of eosinophils and markedly increased numbers of plasma cells have been recorded; these can be correlated with the presence of hypergammaglobulinemia in 83% of patients.[1,2,4,5,6,11] Proliferation of reticulin fibers in various amounts is consistently observed, and excessive proliferation of blood vessels has been recorded as well.[4,5,8] Iron stores are increased, serum iron is low, and ferritin levels are increased.[1] Focal deposits of hemosiderin can frequently be seen, indicating the occurrence of hemolysis.

The cellular maturational abnormalities and morphologic changes resemble those of myelodysplasia, a syndrome that is considered to represent a preleukemic state;[9] however, flow cytometry examination of seven bone marrow specimens from such patients did not reveal the presence of aneuploid clones.[6]

The pathogenesis of bone-marrow abnormalities associated with AIDS is not well understood. They cannot be attributed to the various complications of AIDS patients, because they often occur in the absence of any apparent opportunistic infection. Nor can they be explained as effects of drug administration, because they have been noted in patients who were under no treatment. Although no direct evidence is yet available, it appears probable that the peripheral pancytopenia and the hematopoietic bone-marrow dysplasia are direct effects of the HIV infection.[9] New evidence indicates the potential pathogenicity of HIV for a variety of organs and tissues that are direct targets for this virus. Thus, HIV may affect hemopoietic cells directly, through deregulation of intercellular functions or through release of damaging cellular mediators.

BONE MARROW AND PERIPHERAL BLOOD ABNORMALITIES

Anemia, granulocytopenia, thrombocytopenia, or pancytopenia

Local involvement in the course of systemic infections and neoplasias

Hypercellularity of hematopoietic bone marrow

Myeloid hyperplasia and dysplasia

Myeloid/erythroid ratio increased

Megakaryocytic hyperplasia and dysplasia

Lymphocytic nodules

Plasmacytosis

Eosinophilia

Reticulin fibers increased

Blood-vessel hyperplasia

Hematopoietic changes attributed to direct HIV effect

REFERENCES

1. Castella A, Croxson TS, Mildvan D, et al: The bone marrow in AIDS: A histologic, hematologic and microbiologic study. *Am J Clin Pathol* 1985; 84:425–432.

2. Osborne B, Guarda LA, Butler JJ: Bone marrow biopsies in patients with the acquired immunodeficiency syndrome. *Hum Pathol* 1984; 15: 1048–1053.

3. Ioachim HL, Cooper MC, Hellman GC: Lymphomas in males at high risk for the acquired immune deficiency syndrome (AIDS): A study of 21 cases. *Cancer* 1985; 56:2831–2842.

4. Franco CM, Hendrix LE, Lokey JL: Bone marrow abnormalities in the acquired immunodeficiency syndrome. *Ann Intern Med* 1984; 101:275–276.

5. Geller, SA, Muller R, Greenberg ML, et al: Acquired immunodeficiency syndrome: Distinctive features of bone marrow biopsies. *Arch Pathol Lab Med* 1985; 109:138–141.

6. Hromas RA, Murray JL: Bone marrow in the acquired immunodeficiency syndrome. *Ann Intern Med* 1984; 101:877.

7. Lake JP, Lee S, Spira S: Bone marrow findings in AIDS patients. *Am J Clin Pathol* 1984; 81:799–800.

8. Pehta J, Cooper MC, Ioachim HL: Abnormal hematopoesis in acquired immune deficiency syndrome (AIDS) and AIDS-related complex (ARC), abstract. *Am Soc Clin Pathol* Orlando, FL, National Conference, Sept 27–Oct 3, 1986.

9. Schneider DR, Picker LJ: Myelodysplasia in the acquired immune deficiency syndrome. *Am J Clin Pathol* 1985; 84:144–152.

10. Spivak JL, Selonick SE, Quinn TC: Acquired immune deficiency syndrome and pancytopenia. *JAMA* 1983; 250:3084.

11. Zon LI, Arkin C, Groopman JE: Haematologic manifestations of the human immune deficiency virus (HIV). *Br J Haematol* 1987; 66:251–256.

IMMUNE THROMBOCYTOPENIC PURPURA

Thrombocytopenia is an important and severe hematologic abnormality associated with AIDS.[1] In addition, idiopathic thrombocytopenic purpura has been reported to occur in sexually active young homosexual men, narcotic addicts, and hemophiliacs who did not have symptoms of AIDS at the time of the examination.[2,3] The immune thrombocytopenia purpura (ITP) seen in homosexual men is clinically similar to idiopathic thrombocytopenic purpura unrelated to AIDS. Some patients experience epistaxis, gingival bleeding, and rectal bleeding whereas others suffer no bleeding episodes before the diagnosis of thrombocytopenia.[2] Patients in both groups show evidence of increased platelet turnover manifested by thrombocytopenia, megakaryocytosis and megathrombocytosis, absence of manifest splenomegaly, absence of antinuclear antibody, and clinical response to steroids and splenectomy.[3,4] Homosexual males with ITP also have lymphopenia, hypergammaglobulinemia, and increased levels of circulating immune complexes, changes that are commonly found in AIDS and ARC patients. Studies of the causes of thrombocytopenia have reached different conclusions. Data from one laboratory showed that IgG deposited on the platelets of homosexual ITP patients is due to elevated levels of circulating immune complexes, which bind to platelet F_c receptors.[4,5] Another study, however, has identified an antiplatelet antibody in the serum of 29 of 30 homosexual men with ITP.[1] The antibody binds to a platelet membrane antigen that is not found on any other hematopoietic cells and is distinct from the core protein of HIV. The existence of autoimmune mechanisms associated with AIDS, as suggested by the formation of autoantibodies against platelets, is not unique: the presence of circulating antibodies directed against T_4 lymphocytes has also been demonstrated in AIDS and ARC patients.[6] Regardless of the origin of IgG on the surface of platelets, its presence has been shown to induce accelerated destruction of antibody-coated platelets through phagocytosis by leukocytes and macrophages.[1]

As in the classic idiopathic thrombocytopenic purpura, the spleen plays a major role in the removal of abnormal platelets through active phagocytosis by the cells of the reticuloendothelial system. The beneficial effect of splenectomy on AIDS-associated ITP is evidence for this role. In two series of patients with AIDS-associated ITP treated by splenectomy, a positive response was obtained in 66% of patients in one series and 100% in another series.[2,5] In one study, spleens removed for the treatment of AIDS-associated ITP were compared with spleens from patients with ITP unrelated to AIDS with the aim of evaluating histologic changes.[7] The AIDS patients had high serum levels of immune complexes, whereas the non-AIDS patients did not. The age of the patients, the clinical manifestations of thrombocytopenic purpura, and the weight of the spleens were comparable. There were, however, certain morphologic differences. Whereas the spleens of the non-AIDS patients showed marked hyperplasia of the white pulp with large trizonal follicles made up of activated lymphoid cells, the spleens of the AIDS-ITP patients had markedly diminished white pulp with small, one-zone follicles containing mature lymphocytes but no activated lymphoid cells (see Figs. II.2.56–59). Deposits of PAS-positive material of variable amount and structure were frequently present within the involuted lymphoid follicles.[7]

IMMUNE THROMBOCYTOPENIC PURPURA (ITP)

Major hematologic abnormality in AIDS and ARC patients

AIDS-related ITP clinically similar to non-AIDS-related idiopathic thrombocytopenic purpura

Circulating immune complexes attached to platelets

Antiplatelet IgG antibody bound to platelets

Active splenic phagocytosis of antibody-coated platelets

Splenectomy beneficial in 66% to 100% of cases

Diminished white pulp

Involuted one-zone follicles composed of small lymphocytes

Deposits of PAS-positive material within involuted follicles

REFERENCES

1. Stricker RB, Abrams DI, Corash C, et al: Target platelet antigen in homosexual men with immune thrombocytopenia. *N Engl J Med* 1985; 313: 1375–1380.

2. Abrams DI, Kiprov DD, Goedert JJ: Antibodies to human T-lymphotropic virus type III and development of the acquired immunodeficiency syndrome in homosexual men presenting with immune thrombocytopenia. *Ann Intern Med* 1986; 104:47–50.

3. Morris L, Distenfeld A, Amorosi E, et al: Autoimmune thrombocytopenic purpura in homosexual men. *Ann Intern Med* 1982; 96:714–717.

4. Karpatkin S: Idiopathic thrombocytopenic purpura in homosexual men; in Friedman-Kien AE, Laubenstein LJ (eds): *AIDS: The Epidemic of Opportunistic Infections.* New York, Masson, 1984.

5. Walsh C, Nardi MA, Karpatkin S: On the mechanism of thrombocytopenic purpura in sexually active homosexual men. *N Engl J Med* 1984; 311:635–639.

6. Dorsett B, Cronin W, Chuma V, et al: Anti-lymphocyte antibodies in patients with acquired immune deficiency syndrome (AIDS). *Am J Med* 1985; 78:621–626.

7. Opher-Iosifescu E, Ioachim HL: The spleen in AIDS-associated thrombocytopenic purpura. Presented at the Annual meeting of the American Society of Clinical Pathologists, Orlando, FL, Sept 27–Oct 3, 1986.

Clinicopathologic Entities Not Classified

CARDIOMYOPATHIES

The heart, like most other organs, may be affected by various infections and neoplasias in the course of AIDS. Cases of nonbacterial vegetative endocarditis; fibrinous pericarditides with cardiac effusions and tamponade caused by *Mycobacterium tuberculosis, Nocardia asteroides,* and *Cryptococcus neoformans;* myocardial infection with *Toxoplasma gondii, Pneumocystis carnii,* and CMV; and multifocal cardiac involvement in Kaposi's sarcoma and non-Hodgkin's lymphoma have been reported.[1-7] In addition, there are well-documented cases in which congestive cardiomyopathy—frequently fatal—developed in AIDS patients who had no diagnosable infections or neoplasias.[7-9]

In one study of 24 patients with AIDS who were evaluated for heart involvement, three exhibited severe cardiac dysfunction with distinct clinical and echocardiographic symptoms of dilated cardiomyopathy.[8] These three patients died within four to eight weeks as a result of acute congestive heart failure. Postmortem examination showed striking four-chamber dilatation with generalized focal myocarditis. Microscopic examination demonstrated the presence of multiple foci of lymphocytic-histiocytic infiltrates with myocytic necrosis and fibrosis.[8] In a review of 15 AIDS patients evaluated by means of echocardiography or subsequent morphologic examination, cardiac abnormalities were found in 73%.[9] These abnormalities included left ventricular hypokinesia, dilated right ventricle, and cardiac tamponade, and in most cases occurred in the absence of an obvious infectious or neoplastic etiology. In a retrospective study of cardiac pathology in AIDS, 82 autopsies were reviewed, and myocarditis, defined as focal areas of necrosis surrounded by monocellular infiltrates, was diagnosed in 50%.[1] Opportunistic myocardial pathogens were seen in only 14 cases. Congestive cardiomyopathy was diagnosed when biventricular dilatation was present in the absence of coronary or valvular heart disease. It occurred in 9% of patients and included cases of dilated cardiomyopathy, with associated congestive heart failure, refractory ventricular tachycardia, and sudden death.

Although the available data on cardiac involvement in AIDS are still insufficient, it appears that myocarditis is a frequent finding at autopsy and may explain the fatal congestive cardiomyopathies that occur in some of these patients.[1] The morphologic picture is that of viral myocarditis. In human beings, infection with a wide range of viruses, predominantly of the RNA type, can lead to myocarditis. About 50% of cases of viral myocarditis are caused by coxsackie viruses, which induce acute and chronic myocarditides with gross and microscopic lesions that are characteristic for all viral cardiopathies, namely, ventricular or global dilatation and softening or absence of noticeable gross abnormalities.[10] On histologic examination, areas of myofibrilar hypereosinophilia, loss of striation, and necrosis, are apparent, and accumulations of lymphocytes, plasma cells, and macrophages, along with eventual focal necrosis can be seen.[10] The morphologic changes described in AIDS patients dying of cardiomyopathy closely resemble those described in patients with viral myocarditis (see Fig.II.3.1–3). These findings suggest that in the cardiomyopathy associated with AIDS, any of the numerous viruses activated by the immune deficiency of these patients—and possibly HIV, the initial pathogenic agent, as well—may play an etiologic role.

CARDIOMYOPATHIES

Congestive cardiomyopathy, frequently fatal

Absence of identifiable infections or neoplasias

Dilated ventricles

Hypokinesia

Acute congestive failure

Focal microfibrilar necrosis with lymphocytic-histiocytic infiltrates and fibrosis

Morphology characteristic of viral myocarditis

REFERENCES

1. Anderson DW, Virmani R, Macher AM, et al: Cardiac pathology and cardiovascular cause of death in patients dying with the acquired immunodeficiency syndrome (AIDS). Presented at the Third International Conference on AIDS, Washington, DC, June 1–5, 1987.
2. Autran GA, Gorin I, Leibowitch M, et al: AIDS in a Haitian woman with cardiac Kaposi's sarcoma and Whipple's disease. *Lancet* 1983; 1:767–768.
3. Cammarosano C, Lewis W: Cardiac lesions in acquired immune deficiency syndrome (AIDS). *J Am Coll Cardiol* 1985; 5:703–706.
4. Goldschmidt RH, Mills J: Cardiomyopathy and AIDS. *N Engl J Med* 1987; 316:1158–1159.
5. Ioachim HL, Cooper MC, Hellman GC: Lymphomas in males at high risk for the acquired immune

deficiency syndrome (AIDS): A study of 21 cases. *Cancer* 1985; 56:2831–2842.
6. Silver MA, Macher AM, Reichert CM, et al: Cardiac involvement by Kaposi's sarcoma in acquired immune deficiency syndrome (AIDS). *Am J Cardiol* 1984; 53:983–985.
7. Sutton MSJ, Fink L: Cardiomyopathy and AIDS. *N Engl J Med* 1987; 316:1160.
8. Cohen IS, Anderson DW, Virmani R, et al: Congestive cardiomyopathy in association with the acquired immunodeficiency syndrome. *N Engl J Med* 1986; 315:628–630.
9. Fink L, Reichek N, Sutton MG: Cardiac abnormalities in acquired immune deficiency syndrome. *Am J Cardiol* 1984; 54:1161–1163.
10. Woodruff JF: Viral myocarditis. *Am J Pathol* 1980; 101:425–485.

FOCAL AND SEGMENTAL GLOMERULOSCLEROSIS

A form of rapidly progressing focal and segmental glomerulosclerosis associated with varying degrees of renal insufficiency has been identified in association with AIDS.[1–4] In a series of 92 patients with AIDS, 11 had severe renal disease leading to nephrotic syndrome and azotemia.[3] Five patients were addicted to heroin, which is a risk factor for nephropathy, but the remaining six had no predisposing factors for renal disease. All patients had opportunistic infections and severely depressed helper/suppressor T-cell ratios. Nine patients had nephrotic syndrome with or without azotemia, and two had azotemia associated with proteinuria. In all the AIDS patients, whether they were drug addicts or not, the renal disease pro-

gressed to severe irreversible uremia in 8 to 16 weeks. The shortness of this interval is striking when compared to the seven to 72 months time from diagnosis to severe renal failure recorded by the same authors in a group of heroin-addicted non-AIDS patients with nephropathy.[3] Similar findings have been reported by other authors who have studied renal disorders in AIDS patients. In one unselected group of patients with AIDS, one third had renal disease, manifested as mild to massive proteinuria, acute tubular necrosis, and renal failure.[1]

A clinicopathologic study of 159 patients (131 adults and 28 children) with AIDS or ARC, detected a nephrotic syndrome in 35.[2] Histologic evaluation of these patients by renal biopsy or autopsy revealed the presence of focal and segmental glomerular sclerosis. Correlated with the risk groups of AIDS patients, the results of this study showed that renal lesions were present in 50% of the intravenous drug users, but in only 2% of homosexuals. These findings confirm the pathogenic role of IV drug use in renal disease; however, it does not entirely explain renal involvement in AIDS. Characteristic glomerular lesions were found in 30% of Haitians, a group at low risk for IV drug abuse, and in 29% of children with no exposure to drugs, which indicates that factors other than drug abuse play an important role in the induction of renal disease in AIDS patients.[2] The rapid progression associated with the AIDS nephropathy remains to be explained; it may be related to the repeated antigenic stimulations suffered by these patients.[4]

The histologic lesions, as observed by renal biopsy, consist of focal and segmental glomerulosclerosis with various degrees of tubular dilatation, tubular atrophy, focal monocellular infiltration, and fibrosis (see Figs. II.6.1–3).[1–4] There is also granular mesangial deposition of IgM and C_3, as well as diffuse mesangial hypercellularity.[1–3] Electron microscopy shows mesangial cell increase with electron-dense mesangial and subepithelial deposits indicative of immune-complex renal disease. Ultramicroscopic studies also reveal the presence of multiple complex inclusions in both the nuclei and the cytoplasm of a variety of cells.[5] Especially remarkable is the increased frequency, size, and complexity of nuclear bodies, particularly the tubuloreticular inclusions observed in interstitial and in tubular epithelial cells.[5]

Renal involvement in AIDS is not yet clearly understood. Whereas intravenous drug abuse is a known cause of glomerulopathy, it has not been a risk factor in a significantly large number of those affected. Circulating immune complexes, along with polyclonal hypergammaglobulinemia, are among the features of deregulated humoral immunity common in AIDS patients. The focal and segmental glomerulosclerosis seen in these patients, however, are not consistent with those seen in patients with immune-complex renal disease, which tend to show diffuse granular capillary depositions of immunoglobulin.[4] The ultrastructural changes—particularly the cellular inclusions, even though they are not specific viral proteins themselves—can be considered morphologic markers of viral infection.[5] Patients with AIDS are affected by a multitude of pathogens, including a variety of viruses in addition to HIV, the etiologic agent of AIDS. Presumably, in the state of severe immune deregulation brought about by AIDS, one of the pathogenic viruses can initiate the rapidly progressive nephropathy observed in these patients.

FOCAL AND SEGMENTAL GLOMERULOSCLEROSIS

Nephrotic syndrome and azotemia

Focal and segmental glomerulosclerosis

Mesangial deposition of IgM and C_3

Tubular dilatation and atrophy

Focal interstitial monocellular inflammatory infiltrates

Complex intranuclear and intracytoplasmic inclusions

Rapid progression to irreversible uremia

REFERENCES

1. Gardenswartz MH, Lerner CW, Seligson GR, et al: Renal disease in patients with AIDS: A clinicopathologic study. *Clin Nephrol* 1984; 21:197–204.
2. Pardo V, Meneses R, Ossa L, et al: AIDS-related glomerulopathy: Occurrence in specific risk groups. *Kidney Int* 1987; 31:1167–1173.
3. Rao TK, Filippone EJ, Nicastri AD, et al: Associated focal and segmental glomerulosclerosis in the acquired immunodeficiency syndrome. *N Engl J Med* 1984; 310:669–673.
4. Rao TKS, Nicastri AD, Friedman EA: Natural history of heroin-associated nephropathy. *N Engl J Med* 1974; 290:19–23.
5. Chander P, Soni A, Suri A, et al: Renal ultrastructural markers in AIDS-associated nephropathy. *Am J Pathol* 1987; 126:513–526.

SALIVARY GLAND LYMPHADENOPATHIES AND LYMPHOMAS

The lymph nodes of the salivary glands may be the primary sites of HIV lymphadenitides and AIDS-associated lymphomas.[1,2] Normally, lymph nodes are intimately associated with the salivary glands, particularly the parotid. Five to 10 lymph nodes are embedded in the parotid gland, several lymph nodes are adjacent to the submaxillary gland, and salivary gland acini and ducts are commonly present in the medulla of upper cervical lymph nodes.[3] The ratio of lymphoid to salivary tissues varies, with the former sometimes reduced to a thin shell around the parotid lobules.[3] Whereas it was once believed that glandular inclusions in lymph nodes represent ectopic salivary glands, sequential studies of human embryos have shown that there are rudimentary lymph nodes arising in the primitive mesenchyme that penetrate the salivary glands and proliferate around their ductal and acinar structures.[4,5] By the 13th week, these formations are already in place, and their association with the salivary glands is a constant feature of normal development.

In the course of HIV infection, salivary gland lymph nodes may be the primary target for the viral infection like any other peripheral lymph nodes that are commonly involved.[1,2,6] In such cases, persons who are at risk for AIDS present with a tumorlike mass of the salivary gland, usually without any other symptoms (see Fig. II.5.14). The mass, which may be unilateral or bilateral, is painless, nodular, and generally large, reaching a diameter of 4 to 7 cm.[1,2,6] When surgically excised, often as a result of a tentative diagnosis of salivary gland tumor, these masses show multiple enlarged lymph nodes and portions of salivary gland that are not easily distinguishable on gross examination (see Fig. II.5.15). Microscopically, the bulk of the tissues excised is made up of lymph nodes showing excessive follicular hyperplasia. The enlarged follicles comprise markedly expanded and irregularly shaped reactive germinal centers that show the typical starry-sky pattern of acute HIV lymphadenitis (see Fig. II.5.17). Cellular lysis, nuclear breakage, tingible-body macrophages with engulfed nuclear debris, and patches of monocytoid lymphocytes can be observed (see Fig. II.5.19).

Other morphologic changes usually seen in the chronic stages of HIV lymphadenopathies—such as lymphocyte depletion, excessive vascular pro-liferation, and atrophic fibrosed germinal centers—are also present. In addition, portions of salivary glands are infiltrated by inflammatory cells, and ducts are lined by metaplastic squamous epithelium. The obliteration of ducts and the accumulation of keratin produced by the newly formed squamous epithelium results in large cystic structures filled with keratin (see Figs. II.5.16, 18).[1,2,6] The leakage of keratin is accompanied by accumulation of foreign body giant cells, as well as large amounts of neutrophils, plasma cells, and lymphocytes. These lesions resemble to some extent those seen in sialolithiases and in Sjögren's syndrome, which may lead to their misinterpretation as cases of Sjögren's disease or of Whartin's tumor associated with AIDS.[7] In the first series of cases of HIV lymphadenitis involving salivary gland lymph nodes, five of six patients had no other manifestations when they presented with salivary gland masses. Two of the five manifested complications of AIDS within the next two years; the other three continued to have only unilateral or bilateral lymphadenopathy.[1,6]

Salivary gland lymph nodes—again, like lymph nodes in other locations—can also be the site of AIDS-related lymphomas as well as of HIV-related lymphadenitides. Three cases of non-Hodgkin's lymphomas were included in a series of cases reporting the involvement of salivary gland lymph nodes in the complications of AIDS.[1,6] The lymphomas were primary at this site, and the patients presented with a salivary tumor mass. Microscopically, the enlarged lymph nodes were partially or totally replaced by sheets of lymphoma cells, in some cases with foci of necrosis that extended deep into the surrounding salivary gland and fibroadipose tissues (see Fig.II.5.20). The histologic appearance was that of undifferentiated Burkittlike lymphoma in two cases and that of large-cell plasmacytoid-type lymphoma in another (see Figs. II.5.21,22). The immunologic phenotype was B-cell in all three cases. Next to the sheets of lymphoma cells were uninvolved areas of lymph nodes and parotid glands that still showed reactive germinal centers as well as keratin-containing cysts lined by squamous epithelium.[1,6] Kaposi's sarcoma, another neoplasm associated with immune deficiency, has also been reported to have affected the lymph nodes of salivary glands primarily.[8]

SALIVARY GLAND LYMPHADENOPATHIES IN HIV INFECTION

Homosexual males, drug addicts, and others at risk for AIDS

Absence of infection or apparent illness

Reversed helper/suppressor T lymphocyte ratio

Positive anti-HIV antibodies test

Intraparotid lymph nodes affected

Presentation as salivary gland tumor mass

Lymphadenitis

    Enlarged lymphoid follicles

    Hyperplastic germinal centers

    Cytolysis

    Tingible-body macrophages

    Obstructed, dilated salivary ducts

    Keratin cysts with squamous cell lining

Non-Hodgkin's Lymphoma

    Primary in salivary gland lymph nodes

    High-grade, undifferentiated cell type

    Residual salivary gland tissues

REFERENCES

1. Ioachim HL, Ryan JR, Blaugrund SM: Parotid gland lymph nodes, the site of lymphadenopathies and lymphomas associated with the human immuno-deficiency virus (HIV) infection. *Lab Invest* 1987; 56:33A.

2. Ryan JR, Ioachim HL, Marmer J, et al: Acquired immune deficiency syndrome-related lymphadenopathies presenting in the salivary gland lymph nodes. *Arch Otolaryngol* 1985; 111:554–556.

3. Thackray AC, Lucas RB: Tumors of the major salivary glands in *Atlas of Tumor Pathology*. Washington, DC, Armed Forces Instit of Pathol 1974, fasc 10, pp 1–3.

4. Brown RB, Gaillard RA, Turner JA: The significance of aberrant or heterotopic parotid gland tissues in lymph nodes. *Ann Surg* 1953; 138:850–856.

5. Marques B, Gay G, Jozan S, et al: Origine embryologique des inclusions salivaires dans les ganglions lymphatiques parotidiens. Bull Assoc Anat 1983; 76:219–228.

6. Ioachim HL, Ryan JR, Blaugrund SM: Salivary gland lymph nodes, the site of lymphadenopathies and lymphomas associated with human immunodeficiency virus (HIV) infection. *Arch Pathol Lab Med* (in press).

7. Ulirsch RC, Jaffe ES: Sjögren's syndrome-like illness associated with the acquired immuno-deficiency syndrome-related complex. *Hum Pathol* 1987; 18:1063–1069.

8. Puterman M, Goldstein J: Primary lymph nodal Kaposi's sarcoma of the parotid gland. *Head Neck Surg* 1985; 5:535–556.

Secondary Viral Diseases Associated with AIDS

chapter
three

CYTOMEGALOVIRUS (CMV) INFECTION

Cytomegalovirus (CMV), the etiologic agent of a wide variety of pathologic lesions in AIDS patients, belongs to the family of herpesviruses. The mature virions are made up of a DNA core and an icosahedral capsid with 162 capsomeres.[1] The characteristic viral inclusion bodies, the largest of any human virus, are present within both the nucleus and the cytoplasm of infected cells. They are composed of a variable number of virus particles in various stages of development, admixed with structurally altered chromatin.[2]

Cytomegalovirus is a ubiquitous pathogenic agent with worldwide distribution. In the United States, complement-fixing antibodies to CMV were present in 44% and 53% of males over 15 years of age in different studies. In homosexual males between 18 and 29 years of age, the presence of anti-CMV antibodies has been reported to be as high as 92%.[3] Transmission by blood transfusion and by transplacental passage have been documented, as well as person-to-person spread through saliva and respiratory secretions. In homosexual males, CMV-infected semen appears to be the main route of infection.[3] In a fairly large part of the population, CMV infection occurs in childhood and manifests itself in the form of a noncharacteristic flu-like syndrome. Subsequently, the infection becomes clinically occult, and the virus is undetectable by any laboratory technique. This is explained by the incorporation of the viral genome into the host genetic material of various cells, particularly leukocytes and renal tubular epithelial cells. A latent infection may thus persist indefinitely.[4]

In immunocompetent adults, CMV infection may take the form of an acute, usually benign, syndrome that is clinically indistinguishable from infectious mononucleosis. The patients, who are generally young adults, have fever, lymphocytosis with atypical lymphocytes, enlarged lymph nodes, and mild hepatitis.[5] Under histologic examination, the lymph nodes show diffuse extensive proliferation of activated lymphocytes, which is similar to what is seen in the lymphadenitis of infectious mononucleosis.[6] On occasion, CMV infection can be transmitted to newborns. In such instances, it results in a severe and frequently lethal syndrome that affects multiple organs, including the central nervous system.[4]

In immunodeficient individuals, either primary CMV infection or reactivation of a latent CMV infection may occur. It is believed that a newly acquired primary infection is the usual cause of opportunistic CMV disease and that reactivation, even if the virus is obviously present, is less likely to have clinical manifestations.[4] CMV infection may be either systemic or localized to a variety of organs (see Figs. I.3.1–2, Figs. II.5.82; II.7.6, 7); the most common manifestations are gastrointestinal ulcers, interstitial pneumonia, glomerulonephritis, and retinitis (see Figs. II.10.7–13). Organ transplant recipients are at high risk for CMV infection: about two thirds show CMV reactivation, and 50% to 60% of seronegative recipients—that is, about one third of the total—can be expected to acquire primary CMV infection.[4]

In almost all the AIDS patients studied at NIH, CMV has been isolated from throat washings, urine, and blood.[7] Patients with AIDS may present with fever, granulocytopenia, lymphocytopenia, thrombocytopenic purpura, maculopapular rashes, interstitial pneumonia, gastrointestinal ulcers (see Fig. II.5.61), chorioretinitis, and encephalitis.[7,8] The pulmonary infection generally appears as a diffuse dissemination of CMV-infected cells, as foci of tissue necrosis, or as diffuse interstitial pneumonitis (**Fig. I.3.1;** see Figs. II.4.10, 11). In the first case, the typical inclusion bodies are noted in endothelial cells, pneumocytes, or alveolar macrophages scattered through pulmonary tissues that are generally unaffected (**Fig. I.3.2**). In the second, infected cells are present in an area of tissue necrosis and are admixed with tissue debris and polymorphonuclear leukocytes.[2,9] In the third, the lungs are wet and dense and have the appearance of a coarse sponge.[4] Microscopic study reveals diffuse interstitial edema with mononuclear cell inflammation and focal intra-alveolar fibrinous exudate with occasional formation of hyaline membranes.[4] The number of inclusion-bearing cells has been found to correlate roughly with the virus titer in the affected tissues.[2] Frequently, in both children and adults, pulmonary CMV infection is associated with *Pneumocystis carinii* pneumonia. This association was noted long before the AIDS epidemic; it was first observed in patients with Hodgkin's disease and those receiving immunosuppressive treatment.[10] In AIDS patients, pulmonary infection with both CMV and *P. carinii* is not uncommon, owing to the background of cellular immune deficiency and possibly to some synergism between the two organisms.

Infection with CMV is common in the gastrointestinal tracts of patients with AIDS, and characteristic inclusions are easily seen in routine paraffin sections (see Figs. II.5.42–45). As in infected tissues of other organs, the CMV-infected cells appear as (1) nuclear amphophilic inclusions surrounded by a clear halo with the typical owl-eye appearance (see Figs. II.5.44–46); (2) cytoplasmic granular amphophilic or acidophilic inclusions; and (3) cells that are markedly enlarged without clearly defined inclusion (see Figs. II.5.43–47).[9] *Candida, Shigella, Mycobacterium avium*, cryptosporidia, and other infections are associated

Fig. I.3.1 CMV intranuclear inclusion bodies within alveolar cells. Small amounts of alveolar exudate and interstitial lymphocytic infiltrate. (HPS stain, ×400)

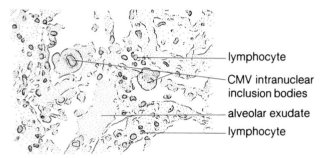
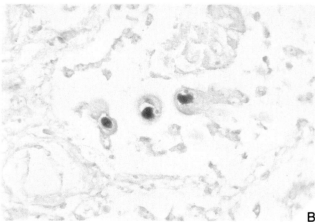

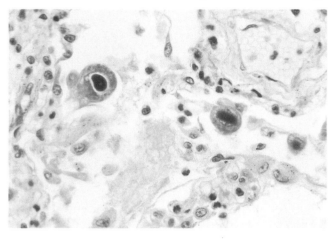

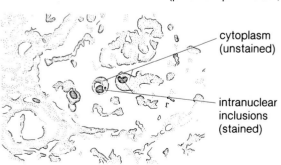

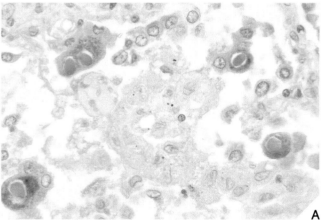

Fig. I. 3.2 A. Intracytoplasmic, brown, granular staining with anti-CMV mononuclear antibody from CMV-infected alveolar cell. Intranuclear inclusions not stained.

(perox-antiperox stain, ×400)

B. Intranuclear CMV inclusion bodies in infected alveolar cells stained after hybridization with CMV probe. Cytoplasm not stained. (perox-antiperox stain, ×400)

with CMV infection. Ulcers are seen in more than 50% of cases; they are usually well-circumscribed and shallow, and may be single or multiple.[11,12] Within the gastrointestinal tract, the colon shows the largest number of CMV inclusions, and the ascending colon shows more than the descending colon or the rectum.[11] The stomach and esophagus are contaminated to a much lesser degree. The inclusions are found predominantly in mesenchymal cells, usually in areas of ulceration and inflammation. Endothelial cells, macrophages, and smooth-muscle cells are common sites of inclusions;[9,12] epithelial cells from colonic crypts (but not from squamous epithelium) are also involved.[11]

The kidneys are frequently affected, with nuclear and cytoplasmic inclusions present in the epithelial cells of proximal, distal, and collecting tubules (see Fig. II.6.4). Such cells may be shed in the urine and detected by urine cytology (**Fig. I.3.3;** see Figs. II.7.6, 7). The cell lesions are usually not associated with inflammation or necrosis;[9] however, the glomeruli may show focal necrosis and lymphocyte infiltration.

In the liver, a mild chronic inflammatory infiltrate, located mostly in the portal areas, may be observed. Inclusion bodies are infrequent. When they do appear, they tend to be located in bile duct epithelial cells and in sinusoidal cells.

The adrenal glands also are commonly involved. Focal areas of necrosis, comprising cells with inclusion bodies, can be seen (see Figs. II.8.3, 4), In some cases, large areas of hemorrhage and infarction have been observed.[13] The medulla seems to be involved earlier, though both the cortex and the medulla usually exhibit the characteristic lesions.[13] The skin may show ulcerations as a result of focal necrosis induced by viral dermal vasculitis.[9]

The eye is frequently affected; CMV chorioretinitis is estimated to occur in more than 25% of AIDS patients.[8] Fundoscopic examination reveals retinal opacification, hemorrhages, exudates, and vascular sheathing. Histologic study shows necrotizing retinitis (see Figs. II.10.7–9), with CMV inclusions possibly present in the retina, the choroid (see Figs. II.10.9,11,12), and the optic nerves (see Fig. II.10.10).[13]

The central nervous system can be affected in systemic CMV infection. Demyelinating lesions have been observed in the hypothalamic region, the spinal cord, and the peripheral nerves of three different patients.[14] These patients also showed occasional microglial nodule formation, as well as typical intranuclear CMV inclusion bodies. No organs are spared from CMV infection; typical lesions have been also observed in lymph nodes, bone marrow, the spleen, the thymus, the heart, the thyroid, and the pituitary.[13]

Finally, CMV has been implicated as a possible etiologic agent in Kaposi's sarcoma, which is known to occur in over 30% of AIDS patients. CMV antigens and genetic material have been identified in Kaposi's sarcoma tissues. Recently it was noted that the incidence of CMV infection among gay men in San Francisco decreased significantly between 1981 and 1984, and that this decrease paralleled a decline in the incidence of Kaposi's sarcoma. This association suggests an etiologic relation.[8]

Fig. I.3.3 CMV infection of prostate. Clusters of desquamated epithelial cells with numerous intranuclear haloed inclusion bodies in lumen of prostatic gland. (HPS stain, ×1,000)

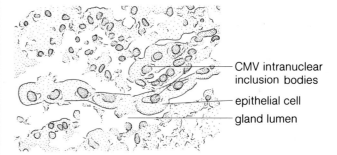

CMV intranuclear inclusion bodies

epithelial cell

gland lumen

CYTOMEGALOVIRUS (CMV) INFECTION

Herpesvirus, DNA core

Intranuclear and intracytoplasmic inclusion bodies

Ubiquitous pathogenic agent

Incidence of CMV antibodies up to 53% in general population

Incidence of CMV antibodies up to 93% in homosexual population

Transmission by blood, by secretions, by semen, and across placenta

Early infections, clinically inapparent

Mononucleosis-like syndrome in immunocompetent hosts

Opportunistic infections in immunodeficient hosts

CMV systemic or localized to various organs

Frequently associated with *P. carinii* pneumonia

Frequently associated with gastrointestinal pathogens

Colon, particularly ascending, most commonly affected

Chorioretinitis in 25% of AIDS patients

Inclusion bodies predominantly in mesenchymal cells

CMV antigens and genetic material in Kaposi's sarcoma cells

REFERENCES

1. Dulbecco R, Ginsberg HS: Cytomegalovirus, in Davis BD, Dulbecco R, Eisen HN, et al: *Microbiology.* New York, Harper & Row, 1974, pp 1249–1252.

2. Craighead JE: Cytomegalovirus pulmonary disease, in Ioachim HL (ed): *Pathobiology Annual 1975.* New York, Appleton-Century-Crofts, 1975, pp 197–220.

3. Drew WL, Mintz L, Miner RC, et al: Prevalence of cytomegalovirus infection in homosexual men. *J Infect Dis* 1981; 143:188–192.

4. Myerowitz RL: Cytomegalovirus, in Myerowitz RL (ed): *The Pathology of Opportunistic Infections.* New York, Raven, 1983, pp 161–176.

5. Klemola E, von Essen R, Wager O, et al: Cytomegalovirus mononucleosis in previously healthy individuals. *Ann Intern Med* 1969; 71:11–19.

6. Ioachim HL: Cytomegalovirus lymphadenitis, in *Lymph Node Biopsy.* Philadelphia, JB Lippincott, 1982, pp 53–57.

7. Fauci AS, Macher AB, Longo DL, et al: Acquired immunodeficiency syndrome: Epidemiologic, clinical, immunologic, and therapeutic considerations. *Ann Intern Med* 1984; 100:92–106.

8. Selwyn PA: AIDS: What is now known: III. Clinical aspects. *Hosp Pract* 1986; 21:119–153.

9. Myerson D, Hackman RC, Nelson JA, et al: Widespread presence of histologically occult cytomegalovirus. *Hum Pathol* 1984; 15:430–439.

10. Symmers WStC: Generalized cytomegalic inclusion-body disease associated with pneumocystis pneumonia in adults. *J Clin Pathol* 1960; 13:1–21.

11. Hinnant KL, Rotterdam HZ, Bell ET, et al: Cytomegalovirus infection of the alimentary tract: A clinicopathological correlation. *Am J Gastroenterol* 1986; 81:944–950.

12. Rotterdam H, Sommers SC: Alimentary tract biopsy lesions in the acquired immune deficiency syndrome. *Pathology* 1985; 17:181–192.

13. Reichert CM, O'Leary TJ, Levens DL, et al: Autopsy pathology in the acquired immune deficiency syndrome. *Am J Pathol* 1983; 112:357–382.

14. Moskowitz LB, Gregorios JB, Hensley GT, et al: Cytomegalovirus. *Arch Pathol Lab Med* 1984; 108:873–877.

HERPES SIMPLEX VIRUS (HSV) AND HERPES ZOSTER VIRUS (HZV) INFECTIONS

Herpes simplex virus (HSV) and Herpes zoster virus (HZV) are members of the family of herpesviruses, which also includes CMV and Epstein-Barr virus (EBV). These morphologically similar, large DNA viruses are all ubiquitous human pathogens.[1,2] There are two genetically and immunologically related types, HSV-1 and HSV-2—which share common nucleotide sequences and antigens.[1,2] Both are capable of producing mucocutaneous and visceral infections; generally, however, HSV-1 causes infections above the diaphragm and HSV-2 infections below.[2] As a rule, therefore, it is HSV-1 that produces lesions of the lips and mouth and HSV-2 that produces anogenital lesions. In healthy, immunocompetent hosts, the infections are superficial, self-limited, and latent for long periods; they may, and sometimes do, recur. In immunosuppressed hosts, the infections tend to expand, ulcerate, and disseminate to deep-seated organs. Herpes zoster virus is morphologically identical to HSV and is similarly widespread. It causes varicella or chickenpox in children and herpes zoster or shingles when reactivated in adults. In immunosuppressed individuals, HZV can also become an opportunistic agent that carries significant morbidity; however, it is less severe than HSV and is not fatal.[2]

Herpesvirus infections are common in patients with malignant diseases and in recipients of transplanted organs.[3] In bone marrow transplant recipients infection with HSV occurs in about 90% during the first two weeks, and infection with HZV in about 30% after a few months.[3] Herpesvirus infections, particularly with HSV, are also common in homosexual men and other persons with HIV infection and AIDS.[3,4] In such cases, the resulting disease is likely to be unusually severe.

The primary infection occurs through direct contact with infected oral or genital secretions from humans, who appear to be the reservoir of infection.[2] The characteristic vesicles on the skin and various mucosal surfaces appear in three to five days. In HSV-1 infections, the face, lips (see Fig. II.1.2), tongue, buccal mucosa, nipples, neck, ear, and cornea show randomly distributed vesicles, singly or in clusters. In HSV-2 infections, the vesicles are randomly distributed in a similar fashion on the perineum, perianal area (see Figs. II.1.8, 9; II.7.11) vulva, vagina, cervix, urethra and penis (see Fig. II.7.4). In HZV infections, vesicles appear on the skin, particularly thoracic, in a dermatome distribution (see Fig. II.1.10). In healthy, immunocompetent individuals, the vesicles remain small (usually less than 1 cm in diameter), with round margins and surrounding erythema. Within one to two days, the vesicles evolve to pustules, which eventually form a crust and heal.[2] In immunocompromised hosts, the vesicles become large, irregularly shaped, and confluent ulcers. These ulcers are long-lasting and are usually accompanied by a secondary bacterial or fungal infection and final scarring.[2]

On microscopic examination (see Figs. II.1.3–7), it can be seen that in the squamous epithelium of skin or mucosae the keratinocytes become edematous and lyse, forming an intraepithelial vesicle. The remaining cells at the periphery show the characteristic changes: cytoplasmic swelling with ballooning degeneration, multinucleated giant cells with nuclear molding, and intranuclear inclusions. The dermis below the lesion shows marked vascular congestion and accumulation of neutrophiles.[2] In the early stages of cellular infection, the nuclear inclusions of HSV and HZV have the appearance of lilac-stained, ground-glass bodies that fill the nucleus entirely (**Figs. I.3.4, 3.5).** In the multinucleated squamous cells, the nuclei with ground-glass inclusions mold against each other like the pieces of a jigsaw puzzle.[2] In later stages, the intranuclear body is eosinophilic and acquires the halo typical of the Cowdry type A inclusion (see Figs. II.5.28, 29). Unlike CMV, HSV and HZV do not induce cytomegaly or produce cytoplasmic inclusions.[2]

An infected individual may actively shed infectious virus or progress to a latent stage in which the infection is entirely inapparent. During this time, HSV or HZV travel in a retrograde fashion along sensory nerves to the neurons of dorsal root ganglia, where they remain latent as complete virions within the nuclei for long periods.[4] Reactivation of the virus infection is associated with stress, fever, or trauma. The mechanism responsible for the induction of reactivation is probably the suppression of cellular immunity, which is known to occur in the various categories of acquired immune deficiency. In such cases, the virus is able to follow the same route in reverse, moving along the sensory nerves from the ganglia back to the mucocutaneous surfaces.[2,4]

Over the past two decades, the incidence of genital herpes simplex virus infection has increased more than that of any other sexually transmitted disease. It is now the most common cause of genital ulcerations.[5] First episodes of genital herpes involve multiple anatomic sites, last about three weeks, and have a high incidence of complications, including aseptic meningitis (in 8% of cases) and extragenital lesions (in 20%).[6] The duration of viral shedding is similar in men and women, but the duration of symptoms is longer and the incidence of complications higher in women.[6] Over 50% of patients with primary genital herpes have constitutional symptoms, several anatomic sites of involvement such as the cervix, urethra, pharynx, and extragenital skin, as well as satellite adenopathy in 80% of cases.[6] Recurrent genital herpes is of milder duration and intensity.

In immunocompromised patients, the vesicles ulcerate early, and for long periods the coalescing lesions do not heal and continue to shed virus. Chronic perianal ulcerative herpetic lesions have been reported in medically immunosuppressed patients, and more recently in homosexual men (see Figs. II.1.8, 9; II.5.58–60).[7,8] Chronic polycyclic friable ulcerations in the sacral area have occasionally been confused with decubitus ulcers (see Fig. II.1.9).[7] In one group of four men with AIDS, perianal ulcers up to 12 cm in diameter gradually developed, which showed no tendency to heal. All four patients died after a prolonged course of illness. At autopsy, HSV-1 dissemination to internal organs, including the colon, adrenals, lungs, and spinal cord was apparent.[8] Primary herpes proctitis has also been reported in 23 of 119 homosexual men who had presented with anorectal pain. These patients had multiple severe friable rectal ulcers with inguinal adenopathy.[9]

Of all the viscera, the esophagus is the one most often affected by herpetic infections, and the distal esophagus is by far the most common site in the gastrointestinal tract.[2,10] Unfortunately, however, because herpetic esophagitis is usually asymptomatic, the diagnosis is rarely made while the patient is alive, and the incidence of the condition is grossly underestimated.[10,11] Autopsy studies have shown that esophageal ulcers with the characteristic histologic features of HSV infection are common in immunosuppressed patients (see Fig. II.5.26).[10,11] On gross examination, the early lesions are multiple, discrete, punched-out ulcers with raised granular margins. Since most of these ulcers occur in immunocompromised patients, the ulcers tend to enlarge and merge, and they often become superinfected with *Candida.* Consequently, if the ulcer margins are not examined histologically with the aim of finding the squamous cells with typical inclusion bodies, the diagnosis of herpetic infection is easily missed.[2,10]

The respiratory tract can be also involved: the larynx, trachea, and bronchi may exhibit ulcerations, and necrotizing bronchopneumonia, characterized by patchy yellow areas of coagulation necrosis due to direct viral cytopathic effect on the pulmonary tissues, may be noted.[2] The liver can be affected by HSV, in which case the result is large foci of coagulation necrosis associated with minor inflammatory reaction.[2] In the lung and the liver, infected cells show the typical haloed inclusion bodies, but not the multinucleated giant cells.[2]

Herpetic encephalitis may occur as a fulminant disease with necrotizing lesions that tend to be located in the medial temporal and inferior frontal regions of the brain (see Figs. II.9.9,10).[10] On microscopic examination, marked lymphocytic infiltration around the necrotic area and proliferation of glial nodules can be observed. In patients with induced immunosuppression (usually for treatment of Hodgkin's disease and other lymphomas), herpetic encephalitis caused by HSV or HZV has been reported.[10,12] The course of the disease was not acute in these cases, and the histologic components of necrosis and inflammation were markedly reduced.[10] Instead, there were multiple yellow-gray granular areas within the white matter of the brain and spinal cord. On microscopic examination (see Figs. II.9.11–13), these areas

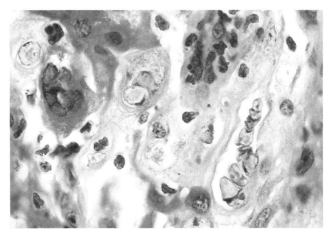

Fig. I.3.4 HSV infection of skin. Ballooning degeneration of squamous cells; lilac-stained, ground-glass, early HSV inclusions without haloes filling the nuclei; and eosinophilic, haloed, late intranuclear HSV inclusion bodies. Nuclei molded around the vacuoles. (HPS stain, ×1,000)

Fig. I.3.5 Herpes simplex vesicle in anus. Ground-glass, lilac-stained, early inclusions and eosinophilic, haloed inclusions in nuclei of enlarged squamous cells. Multinucleated giant cell. (HPS stain, ×100)

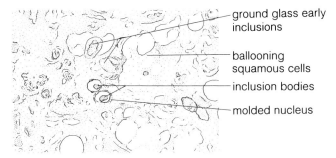

ground glass early inclusions

ballooning squamous cells

inclusion bodies

molded nucleus

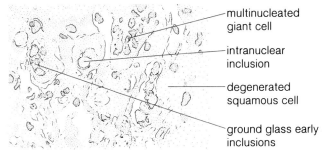

multinucleated giant cell

intranuclear inclusion

degenerated squamous cell

ground glass early inclusions

showed demyelination, focal necrosis, and cells with intranuclear eosinophilic inclusions of Cowdry type A that stained positively with HSV-1 or HZV antibodies in immunohistochemical staining.[10,12,13]

In patients with AIDS or ARC who have CNS complications, the incidence of herpetic encephalitis is about 3%.[13,14] HSV-1 is more often the cause of encephalitis than HSV-2, and displays a rapid progression and severity of lesions which is directly proportional to the degree of immune deficiency.[14] Two patients with HIV lymphadenopathy suffered an acute encephalitis, and a biopsy of the temporal lobe showed typical inflammatory lesions from which herpesvirus was cultured. In contrast, patients with advanced AIDS manifested no neurologic illness and showed no typical pathological changes, though all the biopsied brain tissues proved to be positive for HSV-1.[14]

Herpetic disease can be diagnosed by several means, depending on the presentation. For vesicular lesions, the classical Tzanck preparation, in which a clean slide is pressed against the base of a freshly unroofed vesicle, is prefered. The smear is stained with Giemsa or Papanicolaou stain, and the herpetic multinucleated giant cells or the intranuclear inclusion bodies are identified.[1,2] Biopsy of skin or mucosal lesions, endoscopic biopsy of esophagus or larynx, and brain biopsy are effective means of diagnosis, in that they allow recognition of the characteristic morphologic changes. These methods can be supplemented by electron microscopy, which will demonstrate the herpesvirus particles (see Fig. II.10.18), or by immunohistochemistry using specific antibodies with the direct immunofluorescence or the immunoperoxidase technique. Moreover, HSV can be cultured in vitro on fibroblast lines. The virus grows rapidly on these lines, producing characteristic cytopathic changes within 24 to 48 hours. Serodiagnosis is not a useful approach because most adults have antibodies to HSV and therefore the reactivation infections that represent the majority of herpes disease in immunodeficient individuals cannot be recognized.[2]

HERPES SIMPLEX VIRUS (HSV) AND HERPES ZOSTER VIRUS (HZV) INFECTIONS

HSV-1, infections above diaphragm; HSV-2, below diaphragm; HZV, dermatome distribution

Self-limited mucocutaneous vesicular lesions in primary infections

Virions within sensory ganglia during latency periods of variable duration

Milder, recurrent lesions during reactivation

Coalescing ulcers, severe disease, visceral involvement in immunodeficient hosts

Multinucleated giant cells with molding nuclei and ground-glass inclusions

Haloed, Cowdry type A, intranuclear inclusion bodies

HSV infection most common cause of genital ulcerations

HSV perianal ulcerations and proctitis frequent in homosexual males

HSV esophagitis most common visceral involvement

Herpetic encephalitis, 3% of CNS complications in AIDS patients

Severity of disease and rapidity of progression proportional to immunodeficiency in all HSV infections

Diagnosis by cytology of vesicle fluid, tissue biopsy, tissue culture

REFERENCES

1. Kaplan M, Swenson PD: Herpes virus infection, in Sun T: *Sexually Related Infectious Diseases.* New York, Field, Rich & Assoc, 1986, pp 85–97.
2. Myerowitz RL: Diseases caused by herpes simplex virus, in Myerowitz RL (ed): *The Pathology of Opportunistic Infections.* New York, Raven, 1983, pp 177–198.
3. Quinnan GV, Masur H, Rook AH, et al: Herpesvirus infections in the acquired immune deficiency syndrome. *JAMA* 1984; 252:72–77.
4. Resnick L, Herbst JS: Dermatological (non-Kaposi's sarcoma) manifestations associated with HTLV-III/LAV infection, in Broder S (ed): *AIDS.* New York, Marcel Dekker, 1987, pp 285–303.
5. Corey L, Holmes KK: Genital herpes simplex virus infections: Current concepts in diagnosis, therapy, and prevention. *Ann Intern Med* 1983; 98:973–983.
6. Corey L, Adams HG, Brown ZA, et al: Genital herpes simplex virus infections: Clinical manifestations, course, and complications. *Ann Intern Med* 1983; 98:958–972.
7. Kalb RE, Grossman ME: Chronic perianal herpes simplex in immunocompromised hosts. *Am J Med* 1986; 80:486–490.
8. Siegal FP, Lopez C, Hammer GS, et al: Severe acquired immunodeficiency in male homosexuals, manifested by chronic perianal ulcerative

herpes simplex lesions. *N Engl J Med* 1981; 305:1439–1444.

9. Goodell SE, Quinn TC, Mikrtichian PAC, et al: Herpes simplex proctitis in homosexual men. *N Engl J Med* 1983; 308:868–871.
10. Buss DH, Scharyl M: Herpesvirus infection of the esophagus and other visceral organs in adults. *Am J Med* 1979; 66:457–462.
11. Nash G, Ross JS: Herpetic esophagitis: A common cause of esophageal ulceration. *Hum Pathol* 1974; 5:339–345.
12. Horten B, Price RW, Jimenez D: Multifocal varicella-zoster virus leukoencephalitis temporally

remote from herpes zoster. *Ann Neurol* 1981; 9:251–266.
13. Petito CK, Cho ES, Lemann W, et al: Neuropathology of acquired immunodeficiency syndrome (AIDS): An autopsy review. *J Neuropathol Exp Neurol* 1986; 45:635–646.
14. Levy RM, Bredesen DE, Rosenblum ML: Neurological manifestations of the aquired immunodeficiency syndrome (AIDS): Experience at UCSF and review of the literature. *J Neurosurg* 1985; 62:475–495.

CONDYLOMATA

Condylomatous lesions are not considered to be among the diseases associated with AIDS; however, they are sexually transmitted, and they are frequently seen in individuals at high risk for AIDS. In females, they occur on the vulva, vagina, and cervix; in males, on the glans and shaft of the penis; in both sexes, in perineal and perianal skin, in the urethra, and in the oral cavity. Juvenile laryngeal papillomatosis is caused by a virus of the same group, and infants may have condylomata as a result of transmission during childbirth. Condylomatosis is one of the most common sexually transmitted diseases in the United States. Individuals affected range in age from 14 to 55 years and the highest risk is in the 20 to 24 year age group.[1,2] About two thirds of the partners of individuals with genital condylomata are also affected. The incubation period is from one to three months.[2]

In recent years, much progress has been made toward understanding the biology and the pathogenic role of human papillomaviruses (HPVs) in a variety of benign and malignant processes.[3,4] The HPVs belong to a larger group, the papovaviruses, which also include SV_{40} and polyomavirus, both of which are animal viruses with demonstrated oncogenic potentials in vitro and in vivo. About 12 different types of HPV have been isolated so far, each associated with characteristic lesions in various parts of the body. The HPVs are DNA viruses with large (50 to 55 nm in diameter) nonenveloped particles composed of double-stranded DNA enclosed in an icosahedral nucleocapsid made up of 72 capsomeres.

On colposcopy, genital condylomatous lesions take one of four forms: (1) flat, white, granular lesions that are usually multifocal (the most com-

mon form) (see Fig. II.7.2); (2) thick, papillary lesions with finger-like projections or large cauliflower lesions (see Fig. II.7.9); (3) spiked, fine, white asperities, or (4) condylomatous cervicovaginitis with a rough mucosal surface covered by numerous fine excrescences.[5,6] On histologic examination, the lesions follow one of three morphologic patterns: condyloma planum, or flat condyloma (the most common type); (2) condyloma acuminatum (the papillomatous type) (see Fig. II.7.9); and (3) endophytic condyloma (the inverted type) (see Fig. II.7.2).[5,7]

Regardless of their architecture, all types exhibit the single most characteristic feature, koilocytotic atypia (see Figs. II.7.3, 10).[6–9] The koilocytotic cells are generally confined to the upper third of the squamous epithelium, which also shows moderate acanthosis and a thin layer of parakeratotic cells in the stratum corneum.

Koilocytes are enlarged squamous cells with totally vacuolated cytoplasms and degenerating nuclei that appear hyperchromatic, crinkled, and pyknotic. They are a prime characteristic of condyloma and can be used to differentiate condyloma from carcinoma in situ.[5,6,9]

The second most common morphologic change in condyloma is dyskeratosis in the form of individual cell keratinization.[7] In a cytologic smear from a condylomatous lesion stained by the Papanicolaou technique, the two predominant cell types are the koilocytes, which have sharp cellular borders, clear cytoplasm, and pyknotic nuclei, and the dyskeratocytes, which occur singly or in small clusters and have orange cytoplasm and small, dense nuclei.[2] The combination of the two types of desquamated cells in a Papanicolaou smear is diagnostic of condyloma.[5,8,9] In a flat condyloma, the lesion appears as an area of acanthosis with elongated rete pegs, dyskeratosis, and koilocytosis; the most striking feature is the contrast between the upper third, which is koilocytotic, and the two lower thirds, which are uninvolved. In classic condyloma acuminatum, papillomatosis, acanthosis, and koilocytosis are observed. Endophytic condyloma, the least common form, resembles an inverted papilloma with inward growth and occasional gland involvement.[2]

Electron microscopy has identified HPV particles in the nuclei of the koilocytotic cells of condylomas, but not in those of the normal-appearing cells. The particles are abundant, are confined to the nuclei and sometimes to the nucleoli, and are distributed in crystalline arrays or scattered throughout the nucleoplasm.[7] Use of specific sera and the immunoperoxidase technique has made it possible to identify the antigen-containing nuclei, which are generally located within the koilocytotic cells. In a study employing parallel ultrastructural and immunohistochemical analysis of 97 cervical condyloma specimens, viral particles were detected in 25% of cases by electron microscopy and in 48% of cases by the immunological technique.[7] The antigen was always detected when the particles were visible, but, as the additional number of positive cases shows, immunohistochemistry was almost twice as sensitive as electron microscopy. Both techniques detected HPV more often in flat than in papillary condylomas.[7]

The current prevalence of genital condylomata can be attributed not only to their increased frequency but also in large part to better recognition of these lesions, which in the past were often diagnosed as mild and moderate degrees of cervical intraepithelial neoplasia (CIN I and II).[7] Condylomatous lesions may, however, occur in association with dysplastic and neoplastic lesions of the genital organs. In a study of 169 women with histologically confirmed dysplasias and neoplasias of the uterine cervix, condylomatous lesions were also present in 50% of cases.[10] Those women who had condylomatous lesions in addition to neoplasia were significantly younger than those who did not; moreover, in patients who were less than 20 years of age, dysplastic cervical changes were never present without coexistent condylomatous lesions.

These and other recent studies suggest that in human beings some papillomaviruses, like some papovaviruses in other animal species, may be associated with benign lesions capable of progressing to malignancy.[3] The association of condyloma with epithelial dysplasia has led to the prevailing opinion that condylomatous lesions could, under special conditions, be precursors of carcinoma.[5,9,10] Such conditions are created by the various immunodeficient states, which are associated with markedly higher rates of neoplasias of genital organs (as indeed they are with higher rates of neoplasia in general).[11]

In a group of 20 women with immunosuppression induced by prednisone therapy or various immune disorders who also had genital (cervical, vaginal, vulvar) neoplasia, evidence of HPV infection was found. Koilocytotic atypia was present in all patients, virus particles were detected in 50%, and HPV antigen was identified in 60%. The helper/suppressor T-cell ratios were reversed, and patients exhibited deficient responses to mitogenic stimulation.[12] Like many other neoplastic processes associated with immune suppression, the HPV-related neoplasias in these patients were more aggressive and resistant to treatment. In 12 of the 20 patients, intraepithelial neoplasia was recurrent, and in one it progressed to invasive squamous carcinoma.[12] In immunosuppressed renal transplant patients, the frequency of cervical carcinoma in situ is increased 14-fold.[11] In a group of 105 immunosuppressed kidney transplant recipients, 18 showed evidence of HPV infection, and 9.5% had lower genital neoplasia.[13] The frequency of HPV infection in this group of patients was ten times higher than in a comparable population of normal women, and that of lower genital neoplasia was 16 times higher. These studies provide valuable evidence regarding the association of HPV with condylomatous lesions, their relationship with neoplasia of genital organs, and the role of immunodeficiency in accelerating and aggravating the neoplastic progression.

CONDYLOMATA

Common in populations at high risk for AIDS

Genital, perianal, and oral distribution

Sexually transmitted, viral-induced

Human papillomaviruses, characterized according to lesions and locations

Three morphologic patterns: condyloma planum, condyloma acuminatum, and endophytic condyloma

Koilocytosis and dyskeratosis

HPV particles and antigen in nuclei of koilocytotic cells

Condylomata associated with squamous epithelial dysplasia and neoplasia

Immunosuppression favors extension and recurrence

REFERENCES

1. Centers for Disease Control: Condyloma acuminatum: United States 1966–1981. *MMWR* 1983; 32:300.
2. Szabo K: Condyloma acuminatum (infection by human wart virus), in Sun T (ed): *Sexually Related Infectious Diseases.* New York, Field, Rich & Assoc, 1986, pp 129–134.
3. Howley PM: The human papillomavirus. *Arch Pathol Lab Med* 1982; 106:429–432.
4. Zur Hausen H: Condylomata acuminata and human genital cancer. *Cancer Res* 1976; 36:794.
5. Meisels A, Fortin R, Roy M: Condylomatous lesions of the cervix: II. Cytologic colposcopic and histopathology study. *Acta Cytol* 1977; 21:379.
6. Roy M, Meisels A, Fortier M, et al: Vaginal condylomata: A human papilloma virus infection. *Clin Obstet Gynecol* 1981; 24:461.
7. Ferenczy A, Braun L, Shah KV: Human papillomavirus (HPV) in condylomatous lesions of cervix. *Am J Surg Pathol* 1981; 5:661–670.
8. Koss LG, Durfee GR: Unusual patterns of squamous epithelium of uterine cervix: Cytologic and pathologic study of koilocytotic atypia. *Ann NY Acad Sci* 1956; 63:1235–1261.
9. Meisels A, Fortin R: Condylomatous lesions of the cervix and vagina: I. Cytologic patterns. *Acta Cytol* 1976; 20:505.
10. Syrjänen KJ: Condylomatous lesions in dysplastic and neoplastic epithelium of the uterine cervix. *Surg Gynecol Obstet* 1980; 150:372–376.
11. Penn I: Malignancies associated with immunosuppressed organ or cytotoxic therapy. *Surgery* 1978; 83:492.
12. Sillman F, Stanek A, Sedlis A, et al: The relationship between human papillomavirus and lower genital intraepithelial neoplasia in immunosuppressed women. *Am J Obstet Gynecol* 1984; 150:300–308.
13. Halpert R, Butt KMH, Sedlis A, et al: Human papillomavirus infection and lower genital neoplasia in female renal allograft recipients. *Transplant Proc* 1985; 17:93–95.

ORAL HAIRY LEUKOPLAKIA

Oral hairy leukoplakia, or condyloma planum, is a newly described lesion of the tongue and oral mucosa observed in immunosuppressed individuals with HIV infection.[1-4] It consists of slightly whitish raised areas, ranging in size from a few millimeters to a few centimeters, that have a corrugated, hairy-appearing surface **(Fig. I.3.6;** (see Figs. II.5.1, 2).[2] In 86% of cases, the lesions are located on the tongue (72% on the lateral border and 14% on the ventral aspect); occasionally they are found on the buccal mucosa.[1,2] The lesions are generally asymptomatic. They are firmly adherent and cannot be scraped off with a tongue blade.[1] *Candida* frequently colonizes the lesions with spores and hyphae growing into the parakeratin layer.[1,5]

On histologic examination, fine hairy keratin projections can be seen on the surface of the squamous epithelium of the tongue, which shows acanthosis, parakeratosis, and focal ballooning of squamous cells (see Figs. II.5.3–5). Some of the ballooning cells contain the clear cytoplasm and eccentric, pyknotic nuclei that are characteristic of koilocytotic atypia. There is also mild nuclear atypia and a slight increase in the number of mitoses. Inflammation in the form of lymphocytic infiltrates is minimal. In all, the microscopic picture is similar to that of flat condylomata commonly seen in genital and anal areas. Like some of these, the oral lesions also regress and recur spontaneously on occasion.

Several studies have been undertaken to investigate whether oral hairy leukoplakia, like anogenital condylomata, is etiologically related to spe-

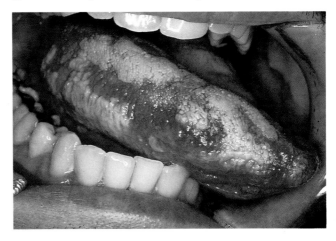

Fig. I.3.6 Hairy leukoplakia of tongue. White, confluent, corrugated, adherent plaques, which bleed when detached, on lateral aspect of tongue.

cific viruses. In one, 49 (73%) of 67 biopsy specimens of tongue hairy leukoplakia showed positive intranuclear immunohistochemical staining for the core antigen of papillomavirus.[6] Electron microscopic examination revealed papillomaviruslike particles in all 25 biopsies examined; however, there was also a herpeslike virus in 23 of these specimens. In some specimens, both types of particles were found within the same individual squamous cell. Immunofluorescence studies using specific antibodies yielded negative results for HSV, HZV, and CMV, but positive intense nuclear staining in the squamous epithelial cells for the viral capsid antigen of EBV. Similarly, DNA hybridization in Southern blots demonstrated the presence of EBV DNA in the same type of cells. The presence of papillomavirus and EBV, two viruses associated with dysplasia and neoplasia in the tissues of other organs, suggests a possible viral etiology for the lesions of oral hairy leukoplakia.

In addition, patients with oral hairy leukoplakia also demonstrate ample evidence of HIV infection. One study examined 155 homosexual men with oral hairy leukoplakia who for the most part were healthy at the time of presentation but who showed the characteristic signs of T-cell deficiency.[3] Of 101 patients tested in this group, 100 had antibodies to HIV, and in 22 of 28 tested HIV was recovered from peripheral blood mononuclear cells. Follow-up of these patients with hairy leukoplakia revealed that AIDS developed in 48% by 16 months and in 83% by 31 months.

The high proportion of patients with hairy leukoplakia who progress to AIDS makes this lesion an important early prognostic sign in the course of the HIV infection.[3] Oral hairy leukoplakia has been also reported in recipients of transfused blood and in women at risk for HIV infection, but so far not in individuals with forms of immunosuppression unrelated to AIDS.[3]

ORAL HAIRY LEUKOPLAKIA

Raised, corrugated, white patches with striated margins

Lateral borders and ventral aspect of tongue and buccal mucosa

Acanthosis, parakeratosis, and koilocytotic atypia

Minimal inflammatory reaction

Papilloma virus particles and intranuclear core antigen in squamous cells

EBV DNA, EBV capsid antigen, and EBV particles in squamous cells

HIV and HIV antibodies in peripheral blood

Cellular immune deficiency

High incidence of progression to AIDS

REFERENCES

1. Eversole LR, Jacobsen P, Stone CE, et al: Oral condyloma planum (hairy leukoplakia) among homosexual men: A clinicopathologic study of thirty-six cases. *Oral Surg Oral Med Oral Pathol* 1986; 61:249–255.
2. Greenspan D, Conant M, Silverman S Jr, et al: Oral "hairy" leukoplakia in male homosexuals: Evidence of association with both papillomavirus and a herpes-group virus. *Lancet* 1984; 2:831–834.
3. Greenspan D, Greenspan JS, Hearst NG, et al: Relation of oral hairy leukoplakia to infection with the human immunodeficiency virus and the risk of developing AIDS. *J Infect Dis* 1987; 155:475–481.
4. Silverman S Jr, Migliorati CA, Lozada-Nur F, et al: Oral findings in people with or at high risk for AIDS: A study of 375 homosexual males. *J Am Dent Assoc* 1986; 112:187–192.
5. Lozada F, Silverman S, Migliorati CA, et al: Oral manifestations of tumor and opportunistic infections in the acquired immunodeficiency syndrome (AIDS): Findings in 53 homosexual men with Kaposi's sarcoma. *Oral Surg* 1983; 56:491–494.
6. Greenspan JS, Greenspan D, Lenette ET, et al: Relation of Epstein-Barr virus within the epithelial cells of oral "hairy" leukoplakia, an AIDS-associated lesion. *N Engl J Med* 1985; 313:1564–1571.

PROGRESSIVE MULTIFOCAL LEUKOENCEPHALOPATHY (PML)

Progressive multifocal leukoencephalopathy (PML), a subacute, progressive demyelinating disease of the central nervous system, was originally described as a complication of leukemia and Hodgkin's disease. It occurs almost exclusively in patients that are debilitated, chronically ill, or immunosuppressed.[1-3] Approximately 40% to 50% of AIDS patients have neurologic symptoms, and at autopsy as many as 80% show lesions of the central nervous system.[4] The incidence of PML in patients with AIDS was 2% to 4% in four separate series of autopsies in which the brains were systematically examined.[4-7]

The etiologic agent of PML is a small DNA virus called JC, which belongs, along with the viruses BK and SV-40, to the family of papovaviruses. It appears that JC is virtually ubiquitous, considering that more than 70% of adults worldwide have hemagglutination-inhibition antibodies to it.[3] The primary infection probably occurs in childhood and remains latent, possibly within the CNS, until conditions of deficient immunity permit its reactivation.[3] The infection seems to be age-related: cases of PML have not been reported in children, and the prevalence of JC antibodies generally increases with age.[3]

Other papovaviruses may be also human pathogens: two cases of PML have been shown to be caused by SV-40.[8] The viruses BK and JC have frequently been isolated from the urine of renal transplant recipients, though they had not been associated with any disease under those circumstances.[9] Humoral immunity is not effective against JC: antibody titers are no higher in patients with PML than in normal individuals.[10] It is cell-mediated immunity that determines the reactivation and pathogenicity of JC virus: in all reported cases of PML, cell-mediated immunity has been deficient.[2] The occurrence of this rare neurologic disease in AIDS patients is further proof of its dependence on cellular immune deregulation.

Clinically, PML presents as an insidious, subacute disease that is not accompanied by fever or other signs of infectious inflammatory disease. The patients manifest progressive dementia and focal neurologic deficits, which may include motor weakness, hemiparesis, ataxia, aphasia, and sensory and visual disturbances.[2,3,10-12] The lesions can be detected radiologically by means of CT scanning (see Fig. II.9.14). They appear as lucent areas of low density with no enhancing effect. The affected areas have irregular borders and do not appear as masses; these features distinguish them from tumors, abscesses, or toxoplasmic cysts.[10-12] The cerebrospinal fluid shows no significant changes and is therefore nondiagnostic. Serologic study is also noncontributory, since antibody titers do not reflect the disease process.[2,10,11] The definitive diagnosis can be only made through brain biopsy and recognition of the characteristic histologic lesions.[3,13]

The pathology of PML was described in detail before the AIDS epidemic. It has since been confirmed, after the association between PML and AIDS was recognized.[1-7,11,12] On examination of the brain, there are usually multiple PML lesions that appear to be randomly distributed within the white matter of the cortex (see Fig. II.9.15). In 10% of cases, the lesion is unifocal and involves the cerebellum and the pons (see Fig. II.9.19).[10,12] There are multiple asymmetric foci with irregular borders that vary in size from a pinpoint to 1.5 cm.[11] Sometimes, the foci in the white matter of the frontal, parietal, or occipital lobes or of the internal capsule encroach on the grey matter along the borders.[11]

On histologic examination, the lesions consist of large areas of demyelination (see Fig. II.9.17), sometimes with foci of infarct-like necrosis (see Fig. II.9.23).[5] The areas of demyelination have few oligodendrocytes and lack inflammatory cells entirely (**Fig. I.3.7;** see Fig. II.9.16). Enlarged, bizarre, hyperchromatic astrocytes are scattered

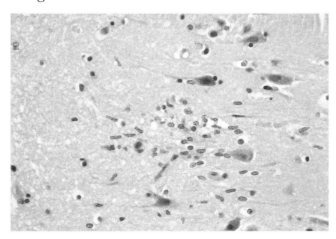

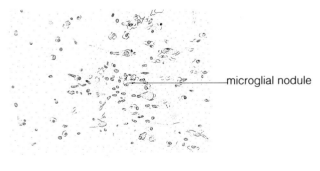

Fig. I.3.7 Progressive multifocal leukoencephalopathy. Microglial nodule. (HPS stain, ×400)

microglial nodule

in the affected areas **(Fig. I.3.8;** see Figs. II.9.18, 21). These cells, with strongly basophilic and pleomorphic nuclei, are gemistocytic astrocytes which often resemble neoplastic cells. There are also mononuclear phagocytes that have engulfed products of myelin degradation (see Fig. II.9.18). Finally, there are oligodendrocytes (mainly outside the demyelinated necrotic areas) (see Figs. II.9.16, 20) that contain the characteristic viral inclusion bodies (see Fig. II.9.22).[4,14] These are intranuclear, hyaline, eosinophilic, or amphophilic type A Cowdry bodies without surrounding haloes.[2,3] Under the electron microscope, the nucleus of an infected oligodendrocyte shows marginated chromatin and numerous scattered virus particles in the form of virions or filamentous viral bodies.[6,10]

The clinical diagnosis of PML must be considered in the presence of any slowly progressive, multifocal cerebral process that is not associated with fever and occurs in an immunodeficient patient.[3] Microscopic confirmation is accomplished by means of brain biopsy using a regular hematoxylin-eosin stain, which is sufficient to highlight the characteristic histologic features. Unfortunately, the diagnosis is useful only in ruling out other cerebral pathologic processes. There is no effective treatment for PML; the disease usually progresses relentlessly to a fatal outcome in three to six months.[2,12] A few cases of unexplained spontaneous remission have been reported.[2,11]

Fig. I.3.8 Progressive multifocal leukoencephalopathy. Extensive demyelination. Bizarre, hyperchromatic astrocyte (gemistocyte) and inflammatory cells.   (HPS stain, ×400)

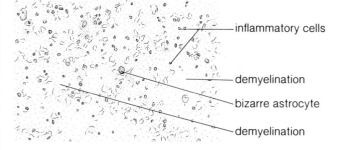

inflammatory cells

demyelination

bizarre astrocyte

demyelination

PROGRESSIVE MULTIFOCAL LEUKOENCEPHALOPATHY (PML)

Subacute, progressive, demyelinating disease of CNS

Almost exclusively in patients with deficient cellular immunity, including AIDS patients

Caused by JC, a small DNA human papovavirus

Ubiquitous, worldwide distribution

Childhood asymptomatic infection, with subsequent JC latency and potential reactivation

Insidious onset of disease, lack of fever, and slow course

Progressive dementia and focal neurologic deficits

Lucent, irregular, nonenhancing areas on CT scan

Multiple asymmetric lesions in white matter

Areas of demyelination, phagocytes with degraded myelin

Atypical hyperchromatic astrocytes

Oligodendrocytes with intranuclear inclusion bodies

Definitive diagnosis by brain biopsy

Treatment inefficient, survival short

REFERENCES

1. Astrom KE, Mancall EL, Richardson EP: Progressive multifocal leukoencephalopathy: A hitherto unrecognized complication of chronic lymphatic leukemia and Hodgkin's disease. *Brain* 1958; 81:93–111.
2. Mathews T, Wisotzkey H, Moossy J: Multiple central nervous system infections in progressive multifocal leukoencephalopathy. *Neurology* 1976; 26:9–14.
3. Myerowitz RL: Progressive multifocal leukoencephalopathy, in Myerowitz RL (ed): *The Pathology of Opportunistic Infections.* New York, Raven, 1983, pp 199–204.
4. Petito CK, Cho E-S, Lemann W, et al: Neuropathology of acquired immunodeficiency syndrome (AIDS): An autopsy review. *J Neuropathol Exp Neurol* 1986; 45:635–646.
5. Anders KH, Guerra WE, Tomiyasu U, et al: The neuropathology of AIDS: UCLA experience and review. *Am J Pathol* 1986; 124:537–558.
6. Moskowitz LB, Hensley GT, Chan JC, et al: The neuropathology of acquired immune deficiency syndrome. *Arch Pathol Lab Med* 1984; 108: 867–872.
7. Snider WD, Simpson DM, Nielsen S, et al: Neurological complications of acquired immune deficiency syndrome: Analysis of 50 patients. *Ann Neurol* 1983; 14:403–418.
8. Weiner LP, Johnson RT, Herndon RM: Viral infections and demyelinating diseases. *N Engl J Med* 1973; 288:1103–1110.
9. Hogan TF, Borden EC, McBain JA: Human polyomavirus infections with JC virus and BK virus in renal transplant patients. *Ann Intern Med* 1980; 92:373–378.
10. Miller JR, Barrett RE, Britton CB, et al: Progressive multifocal leukoencephalopathy in a male homosexual with T-cell immune deficiency. *N Engl J Med* 1982; 307:1436–1438.
11. Bernick C, Gregorios JB: Progressive multifocal leukoencephalopathy in a patient with acquired immune deficiency syndrome. *Arch Neurol* 1984; 41:780–782.
12. Blum LW, Chambers RA, Schwartzman RJ, et al: Progressive multifocal leukoencephalopathy in acquired immune deficiency syndrome. *Arch Neurol* 1985; 42:137–139.
13. Moskowitz LB, Hensley GT, Chan JC, et al: Brain biopsies in patients with acquired immune deficiency syndrome. *Arch Pathol Lab Med* 1984; 108:368–371.
14. Kleihues P, Lang W, Burger PC, et al: Progressive diffuse leukoencephalopathy in patients with acquired immune deficiency syndrome (AIDS). *Acta Neuropathol* 1985; 68:333–339.

Secondary Bacterial Diseases Associated with AIDS

LEGIONELLA PNEUMONIA

Legionella pneumonia was first observed in the summer of 1976 as an outbreak of febrile respiratory disease among the participants at the American Legion Convention in Philadelphia. In January 1977, the etiologic agent, a new bacterium, was isolated from the lung tissues of four fatal cases and named *Legionella pneumophila.*[1] Retrospective serologic studies showed that this organism had caused previous epidemics as far back as 1947.[2] At present, it is estimated to be the etiologic agent of 5% of sporadically occurring bacterial pneumonias. Occasional outbreaks aside, a total of about 25,000 cases occur in the United States every year; the mortality is 15% to 20%.[3-5] The *Legionella* family includes seven different species, all of which are gram-negative bacilli. The species can be separated by means of specific antisera.

Legionella pneumophila organisms are commonly found in stagnant waters, streams, and ponds and in air-conditioning systems, as in the Philadelphia epidemic.[3] Although the infection is airborne, it has the potential for person-to-person spread, which makes it a potentially important nosocomial agent in hospitalized immunosuppressed patients.[3] Age appears to play a role in the development of the disease: children are virtually never affected by legionellosis.[5] Responses to infection with *L. pneumophila* cover a wide spectrum from asymptomatic seroconversion to mild, self-limited febrile illness to severe, potentially fatal legionnaire's disease.[2] Legionnaire's disease primarily (often exclusively) affects the lungs. It is manifested by acute pneumonia that begins abruptly with fever, headache, and myalgias and continues with nonproductive cough; extrapulmonary symptoms sometimes occur later.[2,3,5] Chest radiographs show patchy, poorly defined infiltrates that may involve a whole lobe by coalescence and that are bilateral in two thirds of cases.[6]

On gross examination, the lungs are heavy, with large, confluent consolidated areas of red or gray hepatization. Abscesses may occur in 24% of cases, and serous pleural effusions are common.[6] On microscopic examination (**Fig. I.4.1;** see Figs. II.4.12–14), the pattern is that of fibrous purulent pneumonia with abundant alveolar fibrinous exudate containing numerous polymorphonuclear leukocytes and alveolar macrophages in about equal amounts.[5,6] In more than 60% of cases—particularly in immunosuppressed hosts—the central area of consolidation shows extensive leukocytoclasis, which is apparent as a focal area of necrosis with large amounts of bacilli and nuclear debris resulting from fragmented leukocytes.[5,6] The vessel walls show necrotizing vasculitis, and the inflammatory process spreads by extension from one alveolus to the next through the pores of Kohn.[6] In immunocompetent individuals, macrophages may be predominant in the alveolar exudate; in immunodeficient individuals, leukocytes and necrosis are usually present.[3] It has been also noted that in immunosuppressed subjects with *Legionella* pneumonia there are remarkably few inflammatory cells in the abundant serofibrinous exudate.[7] In those who survive, the exudate becomes focally organized, with patches of fibrosis.[8] Extrapulmonary hematogenous and lymphatic spread of inflammation have been observed in sporadic cases of legionellosis occurring in immunosuppressed patients. One study of 23 such patients found involvement of hilar lymph nodes in 44%, of the spleen in 25%, of bone marrow in 13%, and of the kidneys in 3.5%.[7] Demonstration of the presence of *Legionella* in the affected tissues can be achieved by staining smears and sections with Giemsa, Gram, or Gimenez stains; however, none of these routine stains is consistently positive. Silver impregnation by the Dieterle method is generally regarded as reliable for formalin-fixed, paraffin-embedded sections.[3,5,6] When stained with the Dieterle stain, *Legionella* organisms appear as short, black rods 1 to 3 μm in length, generally clustered inside the macrophages and occasionally within the neutrophils (see Fig. II.4.14).[3,6] Electron microscopic observation has revealed as many as 23 bacilli within a single macrophage.[8] In immunosuppressed patients, free bacilli can be also seen in the tissues, including the interalveolar septae.[6]

Although the Dieterle stain is highly sensitive, it is totally nonspecific. The only specific staining method for any species of *Legionella* is the staining of smears or sections with anti-*Legionella* antibodies in a direct immunofluorescent antibody (DFA) stain.[5] Tissue-section diagnosis, though reliable, either is retroactive or requires invasive procedures for the collection of samples. Clinical diagnosis can be achieved through use of an indirect immunofluorescent antibody (IFA) assay to detect serum antibodies or through cultivation of bacteria from sputum or pleural effu-sions. These methods, however, are not rapid enough to permit successful therapy of an acute disease; accordingly, new serologic tests for the detection of antigens are being developed.[3,5] Erythromycin is the treatment of choice for controlling the infection.[2]

Unfortunately, *Legionella* infection has a predilection for immunodeficient hosts, and it can give rise to severe disease with a poor prognosis in such patients. In a study of 241 cases of legionnaire's disease, 151 patients (36%) had significant underlying disease, and 47 (31%) of the 151 were seriously immunocompromised.[2] As an intracellular pathogen, *Legionella* is particularly efficient in individuals with cellular immune deficiency, such as recipients of organ transplants or patients treated with corticosteroids and alkylating agents, in whom legionellosis has been recorded with increasing frequency.[5] Because of their pronounced cellular immune deficiency, AIDS patients are also at risk for this infection. *Legionella* pneumonia should be suspected when fibrinous lobular or lobar pneumonia develops in a patient with severe immunodeficiency and when an alveolar leukocytoclastic inflammatory infiltrate is apparent.[3]

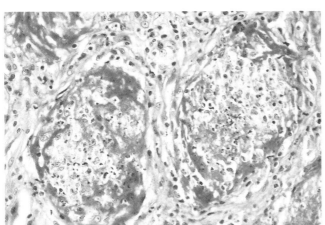

Fig. I.4.1 *Legionella* pneumonitis with alveoli filled by fibrinous exudate and nuclear leukocytic debris.   (HPS stain, $\times$400)

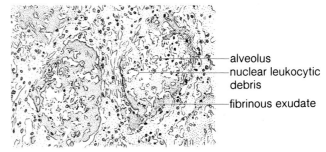

alveolus
nuclear leukocytic debris
fibrinous exudate

LEGIONELLA PNEUMONIA

Sporadic or occasional outbreaks

Gram-negative bacillus growing in stagnant waters

Mild febrile infection or severe, acute pneumonia

Bilateral nodular or lobar consolidation

Fibrinous exudate with polymorphonuclear leukocytes and macrophages

Focal tissue necrosis with leukocytoclasis

Clusters of bacilli within macrophages

Dieterle silver stain, best tissue diagnosis

Cellular immune deficiency, most significant risk factor for infection and poor prognosis

REFERENCES

1. Blackmon JA, Hicklin MD, Chandler FW, et al: Legionnaires' disease. *Arch Pathol Lab Med* 1978; 102:337–343.
2. Kirby BD, Snyder KM, Meyer RD, et al: Legionnaires' disease: Report of sixty-five nosocomially acquired cases and review of the literature. *Medicine* 1980; 59:188–205.
3. Blackmon JA, Chandler FW, Cherry WB, et al: Legionellosis. *Am J Pathol* 1981; 103:429–465.
4. Centers for Disease Control: Legionnaires' disease: United States. *MMWR* 1978; 27:439–441.
5. Myerowitz RL: The *Legionella* pneumonias, in Myerowitz RL (ed): *The Pathology of Opportun-* *istic Infections.* New York, Raven 1983, pp 83–94.
6. Winn WC, Myerowitz RL: The pathology of the *Legionella* pneumonias. *Hum Pathol* 1981; 12:401–422.
7. Weisenburger DD, Helms CM, Renner ED: Sporadic legionnaires' disease. *Arch Pathol Lab Med* 1981; 105:130–137.
8. Hernandez FJ, Kirby BD, Stanley TM, et al: Legionnaires' disease: Postmortem pathologic findings of 20 cases. *Am J Clin Pathol* 1980; 73:488–495.

TUBERCULOSIS

The working definition of AIDS includes disseminated infection with *Mycobacterium avium-intracellulare* (MAI) among the opportunistic infections that characteristically occur in AIDS patients.[1] In contrast, tuberculosis, a disease that is common in the general population, is not considered to be characteristic for AIDS. The evidence shows, however, that in populations with high rates of endemic tuberculosis individuals affected by AIDS are more likely to present with the manifestations of tuberculosis than with those of mycobacteriosis.[2-4] One study determined that the incidence of tuberculosis is very high among Haitian immigrants entering southern Florida: 650/100,000, compared with only 11/100,000 in the United States population as a whole.[2] This same study found that tuberculosis was diagnosed in 27 of 45 Haitians with AIDS but in only one of 37 non-Haitians with AIDS. Conversely, there was only one case of mycobacteriosis among the 45 Haitians with AIDS, compared with an incidence of over 50% in the AIDS population at large.[2,3] The high incidence of tuberculosis in Haitians with AIDS resembles the high incidences of disseminated histoplasmosis and coccidioidomycosis observed in AIDS patients from areas endemic for these fungal diseases; these conditions are also relatively rare in the general AIDS population.

Another AIDS population group showing a high frequency of tuberculosis is intravenous drug abusers.[3,4] One study found that tuberculosis was diagnosed in 24 of 102 intravenous drug abusers with AIDS, but not in any of 22 homosexual AIDS patients who were not drug abusers.[4] Conversely, there appears, however, to be no differences in the incidence of mycobacteriosis among the various populations at risk for AIDS. In New York City, a significant increase in the incidence of tuberculosis has been noted over the past five years. This increase is concentrated in nonwhite men aged 25 to 44 years and is associated with AIDS and IV drug abuse.[3]

Tuberculosis in AIDS patients differs from that seen in the general population: it is more aggressive, more often found in extrapulmonary locations, and more prone to generalization.[2-5] As the impaired cellular immune deficiency of AIDS patients would suggest, AIDS-associated tuberculosis manifests a greater degree of pathogenicity, much as it does in individuals who have lupus erythematosus, who are undergoing therapeutic immunosuppression, or are immunocompromised in some other fashion.[6] In most of these instances, the generalized tuberculosis probably reflects reactivation of old latent disease, through shedding of microorganisms from a cavity, erosion from an involved lymph node, or development of tuberculous bronchitis with bronchogenic or lymphatic spread.[5,6] Progressive primary tuberculosis is also seen in AIDS patients, however; it is manifested by lower lobe infiltrates and considerable involvement of hilar and mediastinal lymph nodes.[4] Classic apical infiltrates are found infrequently.

Extrapulmonary and disseminated tuberculosis are more prevalent in AIDS patients than in the general population. In one study of 48 cases of tuberculosis in AIDS patients in Newark, New Jersey, tuberculosis was extrapulmonary in 72% of cases, an unusually high rate when compared with the rates of extrapulmonary tuberculosis in the general population in Newark and in the

United States: 27% and 16%, respectively.[4] In AIDS patients, tuberculosis is rarely associated with granuloma formation or the presence of epithelioid cells and giant cells. More often, particularly when it is in the lungs, it is exudative, with air spaces consolidated by fibrin, neutrophils, and histiocytes. Necrosis is extensive, and acid-fast tubercle bacilli, usually sparse in the lesions of immunocompetent persons, are present in large numbers.[4,6] In the liver (see Figs. II.5.69–71), the spleen, the kidneys, and the bone marrow, the lesions are miliary, sometimes with larger confluent, necrotic nodules containing abundant mycobacteria. Involvement of the CNS is more common in the form of tuberculous meningitis or tuberculous brain abscess (see Figs. II.9.24–30).[7] Disseminated tuberculosis involving most organs is frequent in immunodeficient hosts, and it is often the first sign of AIDS in patients from developing countries.[5]

Tuberculosis may precede the diagnosis of AIDS or may coexist with other manifestations. In one study of 29 patients with both syndromes, tuberculosis was diagnosed four months to five years before AIDS in 14, and the two diagnoses were concurrent in 13.[4] In another study, tuberculosis coexisted with *Pneumocystis carinii* pneumonia in 15 patients.[8] Predictably, tuberculosis in AIDS is particularly aggressive, and there is massive involvement of organs that are otherwise rarely affected; examples of such involvement include cold abscesses in the ribs, rectal abscesses, multiple brain abscesses, and pericardial effusions with acute cardiac tamponade.[4]

Despite the background of immune deficiency, tuberculous AIDS patients respond well to the usual antituberculous drugs.[2,4,7] Unlike MAI, which is generally resistant, *M. tuberculosis* is sensitive to isoniazid and rifampin, and the therapeutic results are generally good.[2,4] Because of the availability of efficient treatment, early diagnosis is of particular importance. Unfortunately, tuberculin skin tests are not revealing, because of the immune deficiency induced by AIDS. In some studies, radiographic and sputum examinations have not been productive either, leaving the invasive approach of a lung biopsy the most effective mode of diagnosis.[4]

TUBERCULOSIS

Common in AIDS patients from developing countries and IV drug abusers

Often precedes the manifestations of AIDS by months

Extrapulmonary locations common in AIDS patients

Aggressive, tendency to dissemination

Frequent necrosis

Granulomas and giant cells uncommon

Acid-fast tubercle bacilli in large numbers

Tuberculin skin tests inefficient; tissue biopsy often necessary for diagnosis

Responsive to antituberculous treatment

REFERENCES

1. Centers for Disease Control: Revision of case definition of AIDS for national reporting—United States. *MMWR* 1985; 34:373–375.
2. Pitchenik AE, Cole C, Russell BW, et al: Tuberculosis, atypical mycobacteriosis and the acquired immunodeficiency syndrome among Haitians and nonHaitian patients in South Florida. *Ann Intern Med* 1984; 101:641–645.
3. Selwyn PA: AIDS: What is now known: III. Clinical aspects. *Hosp Pract* 1986; 21:119–153.
4. Sunderam G, McDonald RJ, Maniatis T, et al: Tuberculosis as a manifestation of the acquired immunodeficiency syndrome (AIDS). *JAMA* 1986; 256:362–366.
5. Lane HC, Fauci AS: Infectious complications of AIDS, in Broder S (ed): *AIDS*. New York, Marcel Dekker, 1987, pp 185–203.
6. Laurenzi GA, Mark EJ: A 20-year-old Cambodian immigrant with systemic lupus erythematosus and respiratory distress. *N Engl J Med* 1986; 315:1469–1477.
7. Fischl MA, Pitchenik AE, Spira TJ: Tuberculous brain abscess and *Toxoplasma* encephalitis in a patient with the acquired immunodeficiency syndrome. *JAMA* 1985; 313:3428–3430.
8. Murray JF, Felton CP, Garay SM: Pulmonary complications of acquired immunodeficiency syndrome. *N Engl J Med* 1984; 310:1682–1688.

MYCOBACTERIOSIS

The genus *Mycobacterium* includes multiple species that range from widespread innocuous inhabitants of soil and water to organisms that are highly pathogenic for man, such as *Mycobacterium tuberculosis* and *Mycobacterium leprae*.[1] Besides the classic mammalian tubercle bacilli, other acid-fast bacilli, usually with little or no virulence for humans, have been identified; these are referred to as atypical mycobacteria. Lately, however, the importance of nontuberculous mycobacteria as agents of human disease has come to be increasingly recognized, particularly in persons with cellular immune deficiency. The most common of these nontuberculous mycobacteria are two related species, *M. avium* and *M. intracellulare*, both of which are nonphotochromogens classified as belonging to Runyon group III. Because these two species closely resemble each other in laboratory tests, they are collectively known as the *Mycobacterium avium-intracellulare* (MAI) complex.

Before the AIDS epidemic, a literature search revealed only 14 published cases of disseminated MAI infection in adults;[2,3] however, sporadic cases of solitary pulmonary nodules and of chronic lymphadenitis caused by MAI have been observed in immunocompromised patients.[4-7] In a review of 20 resected solitary pulmonary nodules in which granulomas and acid-fast bacilli were identified, 12 (60%) were due to MAI.[4] This finding raises the possibility that a substantial number of pulmonary granulomas are not caused by *M. tuberculosis*, as is generally believed, but by MAI, which may also be rising in incidence at present.[4]

In AIDS patients, mycobacteriosis, the disseminated infection with MAI, has been recognized as one of the common opportunistic infections whose development is favored by the immune deficiency of the host, and it is included in the definition of the syndrome.[3,8-12] It is remarkable, however, that opportunistic infection with MAI, now commonly seen in the immunodeficiency induced by HIV, is not one of the opportunistic infections occurring in non-AIDS immunosuppressed patients with neoplasias.[12] Furthermore, it has been noted that in non-AIDS patients, even those who have been medically immunosuppressed, the bacilli are far less abundant and the macrophages less numerous than in AIDS patients with mycobacteriosis lesions.[5,13,14] This would indicate that a special population of T lymphocytes is responsible for the control of MAI infections and that AIDS directly affects these particular lymphocytes.[14] The MAI complex has been isolated ante mortem from sputum, blood, bronchial washings, CSF, and aspirates of bone marrow and lymph nodes in as many as 50% of AIDS patients; at autopsy, it is easily cultured from the affected organs.[10,12,14] In disseminated mycobacteriosis, the lymph nodes (see Figs. II.2.32–37), spleen (see Figs. II.2.61, 62), and lungs (see Fig. II.4.15) are most commonly involved; the characteristic lesions are also identified in the liver (see Figs. II.5.72–74), adrenals,

small intestine (see Figs. II.5.36, 37), and skin.[10,12]

On gross examination, miliary granulomas are sometimes visible on the cut surfaces of the spleen, liver, lymph nodes, heart, and kidney.[14] They range in size from 0.1 to 1 cm and in color from yellow to tan. When the small bowel is involved, the mucosa has prominent folds and shows elevated yellowish nodules on the surface of the villi.[15]

On microscopic examination (see Figs. II.2.32–34, 61–62; II.5.72–74), the local structures in all organs are replaced with masses of highly distended histiocytes with striated or foamy, yellow or bluish cytoplasm and small, dark nuclei without pleomorphism or mitoses. Although these macrophages are derived from histiocytes, they do not resemble the epithelioid cells of tuberculosis, and they rarely form giant cells that are not of the classical Langhans type. Necrosis is minimal or absent, and calcification and fibrosis are not present.[5,14-16] Staining for acid-fast organisms shows that the macrophages are filled and distended by enormous amounts of MAI bacilli (**Fig. I.4.2;** see Figs. II.2.7, 34, 37 and II.5.74). In the spleen, which may enlarge to ten times its normal weight, the MAI-filled macrophages aggregate selectively around arterioles, producing a characteristic pattern (see Figs. II.2.61–2.62).[17] The tropism of macrophages for these T-cell areas is so far unexplained. The intestinal mucosa is infiltrated by MAI-laden macrophages (see Figs. II.5.36–5.37), yielding a histologic appearance that is very similar to that of Whipple's disease.[15] The lymph nodes are moderately enlarged, the architecture is effaced, follicles are inapparent, and lymphocytic depletion is noted. Sheets of foamy macrophages replace the cortex and part of the medulla (see Figs. II.2.33–37). In the lungs, the infiltrates are located in the interalveolar septae, frequently in the form of ill-defined granulomas. The bone marrow (see Figs. II.2.6,7) shows granulomas or subtle, small clusters of macrophages, which are easily overlooked unless acid-fast staining is routinely performed on patients suspected of AIDS.[18]

The macrophages filled with MAI bacilli commonly seen in mycobacteriosis closely resemble the globi of lepromatous leprosy (Fig. I.4.2; see Figs. II.2.34, 62). This is to be expected, since both are mycobacterial infections occurring in individuals lacking proper immunity. In leprosy, between the two ends of the microscopic spectrum— namely, lepromatous and tuberculoid lesions— there is an intermediate form, known as histoid pattern, which now has also been reported to occur in mycobacteriosis.[19] This consists of a proliferation of spindle-shaped histiocytes in bundles and whorls in a pattern resembling the patterns of a connective tissue tumor (see Figs. II.2.35–37). It has been reported to form nodules in the soft tissues of the hand, but it can be also seen in the lymph nodes, lungs, and skin.[19] When stained, the spindle-shaped histiocytes show abundant intracytoplasmic MAI.

The diagnosis of mycobacteriosis is made through culture of infected fluids and tissues. It can be made far more rapidly through staining of involved tissues with the Kinyoun or Ziehl-Neel-sen stains for acid-fast organisms. The MAI complex also stains strongly with the periodic acid–Schiff (PAS) stain and with silver stains of the GMS type.

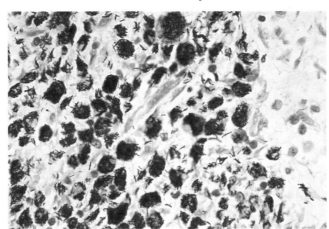

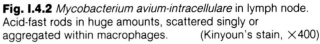

Fig. I.4.2 *Mycobacterium avium-intracellulare* in lymph node. Acid-fast rods in huge amounts, scattered singly or aggregated within macrophages.   (Kinyoun's stain, ×400)

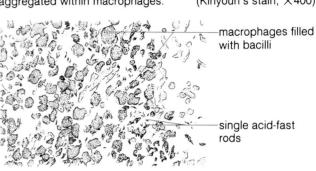

macrophages filled with bacilli

single acid-fast rods

MYCOBACTERIOSIS

MAI complex widespread in soil and water

Acid-fast bacilli, obligate intracellular

Organisms resistant to antituberculosis drugs

Innocuous in immunocompetent

Sporadic focal lesions in immunosuppressed

Disseminated mycobacteriosis in AIDS

Visible miliary lesions in most organs

Ill-formed granulomas or cell sheets without necrosis

MAI-filled striated or foamy macrophages

No epithelioid cells, giant cells, caseation, or calcification

MAI cultured from body fluids and tissues

Strong staining with PAS, with GMS, and specifically with acid-fast stains

REFERENCES

1. Wolinsky E: Mycobacteria, in David BD et al (eds): *Microbiology.* New York, Harper & Row, 1973, pp 861–865.
2. Greene JB, Sidju GS, Lewin S, et al: *Mycobacterium avium-intracellulare:* A cause of disseminated life-threatening infection in homosexuals and drug abusers. *Ann Intern Med* 1982; 97:539–546.
3. Masur H: *Mycobacterium avium-intracellulare:* Another scourge for individuals with the acquired immunodeficiency syndrome. *JAMA* 1982; 248:3013.
4. Gribetz AR, Damsker B, Bottone EJ, et al: Solitary pulmonary nodules due to nontuberculous mycobacterial infection. *Am J Med* 1981; 70:39–43.
5. Horsburgh CR, Mason UG, Farhi DC, et al: Disseminated infection with *Mycobacterium avium-intracellulare:* A report of 13 cases and a review of the literature. *Medicine* 1985; 64:36–48.
6. Marchevski A, Damsker B, Gribetz A, et al: The spectrum of pathology of nontuberculous mycobacterial infections in open-lung biopsy specimens. *Am J Clin Pathol* 1982; 78:695–700.
7. Mufarrij AA, Greco MA, Antopol SC, et al: The histopathology of cervical lymphadenitis caused by *Mycobacterium avium–Mycobacterium intracellulare* complex in an immunocompromised host. *Hum Pathol* 1982; 13:78–81.
8. Centers for Disease Control: Revision of the case definition of acquired immunodeficiency syndrome for national reporting—United States. *Ann Intern Med* 1985; 103:402–403.
9. Fauci AS, Macher A, Longo DL: Acquired immunodeficiency syndrome: Epidemiologic, clinical, immunologic and therapeutic considerations. *Ann Intern Med* 1984; 100:92.
10. Mobley K, Rotterdam HZ, Lerner CW, et al: Autopsy findings in the acquired immune defi-

ciency syndrome. *Pathol Annu* 1985; 20(pt 1): 45–65.

11. Reichert CM, O'Leary TJ, Levens DL, et al: Autopsy pathology in the acquired immune deficiency syndrome. *Am J Pathol* 1983; 112:357–382.

12. Zakowski P, Fligiel S, Berlin GW, et al: Disseminated *Mycobacterium avium-intracellulare* infection in homosexual men dying of acquired immunodeficiency. *JAMA* 1982; 248:2980–2982.

13. Farhi DC, Mason UG, Horsburgh CR: Pathologic findings in disseminated *Mycobacterium avium-intracellulare* infection: A report of 11 cases. *Am J Clin Pathol* 1986; 85:67.

14. Klatt EC, Jensen DF, Meyer PR: Pathology of *Mycobacterium avium-intracellulare* infection in acquired immunodeficiency syndrome. *Hum Pathol* 1987; 18:709–714.

15. Strom RL, Gruninger RP: AIDS with *Mycobacterium avium-intracellulare* lesions resembling those of Whipple's disease. *N Engl J Med* 1983; 309:1323–1324.

16. Sohn CC, Schroff RW, Kliewer KE: Disseminated *Mycobacterium avium-intracellulare* infection in homosexual men with acquired cell-mediated immunodeficiency: A histologic and immunologic study of two cases. *Am J Clin Pathol* 1983; 79:247–252.

17. Seshi B: Two cases of AIDS with florid *Mycobacterium avium-intracellulare* infection in the T-cell areas of the spleen. *Hum Pathol* 1985; 16:964–965.

18. Cohen RJ, Samoszuk MK, Busch D, et al: Occult infections with *M. intracellulare* in bone-marrow biopsy specimens from patients with AIDS. *N Engl J Med* 1983; 308:1475–1476.

19. Wood C, Nickoloff BJ, Todes-Taylor NR: Pseudotumor resulting from atypical mycobacterial infection: A "histoid" variety of *Mycobacterium avium-intracellulare* complex infection. *Am J Clin Pathol* 1985; 83:524–527.

Secondary Fungal Diseases Associated with AIDS

CANDIDIASIS

Systemic, life-threatening fungal infections, rarely seen before the introduction of antibiotic and chemotherapeutic agents, have increased in incidence and severity during the past two decades. This increase is related to the frequency of grave immune deficiency induced by aggressive tumor chemotherapy, by immunosuppression in recipients of organ transplants, and, lately, by AIDS. Among the fungi, the common genus *Candida* is the leading cause of opportunistic mycotic infections. Among opportunistic pathogens as a whole, *Candida* is unique in that it is the only one that is part of the normal flora present in the mouth, pharynx, intestine, skin, and vagina.[1,2] There are multiple species of *Candida* that are morphologically indistinguishable in tissue sections and can be identified only by their growth features in vitro. It is known, however, that the majority of infections are caused by *C. albicans.*

On histologic examination, *C. albicans* appears as colonies of yeasts or blastospores and pseudohyphae. The *Candida* yeasts are sharply defined, round or oval bodies 3 to 4 μm in diameter that

may contain one or more vacuoles.[3] The pseudohyphae are rows of yeasts that only resemble real hyphae (as in *Aspergillus*) and can be distinguished from them by the absence of branchings and by the presence of regular points of narrowing that simulate tubular segmentation. The fungi stain well with hematoxylin and PAS, but in poorly fixed tissues may be overlooked in the purulent cellular reaction. In such cases, the best results are obtained with the various types of silver stains, such as Gridley's, Gomori's, or Grocott's methenamine.[2,3]

Because of the normal presence of *C. albicans* as a saprophyte on various mucosal surfaces and its tendency to proliferate during antibiotic therapy, growth of fungi from sputum, throat swabs, and even blood is of uncertain value for diagnosis. Similarly, serologic tests for antibodies to *Candida* species have not been useful in clinical practice.[1] Therefore, diagnosis of invasive candidiasis must rely exclusively on morphologic study, based on the recognition of yeasts and pseudohyphae within the various tissues.[1,2,4,5]

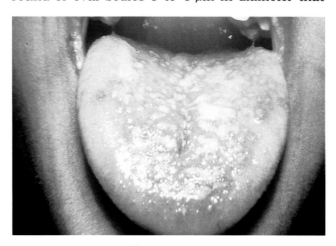

Fig. I.5.1 Confluent, thick, white patches in candidiasis of tongue.

Gastrointestinal candidiasis is most commonly localized in the esophagus, particularly in its distal part; however, any segment of the gastrointestinal tract, contiguous or widely separated, may be involved.[1,6] In oral candidiasis, the tongue is covered by diffuse white patches of exudate (**Fig. I.5.1;** see Fig. II.5.7) or by a thick black or brown coating.[6] Although oral candidiasis is not a sufficient criterion for the diagnosis of AIDS, it has proved to be of prognostic value, in that it indicates progression of the immunodeficiency toward AIDS.[7] Esophageal involvement, however, is included in the definition of AIDS. It is accompanied by dysphagia, odynophagia, and retrosternal pain and can be diagnosed by its characteristic appearance on barium radiography.[7,8] In the esophagus, stomach, and intestine there are gray pseudomembranes covering irregularly shaped ulcers. The pseudomembranes are composed of fibrin and necrotic tissue debris within meshworks of pseudohyphae. When yeasts predominate, the infections tend to be shallow. The pseudohyphae, however, which are the invasive forms of *C. albicans,* may extend deep into the muscular walls of the esophagus or intestines; however, perforations due to *Candida* ulcerations generally do not occur, since the pseudohyphae do not extend beyond the serosae.[1] *Candida* peritonitis, a rare event, has occasionally occurred, but it is the result of direct inoculation during peritoneal dialysis and not of intestinal infection.[6]

Urinary tract candidiasis, usually of the lower part of the tract, is seen in catheterized patients. As a rule, it does not usually progress to involve the kidneys (see Figs. II.6.5–6).

Pulmonary candidiasis (see Figs. II.4.16–20) may be caused by aspiration from mucosal lesions of the upper respiratory tract or by hematogenous spread, particularly in severely immunosuppressed patients.[1,4,5] In the former case, the lesions center on a bronchus and are distributed in patches, usually in the lower lobes.[1] In the latter case, the lesions have a miliary, even, bilateral distribution involving parenchyma and pleura. On microscopic examination, the lesions have the appearance of a target, with a central area of necrotic tissues infiltrated by yeasts and pseudohyphae surrounded by a peripheral area of intraalveolar hemorrhage.[3]

Disseminated candidiasis represents systemic infection with multiple organ involvement, resulting either from vascular invasion by pseudohyphae or from sepsis induced during surgery or intravenous injection (see Figs. II.8.1, 2). In a 1976 study of autopsies performed over 12 years, disseminated candidiasis involved the kidneys in 80% of cases, the brain in 52%, and the heart in 48%.[9] These figures are confirmed by more recent studies, in which the kidneys, heart, liver, and spleen are affected in more than 50% of cases, and the brain, lung, eye, and thyroid in 10% to 50%.[1] Disseminated candidiasis is characterized by the formation of multiple abscesses in the parenchyma of various organs. On gross examination, they resemble miliary granulomas or carcinomatosis, presenting as round white foci 1 to 2 mm in diameter, that are usually surrounded by hemorrhagic areas.[1,2,10] On microscopic examination, the abscesses, located in the kidneys, the liver, the spleen, or the heart, are comprised of a center made up of fungi and tissue necrosis, leukocytes, and peripheral hemorrhage. Epithelioid or giant cells are not usually part of this process.[3]

In the central nervous system, the miliary lesions are distributed randomly in the cerebral cortex and cerebellum, and with increased density in the territory of the middle cerebral artery.[1,9] The eye may be affected in the course of hematogenous fungal dissemination, resulting in *Candida* endophthalmitis. This condition is manifested by multiple white, well-circumscribed, cottonlike exudates with hemorrhagic rims in the chorioretina (see Figs. II.10.28–29) that extend into the vitreous, which becomes hazy and may subsequently show formation of abscesses.[11]

Candida infections are frequently associated with other pathogens, especially bacteria and fungi. Of the infections with multiple fungi, the most common is combined *Candida–Aspergillus* infection.[2]

CANDIDIASIS

Most frequent opportunistic fungal infection

Present in normal flora of mucosae and skin

Candida only fungus to be both saprophyte and pathogen

Yeasts and pseudohyphae

Positive staining with hematoxylin, PAS, and GMS

Histologic diagnosis is the most reliable

Pseudohyphae, the invasive form

Distal esophagus, most common GI localization

Miliary abscesses in disseminated candidiasis

Kidneys, brain, liver, and heart most commonly involved

Common association with *Aspergillus,* other fungi, and bacteria

REFERENCES

1. Myerowitz RL: Localized and disseminated candidiasis, in Myerowitz RL (ed): *The Pathology of Opportunistic Infections.* New York, Raven, 1983, pp 95–114.
2. Rosen PP: Opportunistic fungal infections in patients with neoplastic diseases. *Pathology Annu* 1976; 11:255–317.
3. Binford CH, Dooley JR: Candidiasis, in Binford CH (ed): *Pathology of tropical and extraordinary diseases.* Washington, DC, Armed Forces Inst of Pathol, 1976; vol 2, 568–569.
4. Masur H, Rosen PP, Armstrong D: Pulmonary disease caused by *Candida* species. *Am J Med* 1977; 63:914–925.
5. Rose HD, Sheth NK: Pulmonary candidiasis: A clinical and pathological correlation. *Arch Intern Med* 1978; 138:964–965.
6. Eras P, Goldstein MJ, Sherlock P: *Candida* infection of the gastrointestinal tract. *Medicine* 1972; 51:367–379.
7. Selwyn PA: AIDS: What is now known: III. Clinical aspects. *Hosp Pract* 1986; 21: pp 119–153.
8. Fauci AS, Macher AM, Longo DL, et al: NIH Conference; Acquired immunodeficiency syndrome: Epidemiologic, clinical, immunologic and therapeutic considerations. *Ann Intern Med* 1984; 100:92–106.
9. Parker JC, McCloskey JJ, Knauer KA: Pathobiologic features of human candidiasis: A common deep mycosis of the brain, heart and kidney in the altered host. *Am J Clin Pathol* 1976; 65:991–1000.
10. Reichert CM, O'Leary TJ, Levens DL, et al: Autopsy pathology in the acquired immune deficiency syndrome. *Am J Pathol* 1983; 112:357–382.
11. Edwards JE, Foos RY, Montgomerie JZ, et al: Ocular manifestations of *Candida* septicemia: Review of seventy-six cases of hematogenous *Candida* endophthalmitis. *Medicine* 1974; 53:47–75.

ASPERGILLOSIS

The genus *Aspergillus* is widespread in nature and proliferates rapidly wherever organic material and conditions of moisture and warmth are found.[1] It can be detected on the skin, fingernails, and external ear, as well as in laboratories and in unfiltered hospital air.[1] Owing to their ubiquity, the *Aspergillus* spores are easily inhaled and can cause a variety of infections and clinical syndromes. The species that most often induces opportunistic infections is *A. fumigatus,* which appears as mycelial mats composed of radiating hyphae with a greenish coloration. Identification of *Aspergillus* in tissues is based on the characteristic features of the hyphae: uniformity in size (about 3 to 4 μm in width) and regular septation, with dichotomic branchings at about 45 degrees that advance in the same direction (**Fig. I.5.2;** see Figs. II.4.24, 25).[1,2] The ends of the hyphae develop fruiting heads or vesicles, becoming conidiophores and creating the typical appearance, which resembles that of an aspergillum, from which the name of the organism is derived.[1,3]

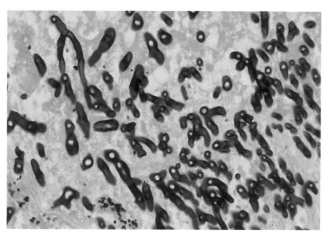

Fig. I.5.2 *Aspergillus fumigatus* in lung. Regularly septated hyphae of uniform width with dichotomic branchings advancing in same direction. (GMS stain, ×1,000)

In nonimmune compromised human beings, *Aspergillus* may cause otitis externa, allergic bronchopulmonary disease, and occasionally fungus balls that develop in preexisting cavitary lesions of the lung.[1,3] In the last instance, aspergillomas—that is, giant three-dimensional fungal colonies several centimeters in diameter—form in pulmonary cavitary lesions attributable to tuberculosis, bronchiectasis, or abscesses that open into a bronchus. These fungi do not, however, invade the tissues; they generally die and are partially expectorated. In contrast, aspergillosis in immunodeficient hosts becomes aggressive, invading the blood vessels and disseminating to distant organs. Often it is fatal. The incidence of invasive aspergillosis has increased continuously over the past 20 years, in parallel with the increased use of corticosteroid and cytotoxic therapy in neoplastic diseases.[4,5] Antibiotics, particularly penicillin and tetracycline, do not appear to increase susceptibility to aspergillosis; this is not true of candidiasis.[5] Patients with acute leukemia are particularly susceptible to aspergillosis: in one study from the early 1970s, it occurred seven times more frequently in leukemia patients than in patients with Hodgkin's disease or lymphoma.[1,4,5] At that time, the incidence of aspergillosis had quadrupled in patients treated for neoplastic diseases, particularly when corticosteroids were part of the immunosuppressive therapy. Recently, in the course of the current epidemic of HIV infection, cases of invasive aspergillosis have been diagnosed in patients with AIDS.

The portal of entry and by far the most common site of infection is the respiratory tract. Unlike candidiasis, which affects the gastrointestinal tract (particularly the esophagus) more often than the lung, aspergillosis is more often pulmonary than esophageal which is rarely of clinical significance.[3] Hematogenous dissemination, an uncommon event, originates in the lung and affects (in order of frequency) the brain, the heart, the kidneys, and the gastrointestinal tract.[3] On gross examination, pulmonary aspergillosis appears as a 2 to 4 cm target lesion with a central gray area of infarction and a peripheralized area of hemorrhage and hyperemia.[1,3] The tendency for infarction is explained by the ability of *Aspergillus* to invade blood vessels and proliferate in their lumina, which leads to vascular thrombosis and tissue infarction. Depending on the size of the artery involved, the infarcts may be either small and nodular or large, with a lobar infiltrate that is usually single but sometimes bilateral.[3]

On microscopic examination (see Figs. II.4.21–25), the thrombosed vessels and infarcted areas contain mats of hyphae admixed with fibrin exudate, necrotic tissue debris, and a limited inflammatory cellular response from neutrophils and lymphocytes. An amorphous, eosinophilic precipitate is sometimes present, coating the *Aspergillus* hyphae. This phenomenon, referred to as the Hoeppli-Splendore phenomenon, is similar to that seen in *Actinomyces* infection and probably represents deposition of antigen-antibody complexes.[1,5] Hyphae and necrotizing inflammation may extend outward into the surrounding lung parenchyma, giving rise to confluent areas of pneumonitis. Granulomas are not formed, though multinucleated giant cells are sometimes seen around the hyphae. Plasma cells and eosinophils are sometimes present at the periphery, which suggests that there is an element of allergy to the reaction.[5]

In general, hematogenous dissemination and secondary foci of involvement develop in about 25 percent of patients with invasive pulmonary aspergillosis.[3] The brain may show several areas of anemic or hemorrhagic infarction located deep in the gray or white matter.[3,4] The meninges are almost never affected, which makes diagnosis by CSF examination inefficient. The heart may have subepicardial or subendocardial lesions made up of areas of necrosis and hyphae crossing the myocardial fibers. Other organs that infarcts and colonies of fungi may involve are the kidneys, the liver, the spleen, the esophagus, and the intestines. Perforations do not occur, because the involvement of the gastrointestinal tract is mostly mucosal.[3] Coinfections with other fungi, particularly *Candida*, and bacteria, most commonly *Pseudomonas aeruginosa*, are not infrequent.[4]

Diagnosis of invasive aspergillosis is difficult and not entirely reliable, except when histologic demonstration, which remains the definitive method, is used. Unfortunately, histologic demonstration requires invasive procedures that are not always possible in severely ill patients. *Aspergillus* hyphae can be occasionally seen on a fresh wet mount of sputum or bronchial washings or stained with Papanicolaou stain in needle aspiration of the lung.[5] Recovery of *Aspergillus*, which is not part of the normal flora, is far more significant than recovery of *Candida*, which is a usual contaminant.[3] Unfortunately, positive cultures are obtained in only 25% to 30% of cases with autopsy-proven aspergillosis.[3,4] Serologic methods for identifying specific antibodies are not standardized and generally are not used. The diagnosis must therefore be based on recognition of the characteristic *Aspergillus* hyphae in tissue sections. These are true septate hyphae, unlike their candidal counterparts, which are pseudohyphae constructed by the apposition of yeasts. *Aspergillus* hyphae are uniform in size, unlike those of *Phycomycetes*, which are of variable thickness, and they are branching, unlike the *Candida* pseudohyphae, which are not. Finally, again unlike *Candida* pseudohyphae, *Aspergillus* hyphae stain poorly with hematoxylin-eosin. Their recognition depends on application of silver stains of the Grocott methenamine type.

ASPERGILLOSIS

Aspergillus fungi widespread in nature

Uniform, septate, branching hyphae

Otitis externa, allergic bronchitis, intracavitary fungal balls in immunocompetent patients

Invasive, disseminated infection in immunodeficient patients

Highest susceptibility in patient with acute leukemia and those undergoing corticosteroid therapy

Vascular invasion and thrombosis with resulting infarctions

Mats of hyphae microscopically apparent in necrotic tissues

Lungs most commonly affected

Brain and heart frequent secondary sites

Histologic recognition of characteristic hyphae, most reliable diagnosis

REFERENCES

1. Schwarz J: Aspergillosis. *Pathol Annu* 1973; 8:85–107.
2. Binford CH, Dooley JR: Aspergillosis, in Binford CH (ed): *Pathology of Tropical and Extraordinary Diseases.* Washington, DC, Armed Forces Inst of Pathol, 1976, vol 2, pp 562–563.
3. Myerowitz RL: Invasive pulmonary and disseminated aspergillosis, in Myerowitz RL (ed): *The Pathology of Opportunistic Infections.* New York, Raven, 1983, pp 115–128.
4. Meyer RD, Young LS, Armstrong D, et al: Aspergillosis complicating neoplastic disease. *Am J Med* 1973; 54:6–15.
5. Rosen PP: Opportunistic fungal infections in patients with neoplastic disease. *Pathol Annu* 1976; 11:255–315.

NOCARDIOSIS

Nocardia asteroides belongs to a group of funguslike bacteria known as actinomycetes. The actinomycetes are gram-positive organisms that grow slowly, by extending branching filaments that form mycelial colonies, like those of fungi. Unlike fungi, however, actinomycetes are prokaryotic, have filaments that are smaller and narrower than those of yeasts and hyphae, contain cell membrane components that are characteristic of bacteria, and are inhibited in their growth by penicillins, tetracyclines, and sulfonamides—antibacterial drugs that have no antifungal activity.[1] *Nocardia* species, unlike *Actinomyces* species, are aerobic, grow on relatively simple media, and are inhabitants of soil, from which infection can spread to animals and human beings. In animals, *Nocardia* causes a suppurative disease of cattle; in human beings, it is a rare, usually self-limited disease, despite its worldwide distribution.[1]

Nocardia organisms are killed by activated macrophages but not by neutrophils, which indicates that immunity to this pathogen is cell-mediated.[2] This explains why *Nocardia* infections are not known to affect immunocompetent hosts and why all reported cases have occurred in immunodeficient patients. Nocardiosis has been reported in patients with leukemia, dysproteinemia, systemic lupus erythematosus, and sarcoidosis.[3] More often, however, Nocardia infection occurred as a complication in patients immunosuppressed by means of radiation or chemotherapy for treatment of underlying neoplastic disease or for organ transplantation.[2,3]

Clinical manifestations include bronchopneumonia, necrotizing pneumonia with multiple abscesses, and hepatic, scrotal, cutaneous, and brain abcesses (see Fig. II.9.31). Not uncommonly, the lesions and the causative agent remain unsuspected and are only discovered at autopsy.[3] During one 22-month period, infections with *N. asteroides* were diagnosed in seven heart transplant patients.[2] In five cases the lesions were confined to the lungs, and in two they extended to the skin, causing extensive destruction of soft tissues—a common tendency of this infection.

Recently, *Nocardia* abscesses and disseminated nocardiosis were reported to have occurred in AIDS patients.[4-6] Thus, in two male intravenous drug abusers with AIDS, *N. asteroides* was isolated from purulent pericardial effusions and diffuse confluent chest abscesses.[4] Disseminated nocardiosis with necrotizing confluent abscesses in the lungs, pericardium, kidneys, spleen, brain, and subcutaneous tissues have also been reported in patients with AIDS.[5,6] On microscopic examination (see Fig. II.9.32), the lesions show extensive tissue necrosis with large accumulations of polymorphonuclear leukocytes, but without formation of giant cells or granulomas.

Identification of the etiologic agent may be difficult. *N. asteroides* appears as fine, branching, beaded filaments that form mycelial colonies in tissue sections, pus smears, and, rarely, in sputum.[3,5] The organisms are gram-positive and weakly acid-fast. Since the Ziehl-Neelsen stain does not stain *Nocardia,* a modified acid-fast stain, such as the Fite-Faraco, must be used.[5] *Nocardia asteroides* is differentiated from *Actinomyces israelii,* the other major member of the Actinomycetales order, by its acid-fast staining property and by the absence of sulfur granules in the purulent infections that it causes.[7]

NOCARDIOSIS

Nocardia asteroides: aerobic, funguslike bacteria growing in mycelial colonies

Gram-positive, acid-fast, branching fine filaments

Rare, self-limiting infections in immunocompetent hosts

Multiple abscesses and disseminated infections in immunosuppressed and AIDS patients

Necrotizing, suppurative lesions in lungs, pericardium, brain, soft tissues, and skin

REFERENCES

1. Kobayashi GS: Actinomycetes: The fungus-like bacteria, in Davis BD et al (eds): *Microbiology.* New York, Harper & Row, 1973, pp 870–879.

2. Krick JA, Stinson EB, Remington JS: *Nocardia* infection in heart transplant patients. *Ann Intern Med* 1975; 82:18–26.

3. Young LS, Armstrong D, Blevins A, et al: *Nocardia asteroides* infection complicating neoplastic disease. *Am J Med* 1971; 50:356–367.

4. Holtz H, Lavery D, Kapila R: Actinomycetales infection in the acquired immunodeficiency syndrome. *Ann Intern Med* 1985; 102:203–205.

5. Macher AM, De Vinatea ML, Daly MJ, et al: AIDS case for diagnosis series: Disseminated nocardiosis and extranodal (renal) non-Hodgkin's lymphoma. *Military Med* 1986; 151:M73–M80.

6. Nelson AM, Macher AM, Neafie RC, et al: AIDS case for diagnosis series: Disseminated nocardiosis and visceral Kaposi's sarcoma. *Military Med* 1986; 151:M80–M88.

7. Robboy SJ, Vickery AL Jr: Tinctorial and morphologic properties distinguishing actinomycosis and nocardiosis. *N Engl J Med* 1970; 282:593–596.

Histoplasma capsulatum, a fungus that is widely distributed in the central regions of the United States, causes asymptomatic, self-limiting disease in normal individuals and severe, disseminated disease in immunodeficient hosts. Its natural habitat is the soil, particularly soil contaminated with the excreta of chicken, birds, or bats.[1] The fungus is dimorphic, taking a mycelial form at room temperature and a yeast form at mammalian body temperatures.[1] Whereas the yeast form has little potential for infection, the hyphae or spores of the mycelial form are infective when inhaled.[1,2] The yeasts are round or oval, measure 2 to 4 μm in diameter, and multiply by budding (**Fig. I.5.3;** see Figs. II.4.32, 34).

It is estimated that in the US 500,000 persons are infected with *Histoplasma* each year, mainly in the endemic areas, where occasional outbreaks are also recorded.[3] Thus, in Indianapolis, a city with a population of 1,000,000, more than 100,000 residents became infected during an outbreak of histoplasmosis in 1978; 300 of them had to be hospitalized, and 15 eventually died of the disease.[3] During this outbreak of histoplasmosis, disseminated disease developed in only 4.2% of immunocompetent persons but in 55.2% of patients who were immunosuppressed.[4] These figures indicate the high risk of virulent histoplasmosis in those individuals with HIV infection and AIDS who reside in endemic areas. This risk has begun to materialize: high incidences of disseminated histoplasmosis in AIDS patients have already been reported from Alabama and Indiana.[4,5]

Inhalation of airborne spores or hyphae causes a primary pulmonary focal infection that in immunocompetent individuals elicits the formation of an epithelioid granuloma. As in tuberculosis, the granuloma may become fibrotic or undergo central caseous necrosis with secondary calcification. Larger collections of coalescing granulomas may form a tumorlike formation known as histoplasmoma. When the initial inoculum is heavy, multiple miliary foci or patches of alveolar pneumonitis accompanied by acute symptoms may result.[2] In contrast, the infection is uncontrolled in immunodeficient hosts; instead of localized lesions that heal spontaneously, disseminated histoplasmosis develops.[2,4,6] In a study of 58 patients in endemic areas who received corticosteroids or cytotoxic drugs for leukemia or Hodgkin's disease and then acquired histoplasmosis, 88% had disseminated histoplasmosis and only 12% the localized form of the disease.[6]

The characteristic histologic picture in the various organs affected by disseminated histoplasmosis consists of large accumulations of histiocytes filled with yeasts (see Figs. II.4.33, 34; II.5.75–77). The intracellular yeasts are viable and apparently multiply inside the macrophages as a result of the loss of the cells' fungicidal capacity.[2] The parasitized histiocytes form sheets of cells that replace normal structures in various organs and often undergo central necrosis, releasing yeasts that can infect newly attracted histiocytes.[1,2] The yeast-laden macrophages have an affinity for vessel walls, which leads to focal lesions, followed by thrombosis and infarction. Such necrotic lesions are frequently seen in the meninges and adrenals.

The organs that are part of the mononuclear phagocyte system (MPS)—e.g., the bone marrow, lymph nodes, spleen, and liver (see Figs. II.5.75–77)—become the site of extensive diffuse histiocytosis with nodules or sheets of viable histiocytes containing huge amounts of viable organisms.[2] The histologic appearance resembles those of lepromatous leprosy, mycobacteriosis, and leishmaniasis; the pathogenic mechanism, nonreactive macrophages, is similar as well.[2] Bone-marrow involvement is common (85% in one study of 102 cases reported from Nashville, Tennessee); bone-marrow biopsy is therefore considered the most useful method of diagnosis.[2,6]

In the lungs (see Figs. II.4.32–34), the principal lesions of disseminated histoplasmosis appear as focal interstitial infiltrates with accumulations of yeast-containing macrophages that thicken the interalveolar septae and encroach on the alveolar spaces ([2]). Parasitized macrophages are also frequently found in the intestinal mucosa—a 70% incidence in one autopsy series—and in the phar-

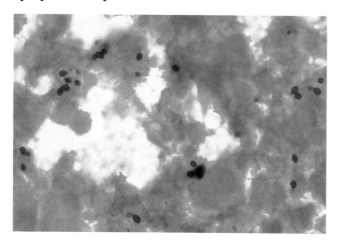

Fig. I.5.3 *Histoplasma capsulatum* in smear of lung brushing. Small ovoid yeasts with narrow-budding forms.

(GMS stain, ×1,000)

ynx and larynx, where they form nodules and ulcers resembling malignant neoplasms.[2] Occasionally, endocarditis with valvular involvement and formation of infective emboli may develop. In the vegetations that develop on the valves, *H. capsulatum* may grow freely, taking hyphal forms not usually seen in the involvement of other organs.[2] Cutaneous manifestations of histoplasmosis are rare; their presence suggests marked immunosuppression.[5]

Diagnosis of histoplasmosis depends on either histologic demonstration or culturing of the fungus from infected tissues. Regular hematoxylin-eosin (H&E) stains can demonstrate the presence of the intracellular yeasts; however, the best results are obtained with silver stains of the GMS type, which can reveal the fungi even in old fibrocaseous, partly calcified lesions that can no longer be stained by other methods (see Fig. II.4.34).[1] Thus, *Leishmania,* which resembles *Histoplasma* in H&E staining, can be easily distinguished from the latter organism in that it is not stained by the special stains for fungi. Another opportunistic agent that may be encountered in AIDS patients and resembles *Histoplasma* is *Toxoplasma,* which is smaller, is not intracellular, and is not stained with silver.[1] *Blastomyces* is multicellular and has broad-based buds, whereas *Histoplasma* is unicellular and has narrow-based buds. *Cryptococcus* is much the same size as *Histoplasma* and, like it, has narrow-based buds; however, it can easily be differentiated by means of a mucicarmine stain, which stains the cell walls strongly.[1]

In disseminated histoplasmosis, organisms can be occasionally detected by means of a Wright-stained smear of peripheral blood or by means of blood or tissue cultures. The culture methods require three to four weeks for recovery and identification of the organisms, which makes them useless in the treatment of these sick patients with rapidly progressing disease.[7] Serologic methods are also inefficient, because in endemic areas a large segment of the population normally has antibodies to *Histoplasma.*[6] The histoplasmin test, in contrast to the test for tuberculosis, requires repeated episodes of infection to remain positive, and therefore is not helpful.[2]

Thus, histopathologic diagnosis remains the preferred method for fast and definitive diagnosis, even if invasive procedures are required.[7] Amphotericin B is the treatment of choice, producing quick resolution of lesions in patients who are not entirely immunosuppressed and in whom an early diagnosis permits administration of a full course of antifungal therapy.[6] In AIDS patients, unfortunately, treatment with amphotericin has not been curative.[4]

HISTOPLASMOSIS

Endemic infection in central US

Histoplasma capsulatum found in contaminated soil

Dimorphic fungus: yeast form has low infectivity, hyphal form has high infectivity

Infection by inhalation of airborne hyphae

Granulomas and localized infections in immunocompetent individuals

Disseminated histoplasmosis in immunosuppressed hosts

High incidence in AIDS patients from endemic areas

Macrophages containing large amounts of viable yeasts

Accumulations of yeast-containing macrophages in most organs

Histologic diagnosis through biopsy and silver staining is most rapid and reliable method

Amphotericin B treatment of choice, but ineffective in immunodeficient patients

---

REFERENCES

1. Binford CH, Dooley JR: Histoplasmosis, in Binford CH (ed): *Pathology of Tropical and Extraordinary Diseases.* Washington, DC, Armed Forces Inst of Pathol, 1976, vol 2, pp 578–581.
2. Goodwin RA, Shapiro JL, Thurman GH, et al: Disseminated histoplasmosis: Clinical and pathologic correlations. *Medicine* 1980; 59:1–33.
3. Wheat LJ, Slama TG, Eitzen HE, et al: Large urban outbreak of histoplasmosis: Clinical features. *Ann Intern Med* 1981; 94:331–337.
4. Wheat LJ, Slama TG, Zeckel ML: Histoplasmosis in the acquired immune deficiency syndrome. *Am J Med* 1985; 78:203–210.

5. Bonner JR, Alexander WJ, Dismukes WE, et al: Disseminated histoplasmosis in patients with the acquired immune deficiency syndrome. *Arch Intern Med* 1984; 144:2178–2181.

6. Kauffman CA, Israel KS, Smith JW, et al: Histoplasmosis in immunosuppressed patients. *Am J Med* 1978; 64:923–932.

7. Paya CV, Roberts GD, Cockerill FR: Laboratory methods for the diagnosis of disseminated histoplasmosis: Clinical importance of the lysis-centrifugation blood culture technique. *Mayo Clin Proc* 1987; 62:480–485.

CRYPTOCOCCOSIS

Cryptococcus neoformans is a monomorphic fungus that forms yeasts but not hyphae. The yeasts are round and are composed of cells surrounded by thick mucopolysaccharide capsules. The cells are 4 to 15 μm in diameter, and the mucopolysaccharide capsules are 3 to 5 μm thick.[1,2] In tissue sections, the capsule appears as a clear space around the yeast that separates the individual cells from one another and from local tissues. Budding is more common in *Cryptococcus* yeasts than in any other yeasts; the process involves formation of characteristic single or double round buds with narrow bases that detach easily reproducing the mother cell **(Fig. I.5.4).**[1,2] Rapidly growing organisms may form short chains of budding cells resembling tubes or hyphae.[1]

Cryptococcus stains well with H&E, PAS, and silver in the GMS stain (see Fig. I.5.4, Figs. II.2.39, II.9.36). India ink preparations can detect the yeasts in sputum or cerebrospinal fluid. Typically, however, diagnosis relies on the mucicarminophilia of the capsule, which appears bright red in Mayer's mucicarmine stain (see Figs. II.4.30-31; II.2.43, 45; and II.9.38). Diagnosis of cryptococcal infection may also involve culture of the organisms on specific media and serologic testing. The antigens of *Cryptococcus* are related to the polysaccharides of its capsule and can be detected by the latex agglutination test, which is simple and rapid. A positive test result, with control tests for rheumatoid factor, is considered conclusive for cryptococcosis; the sensitivity is 90 percent.[3] Serologic tests for the identification of *Cryptococcus* antigens in blood or cerebrospinal fluid are highly reliable and are recommended for evaluation of patients with acute interstitial pneumonia or for monitoring cryptococcal infections.[3,4]

Cryptococcus neoformans has worldwide distribution, infects the soil, and is associated with pigeon excreta. The infection results from inhalation of yeasts, which generates a primary focus of pulmonary cryptococcal infection that subsequently disseminates to the airway and possibly to the blood vessels. Cryptococcosis is one of the few fungal infections that can affect both immunocompetent and immunodeficient individuals.[2] In the former, it usually results in a localized pulmonary lesion that is clinically occult and eventually undergoes fibrosis. In the latter, it may result from reactivation of a latent infection, primary aerogenous infection, or infection by indwelling catheters.[5] Underlying predisposing conditions are malignancies; hepatic cirrhosis

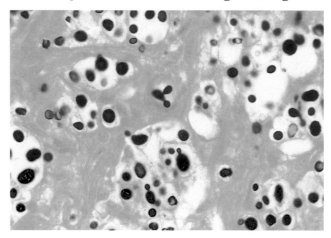

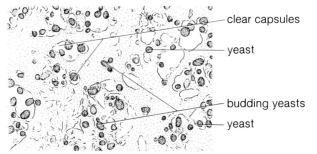

Fig. I.5.4 *Cryptococcus* yeasts with typical round, narrow-based single or double buds and clear capsules.

(GMS stain, ×100)

clear capsules

yeast

budding yeasts

yeast

and other debilitating conditions; radiation; chemotherapy, particularly with corticosteroids; and HIV infection. The clinicopathologic form cryptococcosis takes may be fulminant, chronic, or occult and may include pulmonary, disseminated, meningoencephalitic, cutaneous, and osseous varieties of the disease.[2]

In the lung (see Figs. II.4.26–31) and in lymph nodes (see Figs. II.2.38–45), the lesions usually consist of scattered or confluent granulomas. These are generally noncaseous and consist of aggregates of lymphocytes, epithelioid cells, and multiple multinucleated giant cells containing phagocytized yeasts. When confluent, the granulomas form nodules that become visible on radiologic examination (see Fig. II.4.26).[6] A much less common manifestation of lung cryptococcosis is that of pneumonia in which alveoli are filled with a fibrinous exudate containing numerous yeasts and polymorphonuclear leukocytes.[2] In disseminated cryptococcosis, invasion of blood vessels and fungemia take place, followed by colonization of multiple organs, particularly the meninges, lungs, and kidneys.[6] In the lungs, the result is cryptococcal pneumonia; in the kidneys the result is proliferation of yeasts in glomeruli and tubules. In general, the lesions of disseminated cryptococcosis are acute and unaccompanied by a cellular reaction. This is a reflection of the severe cellular immune deficiency of the host which is the predisposing factor.

In the central nervous system (see Figs. II.9.33–38), the major involvements are of the meninges and, to some extent, of the cerebral tissues around sulci and blood vessels (see Fig. II.9.33). In the acute, fulminant form (the less common one), the meninges covering the cerebral hemispheres are thickened and contain a cloudy, gelatinous, opaque fluid. Microscopic examination (see Figs. II.9.34–38) shows numerous free yeasts, lymphocytes, and plasma cells. In chronic meningoencephalitis (the more common form), the lesion is localized at the base of the brain, and the subjacent cerebral tissues are usually involved. The yeasts, accompanied by the inflammatory reaction, are located in the periarterial Virchow-Robin spaces, which become distended and form small cystic spaces 1 to 2 mm in diameter, known as "soap bubbles."[2] Such cysts are more often found in the basal ganglia, since they develop along the lenticulostriate perforating arteries, which come from the base of the brain, where cryptococcal meningitis is particularly severe.[2] If meningoencephalitis persists long enough, hydrocephalus may also develop.

Disseminated cryptococcosis is characteristically associated with the severe forms of immune deficiency. In AIDS patients, cryptococcal infection takes the form of meningoencephalitis or of disseminated disease, generally with a fatal outcome.[7–9] The course of the disease is fulminant, usually developing from a preexistent latent pulmonary infection. Yeasts are found in various organs, most often in the meninges and in the glomerular capillaries and convoluted tubules of the kidneys.[2] Cellular reactions in this form of acute infection are almost nonexistent. In chronic forms of cryptococcosis, however, localizations in lung, bones, skin, and other organs are commonly accompanied by the formation of granulomas and eventually by fibrosis.[2,6] Cutaneous cryptococcosis is farily common in immunosuppressed patients with disseminated disease. It appears as an erythematous area with herpeslike vesicles or as cellulitis with edema and tenderness.[6] Fluid aspirated from vesicles or scraped from an ulcerated area contains typical yeasts that can be identified on an India ink wet preparation.[6]

CRYPTOCOCCOSIS

Monomorphous fungi with yeasts and no hyphae

Round yeasts of variable sizes with single buds

Thick mucopolysaccharide capsule

Positive staining with India ink, PAS, silver, and mucicarmine

Worldwide distribution

Found in soil infected by pigeons' excreta

Infection by inhalation of yeasts

Both immunocompetent and immunodeficient patients may be affected

Pulmonary occult infections or localized organ lesions in the immunocompetent patient

Meningoencephalitis or fulminant disseminated infections in the immunodeficient patient

Latex agglutination test reliable for capsular antigens in blood and CFS

REFERENCES

1. Binford CH, Dooley JR: Cryptococcosis, in Binford CH (ed): *Pathology of Tropical and Extraordinary Diseases*, Washington, DC, Armed Forces Inst of Pathol 1976; vol 2, 572–574.
2. Myerowitz RL: Local and disseminated cryptococcosis, in Myerowitz RL (ed): *The Pathology of Opportunistic Infections*. New York, Raven, 1983, pp 145–160.
3. Fisher BD, Armstrong D: Cryptococcal interstitial pneumonia. *N Engl J Med* 1977; 297:1440–1441.
4. Drutz DJ: Antigen detection in fungal infections. *N Engl J Med* 1986; 314:115–117.
5. McDonnell JM, Hutchins GM: Pulmonary cryptococcosis. *Hum Pathol* 1985; 16:121–128.
6. Kerkering TM, Duma RJ, Shadomy S: The evolution of pulmonary cryptococcosis. *Ann Intern Med* 1981; 94:611–616.
7. Reichert CM, O'Leary TJ, Levens DL, et al: Autopsy pathology in the acquired immune deficiency syndrome. *Am J Pathol* 1983; 112:357–382.
8. Selwyn PA: AIDS: What is now known: III. Clinical aspects. *Hosp Pract* 1986; 21:119–153.
9. Fauci AS, et al: Acquired immunodeficiency syndrome: Epidemiologic, clinical, immunologic, and therapeutic considerations. *Ann Intern Med* 1984; 100:92–106.
10. Schupbach CW, Wheeler CE, Briggaman RA, et al: Cutaneous manifestations of disseminated cryptococcosis. *Arch Dermatol* 1976; 112:1734–1740.

COCCIDIOIDOMYCOSIS

The dimorphic fungi *Coccidioides immitis*, common in the southwestern United States, and *Histoplasma capsulatum*, common in the Midwest, are the most common pathogenic agents of solitary pulmonary nodules.[1] Both are capable of producing lesions in immunocompetent individuals; however, they are particularly virulent in immunodeficient subjects, especially individuals with HIV infection, in whom they induce severe, disseminated disease. In the United States, it is estimated that there are about 100,000 clinical cases of coccidioidomycosis and 70 deaths annually. In endemic areas, the infection is very common but remains clinically occult, with the possibility of later reactivation. In these areas, symptomatic illness develops in university students at a rate of 0.4% per year, and coccidioidal infection is detected in renal and cardiac transplant recipients at a rate of 3% to 6% per year.[2] In AIDS patients in Tucson, Arizona, a highly endemic area, coccidioidomycosis has been reported to occur at a rate of 27%, compared with an annual incidence of 4% in the general population.[3]

C. immitis exists in a yeast form that is commonly found in contaminated tissues and in a hyphal form, the arthrospores, that infects soil and airborne dust. High-velocity winds can transport the arthrospore-carrying soil for great distances, causing epidemics of coccidioidomycosis in humans and animals.[4] The characteristic yeasts of the organism seen in tissues are spherules 20 to 60 μm in diameter known as sporangia, which are made up of a thick, brown, double-contoured capsule and multiple small round endospores 2 to 5 μm in diameter (**Fig. I.5.5;** see Figs. II.4.36, 4.37; II.5.86). The development of endospores begins in a narrow zone adjacent to the inner surface of the capsule, which on its outer side shows a precipitate of immune complexes.[5] The spores give rise to thin, branching, septate hyphae, which are only rarely found in tissues (mainly in areas of tissue necrosis).[5,6]

In the majority of cases, the primary pulmonary coccidioidal infection is clinically insignificant, occurring as a flulike syndrome, or inapparent, occurring as a self-healing focus of infection.[6,7] It may remain isolated as a localized persistent lesion that has the appearance of a coin lesion on radiographic examination. Since in the general population coin lesions are caused by carcinoma in 25% of cases, these persistent lesions must be resected surgically so that a histologic diagnosis can be made. The nodule in coccidioidomycosis is 2 to 3 cm in diameter, round, sharply demarcated, and yellowish in color, and it usually has a necrotic or cavitary center.[1,6] Histologic examination (see Figs. II.4.35–38, II.2.63, II.5.83–5.86)[6] reveals it to be composed of coalescing granulomatous collections of epithelioid cells, giant cells of the Langhans or foreign-body type, lymphocytes, and plasma cells (which are sometimes numerous). Sporangia containing endospores, empty degenerated cysts, and free small, round spores are present in the area of central necrosis or within the multinucleated giant cells.

Whereas coccidioidomycosis in immunocompetent individuals is characterized by a single localized nodule, the pulmonary disease in the immunodeficient is bilateral and diffuse. In conditions of massive infestation, acute lobar pneumonia may develop. In AIDS-related coccidioidomycosis, the most common form is that of diffuse bilateral pulmonary nodular infiltrates, which was the principal manifestation in five of seven cases reported from Tucson.[3] Their radiographic appearance is that of bilateral reticulonodular infiltrates, and the diagnosis can be made by detection of spores in sputum, bronchoalveolar lavage, bronchial washings, or transbronchial pulmonary biopsy (the most accurate method).[3] Cysts and spores stain selectively with silver; consequently, the optimal staining is the Grocott methenamine silver stain (see Fig. II.5.86). Communications with bronchi, rupture into the pleura, and bronchopleural fistulae are rare complications.

In the general population, extrapulmonary spread of coccidioidomycosis is rare, but in immunodeficient individuals, dissemination to various organs is frequent. Disseminated coccidioidomycosis is manifested by the presence of single or confluent giant-cell granulomas within the parenchyma of liver, spleen, lymph nodes, bone marrow, and other organs. Coccidioidomycosis of the central nervous system (see Fig. II.9.39) may also develop in immunodeficient patients, with extensive colonization of the meninges by *Coccidioides* cysts accompanied by giant cells and lymphocytes. In one case of an HIV-infected patient with coccidioidomycotic meningitis, formation of multiple *Coccidioides* granulomas in the omentum and peritoneum has been observed subsequent to the placement of a ventriculoperitoneal shunt, which was needed to alleviate the increasing pressure of hydrocephalus (see Figs. II.5.83–5.86; II.2.63). Serologic diagnosis of coccidioidomycosis can be accomplished through detection of complement-fixation antibodies.

Fig. I.5.5 Coccidiomycosis granuloma with sporangia comprising PAS-positive capsule and degenerated endospores, occasionally phagocytosed by giant cells.
(PAS, ×250)

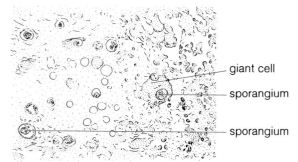

COCCIDIOIDOMYCOSIS

Dimorphic fungus with yeast and hyphal forms

Pulmonary infection by inhalation of airborne spores

Inapparent or localized infections in the immunocompetent patient

Disseminated, extensive infections in the immunodeficient patient

Sporangium with multiple endospores and thick double capsule

Cysts and spores revealed by methenamine silver stains

Serologic diagnosis by complement-fixation antibody tests

Necrotizing giant-cell granulomas in parenchymatous organs

Accumulations of cyst-containing giant cells in effusions

REFERENCES

1. Medeiros AA, Mark EJ: A 51-year-old woman with chest pain and a coin lesion. *N Engl J Med* 1980; 302:218–223.
2. Calhoun DL, Galgiani JN, Zukoski C, et al: Coccidioidomycosis in recent renal or cardiac transplant recipients, in Einstein HE, Catanzaro A (eds): *Coccidioidomycosis: Proceedings of the Fourth International Conference on Coccidioidomycosis.* Washington, DC, National Foundation for Infectious Diseases, 1985, 312:8.
3. Bronnimann DA, Adam RD, Galgiani JN, et al: Coccidioidomycosis in the acquired immunodeficiency syndrome. *Ann Intern Med* 1987; 106:372–379.
4. Flynn NM, Hoeprich PD, Kawachi MM, et al: An unusual outbreak of windborne coccidioidomycosis. *N Engl J Med* 1979; 301:358–361.
5. Binford CH, Dooley JR: Deep mycoses, in Binford CH (ed): *Pathology of Tropical and Extraordinary Diseases.* Washington, DC, Armed Forces Inst of Pathol, 1976, vol 2, 570–572.
6. Deppisch L, Donowho EM: Pulmonary coccidioidomycosis. *Am J Clin Pathol* 1972; 58:489–500.
7. Drutz DJ, Cantanzaro A: A state of the art coccidioidomycosis. *Am Rev Respir Dis* 1978; 117:727–771.

BLASTOMYCOSIS

North American blastomycosis is caused by *Blastomyces dermatiditis,* a fungus found in the soil in Georgia and other southeastern regions of the United States.[1] Sporadic infections and occasional outbreaks have been also reported from Minnesota, Louisiana, and Africa.[1,2] In infected tissues, the organism appears as a round, thick-walled cell 8 to 15 μm in diameter that reproduces by broad-based budding (**Fig. I.5.6;** see Fig. II.4.41). In well-preserved, well-fixed tissues, multiple nuclei are visible within the cell.[1]

The primary lesions, following respiratory infection, are in the lung. The acute form manifests itself in chills, fever, cough, and pleuritic chest pain of several weeks' duration. The chronic form, which may last for years, has a less severe toxicity than the acute form and exhibits a tendency to disseminate, involving the pleura, skin, bones, genitourinary tract, liver, and spleen secondarily.[1,3] In the lungs, the lesions may be unilateral or bilateral, appearing as nodular infiltrates or pneumonic consolidations, with or without cavitation.[3] The characteristic tissue lesions are combinations of granulomas comprising epithelioid and giant cells with neutrophil infiltration and abundant suppuration (see Figs. II.4.39, 40).[1]

The cutaneous and osteoarthritic lesions are accompanied by the formation of sinuses and fistulas.[3] The *Blastomyces* cells are present in the granulomas, either free or engulfed by giant cells. They can also be found in sputum and pleural fluid. Routine examination for this fungus is therefore recommended in patients from endemic areas who have pneumonia or pleural effusions of undetermined origin.[3] In a wet preparation, *B. dermatiditis* can appear as a single or as a broad-based budding spherical cell with thick, refractile walls. On histologic staining, it can be distinguished from *Coccidioides, Cryptococcus,* and *Mucor* because it has multinucleated cells and from *Cryptococcus* because it does not stain with mucicarmine. The lesions of pulmonary blasto-mycosis may resemble neoplasia.

Blastomycosis has not been recorded with increased frequency in patients who have cancer and immune suppression.[4] In AIDS patients, however, blastomycosis may show an increased incidence in individuals from endemic areas, much as other mycoses, such as histoplasmosis and coccidioidomycosis, do.

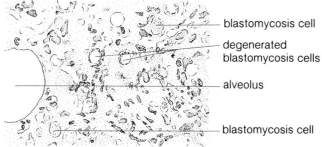

Fig. I.5.6 Blastomycosis cells with thick walls and multiple nuclei, partially degenerated in lung.   (HPS stain, ×400)

blastomycosis cell

degenerated blastomycosis cells

alveolus

blastomycosis cell

BLASTOMYCOSIS

Endemic in southeastern US and regions of Africa

Respiratory infection from contaminated soil

Acute and chronic primary pulmonary lesions

Tendency for dissemination with involvement of skin, bones, and viscera

Spherical, thick-walled, refractile, multinucleated cells with broad-based budding

REFERENCES

1. Binford CH, Dooley JR: Blastomycosis, in Binford CH (ed): *Pathology of Tropical and Extraordinary Diseases.* Washington, DC, Armed Forces Inst of Pathol, 1976, vol 2, pp 565–566.
2. Sarosi CA, Hammerman KJ, Tosh FT, et al: Clinical features of acute pulmonary blastomycosis. *N Engl J Med* 1974; 290:540–543.
3. Cush R, Light RW, George RB: Clinical and roentgenographic manifestations. *Chest* 1976; 69:345 –349.
4. Rosen PP: Opportunistic fungal infections in patients with neoplastic diseases. *Pathol Annu* 1976; 11:255–315.

MUCORMYCOSIS

Phycomycosis, zygomycosis, and mucormycosis are synonymous terms used to designate an acute fungal infection caused by various members of the order Mucorales.[1,2] These fungi are ubiquitous in nature, growing best at temperatures on decaying fruits and vegetable matter around 37° C. Infection results from inhalation of airborne spores into the nose and lung or from deposition of spores on abraded skin.[2] In tissues, the fungi resemble *Aspergillus*; however, they have broader, nonseptate hyphae with thicker walls that, unlike *Aspergillus* hyphae, which branch at regular, acute angles, branch haphazardly at right angles (**Fig. I.5.7;** see Fig. II.4.45).[1,3] The hyphae may be partially collapsed and form folds that can be mistaken for septa, which enhances the possibility of confusion with *Aspergillus*. Similarly, cross-sections of large, empty hyphae can be confused with cross-sections of the spherules of *Coccidioides*.[1] The branching hyphae typical of mucormycosis are deeply stained by hematoxylin; thus, the H&E stain usually gives the best results.

From a pathogenetic viewpoint, mucormycosis also resembles aspergillosis, in that the fungi tend to invade the vessels and cause thrombosis and infarction of tissues (see Figs. II.4.42–44). A characteristic manifestation is the induction of black eschars on the affected mucocutaneous surfaces.[2] The most common underlying condition associated with mucormycosis is diabetes mellitus, though individuals with various forms of immunosuppression—including patients undergoing organ transplantation and chemotherapy and those with leukemias, lymphomas, burns, cirrhosis, and, more recently, AIDS—are also frequently affected.[3]

The usual clinicopathologic forms are rhinocerebral, pulmonary, cutaneous, and gastrointestinal. The rhinocerebral form of mucormycosis is unique among fungal infections. It occurs more often in patients with poorly controlled diabetes and acidosis.[3] It begins as a nasal infection, then spreads to the paranasal sinuses and into the ethmoid, the retro-orbital region, and the brain.[2,3] A black eschar on the palate or nasal mucosa, accompanied by drainage of black necrotic pus, is the diagnostic clue.[3] The cerebral lesions consist of hemorrhagic areas of necrosis at the base of the frontal lobes, without meningitis.[2] Pulmonary mucormycosis is similar to aspergillosis in that it causes pulmonary vascular thrombosis and infarction. The clinical manifestations are patchy infiltrates, areas of consolidation, and occasional formation of cavities. Pleural involvement is uncommon, and allergic pneumonitis in immunocompetent individuals, such as is seen in aspergillosis, does not occur in mucormycosis.[2,3] Disseminated mucormycosis with wide involvement of viscera, including the brain, results from hematogenous spread and may be noted in association with deep immune depression, as occurs in AIDS. Cutaneous mucormycosis can be the result of superinfection in severely burned patients or of vascular spread with formation of nodular lesions resembling ecthyma gangrenosum in severely immunocompromised patients.[3] Finally, gastrointestinal mucormycosis, a rare form, occurs in the stomach as the secondary fungal infection of a peptic ulcer and exhibits the typical black discoloration.[2-4]

Diagnosis by serologic methods is not possible at present, and the isolation of organisms and their identification is not routinely done.[2] The definitive diagnosis, as for candidiasis and aspergillosis, depends on recognition of fungi and their characteristic morphologic features in tissue sections.

Fig. I.5.7 Mucormycosis in lung. Broad, thick-walled, nonseptate hyphae with right-angle branchings. Cross-sectioned empty hyphae resemble yeasts. (GMS stain, ×400)

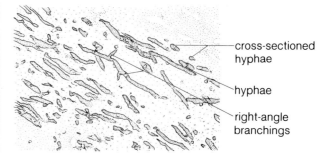

cross-sectioned hyphae

hyphae

right-angle branchings

MUCORMYCOSIS

Ubiquitous in nature

Grows on decaying vegetable matter

Broad, nonseptate, thick-walled hyphae

Irregular, right-angle branching

Diabetes, burns, and immunodeficiency are predisposing conditions

Rhinocerebral lesions unique to mucormycosis

Pulmonary, cutaneous, gastrointestinal locations

Black eschars on skin

Gastric ulcers

Tendency for vascular invasion, thrombosis, and infarction

Diagnosis by biopsy and H&E staining of tissue sections

REFERENCES

1. Binford CH, Dooley JR: Mucormycosis, in Binford CH (ed): *Pathology of Tropical and Extraordinary Diseases.* Washington, DC, Armed Forces Inst of Pathol, 1976, vol 2, pp 564–565.
2. Myerowitz RL: Zygormycosis (mucormycosis), in Myerowitz RL (ed): *The Pathology of Opportunistic Infections.* New York, Raven, 1983, pp 129–137.
3. Lehrer RI, Howard DH, Sypherd PS, et al: Mucormycosis. *Ann Intern Med* 1980; 93:93–108.
4. Parra R, Arnau E, Julia A, et al: Survival after intestinal mucormycosis in acute myelogenous leukemia. *Cancer* 1986; 58:2717–2719.

Secondary Protozoal Diseases Associated with AIDS

chapter

six

PNEUMOCYSTOSIS

Pulmonary infection with *Pneumocystis carinii* (PC) is the most common opportunistic infection of AIDS, as well as the one responsible for most AIDS fatalities. On the whole, the disease was seen sporadically in the past though limited epidemics have occurred in orphanages among premature and debilitated infants.[1] It has also been recorded in patients with neoplasms (particularly lymphomas) who were receiving immunosuppressive therapy, well before the present AIDS epidemic began.[2-4] In an autopsy study of 520 children dying of cancer, 37 were found to have *Pneumocystis* organisms in their lungs, and in 19 of the 37, PC pneumonia was the cause of death.[2] At present, the incidence of PC pneumonia is 65% in AIDS patients and as high as 84% in hemophiliac AIDS patients.[5] In the United States, episodes of PC pneumonia carry a mortality of approximately 30%, and they recur in more than 25% of cases.[6]

The infectious agent is a protozoan parasite of the Sporozoa subphylum. It was first recognized in infected rats in 1907, at which time it was mistakenly considered a form of *Trypanosoma cruzi*.[7] Its separate identity was verified in 1912, but its activity as a human pathogen was only established in 1952, in a study of interstitial plasma cell pneumonia in marasmic children.[1]

In its mature form, the organism is a cyst containing up to eight sporozoites, which appear as tiny nucleated structures. As the sporozoites mature and are eliminated, they become trophozoites, ovoid unicellular organisms 1 to 5 μm in diameter that attach to host cells. The trophozoites develop cyst walls and evolve from precysts to full cysts, exhibiting internal nuclear division and formation of new sporozoites.[8] The life cycle of PC thus alternates between trophozoite form and cyst form, both of which, together with pre-

cysts and empty degenerating cysts, are present in the alveolar pneumonic exudates.[7]

The distribution of PC is worldwide, and it is thought that the infection reservoir is in animals. Though the transmission of organisms from animal to human or from human to human is not well understood, it appears that the route of infection is through the air, since the disease involves the lungs exclusively.[8]

Infections with PC are asymptomatic in most cases. Sometimes occult infections result, from which reactivation occurs in the course of AIDS. The clinical disease develops insidiously in most patients over the course of several days or weeks, typically manifesting itself in low fever, dry cough, and tachypnea.[6,8,9] Less commonly, an acute fulminant form of PC pneumonia with severe hypoxia and cyanosis is seen. The radiographic patterns of PC pneumonia are fairly typical and have been described in detail elsewhere.[3] Commonly, there are early bilateral perihilar infiltrates, described as ground-glass alveolar infiltrates, which are followed by diffuse bilateral reticulonodular infiltrates (see Figs. II.4.46, 49).[3,8] Nodular or lobar infiltrates are rare and are considered atypical. The hilar lymph nodes are usually not involved. Pleural effusions are uncommon; their presence suggests concomitant associated infections.[8] Gallium scintigraphy often reveals diffuse uptake.[6]

In PC pneumonia, the lungs typically are heavy, consolidated, and noncrepitant. Almost invariably, autopsy reveals both lungs to be diffusely and totally involved (see Figs. II.4.47–48). The formalin-fixed cut surface has a typical appearance described as that of a coarse sponge.[8] On microscopic examination, a foamy, eosinophilic, and generally acellular alveolar exudate, sometimes described as having a honey-combed appearance, is characteristic (see Figs. II.4.51–55).[7,8] The alveolar lining cells are prominent and may show cuboidal metaplasia. The interalveolar septae are thickened by an infiltrate made up of lymphocytes, histiocytes, and occasional plasma cells. With H & E stain, the nuclei of PC are faintly stained; with PAS stain, the cyst walls stain, but cannot be easily distinguished from the surrounding PAS-positive exudate.[10] The gomori methenamine silver stain (GMS) clearly demonstrates the parasite cysts, which appear round, ovoid, or collapsed in semilunar forms and have a diameter of 3.5 to 7 μm (**Fig. I.6.1**; see Figs. II.4.54, 55). The trophozoites can best be shown on imprints with the Gram or Giemsa stains; however, the cyst walls are not stained, and thus these stains are not suitable for tissue sections.[10] Within the alveoli filled with the thick, bubbly exudate, the silver-positive PC organisms appear aggregated in small clusters.

Since PC is not an intracellular parasite, the cysts are not found within the inflammatory cells and are rather scarce in the interalveolar septae. The typical microscopic features of PC pneumonia usually seen in autopsy specimens may not always be present in small, lung biopsies. The histologic findings are considered atypical when the foamy alveolar exudate is absent or when there is considerable desquamation of alveolar epithelium. Similarly, the presence of marked interstitial inflammation and fibrosis or of epithelioid granulomata is considered to be atypical.[8] In a study of 36 cases of PC pneumonia, atypical microscopic features were present in 69% and predominated in more than 30%, which indicates the importance of the Gomori methenamine silver stain in reaching the correct diagnosis.[8,11]

For a definitive diagnosis, identification of PC cysts by silver staining is required; the specimens routinely submitted may be obtained through bronchial brushings, bronchoalveolar lavage, transbronchial biopsy, or open-lung biopsy. Because of the adherence of organisms to alveolar walls, the yield from sputum is low, and even bronchial brushings do not give positive results in more than 30% to 40% of cases.[6] In contrast,

transbronchial biopsy has an accuracy of about 90%. It is surpassed in this respect only by open-lung biopsy, with which no false negatives have been recorded.[8]

A positive diagnosis of *P. carinii* infection does not exclude the possibility that one or more of the other organisms with which it is frequently associated may be present.[9,12] The most common association is that between *P. carinii* and CMV in pulmonary involvement.[9,13] Before the present AIDS epidemic, one study reported *P. carinii* pneumonia in 35 of 78 cases of disseminated CMV disease in children aged less than one year,[3] as well as in three adults in whom Hodgkin's disease and Wegener's granulomatosis appeared to be predisposing conditions.[4] The frequent association of pneumocystosis with CMV and herpesvirus infections, candidiasis, and Kaposi's sarcoma reflects the severe cellular immunodeficiency of the host and perhaps, in the case of CMV, a particular biologic synergism between the two pathogenic organisms.[2,4,12]

Unlike CMV and most of the other opportunistic pathogens, *P. carinii* almost never invades other organs outside the lung. Involvement of hilar or retroperitoneal lymph nodes, liver, and spleen has occasionally been reported in children in whom confluent granulomas with epithelioid cells, giant cells, and typical PC cysts were observed.[7,8] This unusual absence of extrapulmonary dissemination for an opportunistic agent is explained by the biology of PC, which is characterized by low motility, lack of invasiveness, and inability to grow intracellularly in monocytes and macrophages that would otherwise assist in its vascular dissemination.[8] Cases of lung infection, if aggressively treated at an early stage, may resolve, and apparently normal pulmonary function and a normal radiographic appearance may be regained; however, autopsies of such patients who die of unrelated causes still reveal the presence of PC cysts in lung tissue. In AIDS patients, unfortunately, the persistence of severe cellular immunodeficiency makes definitive cures impossible. Recurrences of PC infection or secondary infections with other opportunistic agents are the more common course.[6,9,14]

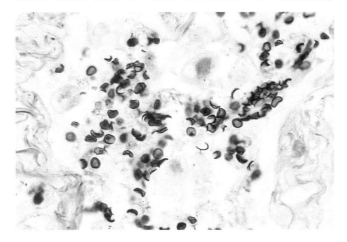

Fig. I.6.1 *Pneumocystis carinii* in lung tissue. Extracellular ovoid cysts, some degenerated and collapsed in interalveolar spaces.   (GMS stain, ×1,000)

PNEUMOCYSTOSIS

Most common, most lethal infection of AIDS

P. carinii, protozoan parasite of Sporozoa subphylum

Cysts and trophozoites are forms of life cycle

Worldwide distribution

Animal reservoir

Lungs involved almost exclusively

Extrapulmonary lesions extremely rare

Insidious onset of clinical disease

Characteristic radiologic image

Massive bilateral pneumonia

Foamy, eosinophilic alveolar exudate

Lung biopsy most reliable diagnostic method

Gomori methenamine silver most reliable stain

Frequent association with other opportunistic agents

Present medication effective

High rate of recurrence

REFERENCES

1. Dutz W: *Pneumocystis carinii* pneumonia. *Pathol Annu* 1970; 5:309–341.
2. Price RA, Hughes WT: Histopathology of *Pneumocystis carinii* infestation and infection in malignant disease in childhood. *Hum Pathol* 1974; 5:737–752.
3. Rosen P, Armstrong D, Ramos C: *Pneumocystis carinii* pneumonia: A clinicopathologic study of twenty patients with neoplastic diseases. *Am J Med* 1972; 53:428–436.
4. Symmers W St C: Generalized cytomegalic inclusion-body disease associated with *Pneumocystis* pneumonia in adults. *J Clin Pathol* 1960; 13:1–21.
5. Centers for Disease Control: Changing patterns of acquired immunodeficiency syndrome in hemophilia patients—United States. *MMWR* 1985; 34:241–243.
6. Selwyn PA: AIDS: What is now known: III. Clinical aspects. *Hosp Pract* 1986; 21:119–153.
7. Frenkel JK: Pneumocystosis, in Binford CH (ed): *Pathology of Tropical and Extraordinary Diseases*. Washington DC, Armed Forces Inst of Pathol, 1976, vol 1, pp 303–307.
8. Myerowitz RL: *Pneumocystis carinii* pneumonitis, in Myerowitz RL (ed): *The Pathology of Opportunistic Infections*. New York, Raven, 1983, pp 213–223.
9. Fauci AS, Macher AM, Longo DL, et al: Acquired immunodeficiency syndrome: Epidemiologic, clinical, immunologic, and therapeutic considerations. *Ann Intern Med* 1984; 100:92–106.
10. Sun T: Pneumocystosis, in Sun, T (ed): *Sexually Related Infectious Diseases*. New York, Field, Rich & Assoc, 1986, pp 217–225.
11. Weber WR, Askin FB, Dehner LP: Lung biopsy in *Pneumocystis carinii* pneumonia. *Am J Clin Pathol* 1977; 67:11–19.
12. Gottlieb MS, Schroff R, Schanker HM, et al: *Pneumocystis carinii* pneumonia and mucosal candidiasis in previously healthy homosexual men. *N Engl J Med* 1981; 305:1425–1431.
13. Hui AN, Koss MN, Meyer PR: Necropsy findings in acquired immunodeficiency syndrome: A comparison of premortem diagnoses with postmortem findings. *Hum Pathol* 1984; 15:670–676.
14. Masur H, Michelis MA, Greene JB, et al: An outbreak of community-acquired *Pneumocystis carinii* pneumonia: Initial manifestation of cellular immune dysfunction. *N Engl J Med* 1981; 305:1431–1438.

TOXOPLASMOSIS

Toxoplasma gondii, the causative agent of toxoplasmosis, is a protozoan capable of infecting a wide variety of mammals and birds. It is prevalent in warm and humid areas, where almost all people show serologic evidence of infection, and rare in cold and dry areas.[1,2] In the United States, toxoplasmosis is the most common parasitic infection; 20% to 70% of Americans have antibody titers indicative of chronic asymptomatic infection, and about 3,000 children are infected at birth annually.[2]

The parasite has a complex life cycle. The cat is the definitive host for the sexual stage of reproduction, during which trophozoites multiply in the intestinal epithelium and produce oocysts that are eliminated in the stool. Human beings and other mammals, the intermediate hosts, are infected through ingestion of oocysts from contaminated soil or from infected, insufficiently cooked meat.[1,2] More unusual modes of infection are transplacental transfer of *T. gondii* from mother to fetus and transmission of *Toxoplasma* with a transplanted kidney to a susceptible immunodeficient recipient.[3] In intermediate hosts, the ingested oocysts are disrupted by digestive enzymes, and the trophozoites are released into the intestine, from which they spread through lymphatics and blood vessels and are carried by macrophages into the internal organs.[4] Within macrophages, particularly in immunodeficient hosts, the trophozoites multiply rapidly, forming large clusters of small (2 to 6 μm in diameter) crescent-shaped forms called tachyzoites. In immunocompetent hosts, as immunity is established, the parasites are segregated in cysts partially synthesized by the host. In these cysts, protected by the cyst walls, they multiply slowly, as the name given to the stage—bradyzoites—indicates, and stay for long periods **(Fig. I.6.2).**[4]

Most commonly, *Toxoplasma* infection in the general population is either asymptomatic or accompanied by mild, nonspecific mononucleosis-like symptoms, such as fever, myalgias, atypical lymphocytosis, lymphadenopathy, and moderate hepatosplenomegaly.[2,3] The lymphadenopathy may be single or multiple and generally involves the posterior cervical lymph nodes.[5] It has been estimated that 15% of lymphadenopathies of unknown origin are caused by *Toxoplasma*.[2] The characteristic histologic features in involved lymph nodes are reactive hyperplastic follicles, clusters of epithelioid cells encroaching on lymphoid follicles, and aggregates of monocytoid cells along vessels and sinuses.[6] These lesions have been found to correlate with positive serologic test results for *Toxoplasma* and to indicate the presence of acute acquired toxoplasmosis.[7]

In immunocompetent hosts, symptoms resolve spontaneously in a matter of weeks or months. In immunologically compromised hosts, however, such as those with leukemias and lymphomas, those receiving immunosuppressive therapy, and those with AIDS, infection with *T.gondii* becomes acutely disseminated, usually proceeding to involve the CNS.[8–11] In a study of brain biopsies in patients with AIDS, toxoplasmic encephalitis was the diagnosis in 71% of cases.[12] It is also reported to be more common in Haitians than in any other risk group, which is consistent with the higher incidence of toxoplasmosis in tropical areas.[13,14]

In the brain (see Figs. II.9.40, 44), *T. gondii* produces foci of coagulative or hemorrhagic necrosis containing few organisms; these foci are surrounded by a zone of vascular congestion

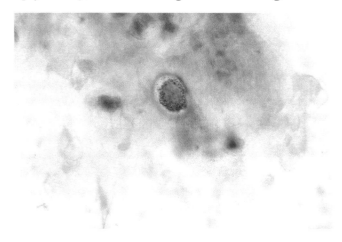

Fig. I.6.2 *Toxoplasma gondii* in smear of lung tissue. Cyst containing numerous bradyzoites among desquamated alveolar cells. (GMS stain, ×1,000)

and endothelial hyperplasia that is intensely inflamed and contains numerous organisms, both free tachyzoites **(Fig. I.6.3;** see Figs. II.2.47; II.9.42, 43) and pseudocysts with bradyzoites **(Fig. I.6.2;** see Fig. II.9.45).[15] The tachyzoites in brain lesions often have a round or oval shape rather than the crescent shape generally seen in other tissues.[12] The periphery of the lesion shows a dense accumulation of astrocytes, pleomorphic microglial cells, and lipid-laden macrophages. Vasculitis with fibrinoid necrosis, thrombi, and perivascular cuffing by inflammatory cells can be seen, sometimes even in the absence of parasites. The lesions can be either diffuse or circumscribed, in the form of abscesses that commonly are localized in the gray matter of the basal ganglia or of the cerebral and cerebellar cortices and sometimes impinge on the overlying subarachnoid spaces.[9] The *Toxoplasma* abscesses have a characteristic appearance on contrast-enhanced CT scans (see Figs. II.9.44, 46), that of single or multiple ring-enhancing cystic structures in the gray matter.[11,13,16] The cerebrospinal fluid examination is usually nondiagnostic, showing only mild elevation of protein level, normal or slightly reduced glucose level, mononuclear pleocytosis, and, on rare occasions, the presence of tachyzoites.[13,17]

After the brain, the lungs **(Fig. I.6.3)** and the heart are the organs most commonly affected by *Toxoplasma*, though in disseminated toxoplasmosis virtually any organ may be involved (see Fig. II.2.47). Pulmonary lesions consist of interstitial pneumonitis with free tachyzoites and lymphocytic infiltrates or of alveolar exudates containing abundant tachyzoites and cysts.[3] In the heart, free tachyzoites are localized within myocardial fibers, as well as in the interstitial spaces, admixed with lymphocytes and eosinophils.[3] Chorioretinitis is also frequent in AIDS patients with toxoplasmic infection. It consists of characteristic white-yellow patches on the retina, pigment deposition, cysts and tachyzoites, inflammation, scarring, and atrophy (see Figs. II.10.25–27).[18]

Congenital infection with *Toxoplasma* occurs in 1 of 1,000 live births in the United States. The chance of transmitting the infection transplacentally is greater during the last trimester; however, the damage to the fetus is greater when transmission occurs in early pregnancy.[4] It is generally a serious systemic illness that produces symptomatic cerebral and ocular lesions. In affected chil-

dren, the brain lesions are usually periventricular, with characteristic focal calcifications.[19]

Diagnosis of toxoplasmosis in tissue imprints and smears is accomplished through identification of the crescent-shaped tachyzoites; the most useful stain is Giemsa.[4] In tissue sections, cysts and pseudocysts can be clearly seen with the help of H & E stains; however, isolated tachyzoites are difficult to recognize. The differential diagnosis involves distinguishing *T. gondii* from *Histoplasma capsulatum*, a fungus, which also is characterized by the presence of multiple organisms within a cell. *Histoplasma* organisms are present only in histiocytes, whereas *Toxoplasma* organisms invade any parenchymal cell; in addition, the cell wall of histoplasma stains strongly with PAS stain.[4] *Leishmania* organisms are differentiated from *T. gondii* by the characteristic presence of a kinetoplast while *Pneumocystis carinii* is differentiated by its failure to stain with hematoxylin and eosin. Intraperitoneal inoculation of mice with infected tissue induces abundant growth of *T. gondii* in peritoneal fluid and is a highly reliable means of diagnosis.

Of the serologic tests, the long used Sabin-Feldman dye test is highly sensitive and specific; however, it requires live *Toxoplasma* organisms. Indirect immunofluorescence tests that use suspensions of purified dried organisms to measure IgM and IgG antibodies to cell-wall antigens are gradually replacing the dye test. Even immunosuppressed patients generally have high titers of IgG antibodies to *Toxoplasma*. The IgM antibodies are first detected a few days after infection; they rise to a peak and decrease over a few weeks or months. A titer of 1:80 or higher is indicative of recent infection.[2,4] The IgG antibodies reach a peak titer of 1:1000 or higher at six to eight weeks after infection; this titer persists for months or years.[2,4] In chronic active infections, complement fixation and indirect hemagglutination tests that reach their peaks at four to six months can also be used.[4] Finally, immunohistochemistry has been employed to identify in situ *T. gondii* by using monoclonal anti-*Toxoplasma* antibodies and the peroxidase-antiperoxidase technique on paraffin-embedded tissue sections.[20] This method permits easier and faster recognition of trophozoites and cysts on smears, imprints, and histologic sections, than H&E or Giemsa stains.[21]

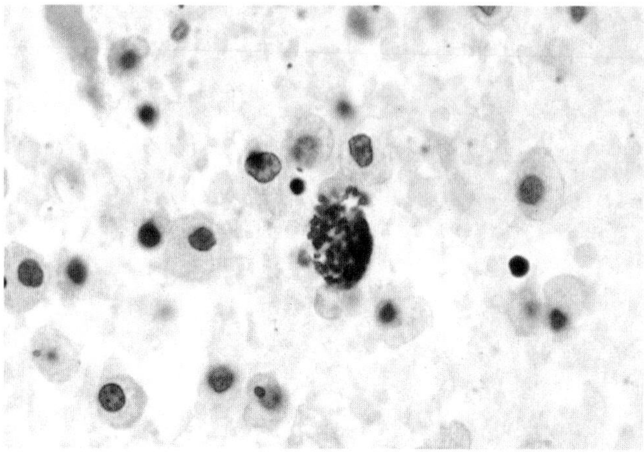

Fig. I.6.3 Free *Toxoplasma* tachyzoites broken out of pseudocyst in cerebral tissue.　　　(HPS stain, ×1,000)

TOXOPLASMOSIS

Worldwide distribution in mammals and birds

Most common parasitic infection in human beings in US

Cat is definitive host and source of contamination by oocysts

Tachyzoites, rapidly multiplying; bradyzoites within cysts, latent forms

Mild, febrile, nonspecific syndrome in immunocompetent individuals

Posterior cervical lymph nodes commonly involved

Acute disseminated infection in immunodeficient

CNS most often affected in immunodeficient individuals

Multiple necrotic foci with abscess formation in gray matter

Characteristic ring-enhancing cystic structures on CT scan

Chorioretinitis; Myocarditis

Pneumonitis, frequent localizations

Congenital toxoplasmosis by transplacental transmission

Tissue diagnosis by identification of trophozoites

Serologic diagnosis by indirect immunofluorescence tests of IgM and IgG antibodies

REFERENCES

1. Frenkel JK: Toxoplasmosis, in Binford CH (ed): *Pathology of Tropical and Extraordinary Diseases.* Washington DC, Armed Forces Inst of Pathol, 1976, vol 1, pp 284–301.
2. Krick JA, Remington JS: Current concepts in parasitology: Toxoplasmosis in the adult: An overview. *N Engl J Med* 1978; 298:550–553.
3. Myerowitz RL: Toxoplasmosis, in Myerowitz RL (ed): *The Pathology of Opportunistic Infections.* New York, Raven, 1983, pp 225–235.
4. Sun T: Toxoplasmosis, in Sun T (ed): *Sexually Related Infectious Diseases.* New York, Field, Rich & Assoc, 1986, pp 227–237.
5. Gray GF, Kimball AC, Kean BH: The posterior cervical lymph node in toxoplasmosis. *Am J Pathol* 1972; 69:349–358.
6. Stansfeld AG: The histological diagnosis of toxoplasmic lymphadenitis. *J Clin Pathol* 1961; 14:565–573.
7. Dorfman RF, Remington JS: Value of lymph-node biopsy in the diagnosis of acute acquired toxoplasmosis. *N Engl J Med* 1973; 289:878–881.
8. Gleason TH, Hamlin WB: Disseminated toxoplasmosis in the compromised host. *Arch Intern Med* 1974; 134:1059–1062.
9. Petito CK, Cho E-S, Lemann W, et al: Neuropathology of acquired immunodeficiency syndrome (AIDS): An autopsy review. *J Neuropathol Exp Neurol* 1986; 45:635–646.
10. Ruskin J, Remington JS: Toxoplasmosis in the compromised host. *Ann Intern Med* 1976; 84:193–199.
11. Snider WD, Simpson DM, Nielsen S, et al: Neurological complications of acquired immune deficiency syndrome: Analysis of 50 patients. *Ann Neurol* 1983, 14:403–418.
12. Moskowitz LB, Hensley GT, Chan JC, et al: Brain biopsies in patients with acquired immune deficiency syndrome. *Arch Pathol Lab Med* 1984; 108:368–371.
13. Levy RM, Bredesen DE, Rosenblum ML: Neurological manifestations of the acquired immunodeficiency syndrome (AIDS): Experience at UCSF and review of the literature. *J Neurosurg* 1985; 62:475–495.
14. Moskowitz LB, Hensley GT, Chan JC, et al: The neuropathology of acquired immune deficiency syndrome. *Arch Pathol Lab Med* 1984; 108:867–872.
15. Anders KH, Guerra WF, Tomiyasu U, et al: The neuropathology of AIDS. *Am J Pathol* 1986; 124:537–558.
16. McLeod R, Berry PF, Marshall WH, et al: Toxoplasmosis presenting as brain abscesses. *Am J Med* 1979; 67:711–714.
17. Alonso R, Heiman-Patterson T, Mancall EL: Cerebral toxoplasmosis in acquired immune deficiency syndrome. *Arch Neurol* 1984; 41:321–323.
18. Selwyn PA: AIDS: What is now known: III. Clinical aspects. *Hosp Pract* 1986; 21:119–153.
19. Best T, Finlayson M: Two forms of encephalitis in opportunistic toxoplasmosis. *Arch Pathol Lab Med* 1979; 103:693–696.
20. Andres TL, Dorman SA, Winn WC Jr, et al: Immunohistochemical demonstration of *Toxoplasma gondii. Am J Clin Pathol* 1981; 75:431–434.
21. Sun T, Greenspan J, Tenenbaum M, et al: Diagnosis of cerebral toxoplasmosis using fluorescein-labeled antitoxoplasma monoclonal antibodies. *Am J Surg Pathol* 1986; 10:312–316.

CRYPTOSPORIDIOSIS

Cryptosporidium is a parasitic protozoan that infects the gastrointestinal tract of animals and human beings. As a member of the order Coccidia, it is closely related to *Toxoplasma, Isospora,* and *Sarcocystis,* other animal parasites that can infect humans, particularly under conditions of immunodeficiency.[1] The life cycle of *Cryptosporidium* is identical to that of *Isospora;* it takes place in a single host, except for the oocyst, which is the infective stage and takes place outside the host.[2] Oocysts become infective after excretion. The main route of transmission is fecal-oral contamination.[3] When oocysts are ingested by a new host, they release sporozoites in the intestine. These attach to the intestinal mucosa, where they multiply in a sexual cycle, eventually forming new oocysts.

Cryptosporidiosis is a well-recognized zoonosis that causes diarrheal illness in a variety of animals, especially calves and lambs (cats and dogs are also affected on occasion).[2,3] It is not species-specific. Animal cryptosporidiosis is usually a short, acute gastrointestinal illness; only rarely is it fatal.[3] In healthy individuals, infection with *Cryptosporidium* is considered a sporadic and infrequent occurrence. In 1982, the Centers for Disease Control recorded only 12 cases in healthy animal handlers. These patients had gastrointestinal symptoms that resolved spontaneously in less than two weeks.[4] Now that more attention is being paid to this infection because of its frequency in AIDS patients, it appears that its incidence in the general population has been underestimated. In one study in Australia, hospitalized patients with gastroenteritis during the summer found that 7% had *Cryptosporidium* oocysts in their stools.[5] Cryptosporidiosis was also a relatively common finding in studies of patients with gastrointestinal symptoms in Finland, Denmark, and Costa Rica; contaminated water or food appeared the most likely cause.[1,5,6] In homosexual men, *Cryptosporidium* is a frequent sexually transmitted pathogen and a cause of gastrointestinal inflammatory disease.[3]

In immunodeficient individuals, cryptosporidiosis causes severe diarrhea, malabsorption, and dehydration. Diarrhea is watery, without blood or mucus, and is accompanied by abdominal cramps. In severe cases, patients may have six to 25 bowel movements and lose 1 to 17 L of fluid per day.[8] Chronic diarrhea accompanied by malabsorption, electrolyte imbalance, and weight loss may persist for months and even lead to death, either directly or through superinfection with other opportunistic agents.[2] The parasites are preferentially located in the small intestine; less frequently, they are found in the cecum, colon, and rectum, and in a few cases they are seen on the mucosa of the biliary (see Fig. II.5.80) and respiratory tracts.[2] The organisms are concentrated primarily along the intestinal surface epithelium (**Fig. I.6.4;** see Figs. II.5.48, 49). They are oval bodies 2 to 6 μm long, located on the brush border of the epithelial cells, lining the tips and the sides of the villi, or on the lumina of the crypts. The organisms stain well with Giemsa, the H & E and the methylene blue counterstain of the Kinyoun stain. They are not acid-fast and stain variably with PAS and Gomori methenamine silver.[3] The crypts and villi appear morphologically normal, though some degeneration and loss of villi may have taken place.[2] The lamina propria below the infected epithelium is infiltrated by numerous lymphocytes and plasma cells.

Cryptosporidium can be distinguished from *Isospora* and *Sarcocystis* on the basis of its superficial location, which may be contrasted with the deep intracytoplasmic location of the two other parasites. The laboratory diagnosis of cryptosporidiosis can be made through conventional stool examination. In mildly infected cases, however, concentration becomes necessary. A higher yield can be obtained with the recently introduced Sheather sucrose flotation technique.[2] It should be noted that the cryptosporidial oocysts are resistant to most common laboratory disinfectants, including glutaraldehyde. Therefore, contaminated instruments should be autoclaved to prevent infection.[9]

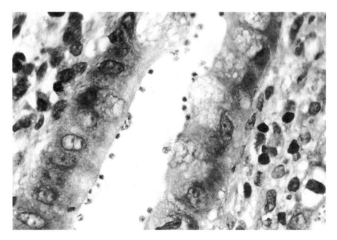

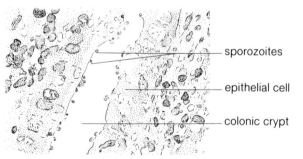

Fig. I.6.4 Sporozoites of cryptosporidiosis in the lumen of a colonic crypt, attached to the apical poles of epithelial cells. (Giemsa stain, ×1,000)

— sporozoites

— epithelial cell

— colonic crypt

CRYPTOSPORIDIOSIS

Protozoan parasite of animals and men

Oocysts transmit infection by fecal–oral route

Short, acute, self-limiting diarrhea in immunocompetent

Chronic, severe, watery diarrhea in immunodeficient

Dehydration and malabsorption, frequently fatal

Organisms on brush border of intestinal epithelium

Cryptosporidium best stained by Giemsa and H&E

Laboratory diagnosis by stool examination

REFERENCES

1. Current WL, Reese NC, Ernst JV, et al: Human cryptosporidiosis in immunocompetent and immunodeficient persons. *N Engl J Med* 1983; 308:1252–1257.
2. Sun T: Cryptosporidiosis, in Sun T (ed): *Sexually Related Infectious Diseases.* New York, Field, Rich & Assoc, 1986, pp 207–217.
3. Soave R, Danner RL, Honig CL, et al: Cryptosporidiosis in homosexual men. *Ann Intern Med* 1984; 100:504–511.
4. Centers for Disease Control: Human cryptosporidiosis—Alabama. *MMWR* 1982; 31:252–254.
5. White WL, Picklo J: Human cryptosporidiosis. *N Engl J Med* 1983; 309:1325.
6. Andersen-Holten W, Gerstoft J, Henriksen S-A: Human cryptosporidiosis. *N Engl J Med* 1983; 309:1325–1326.
7. Current WL: Human cryptosporidiosis. *N Engl J Med* 1983; 309:1326–1327.
8. Centers for Disease Control: Cryptosporidiosis: Assessment of chemotherapy of males with acquired immunodeficiency syndrome (AIDS). *MMWR* 1982; 31:589–592.
9. Weber J, Philip S: Human cryptosporidiosis. *N Engl J Med* 1983; 309:1326.

ISOSPORIASIS

Chronic diarrhea is a common symptom in homosexual men with HIV infection and in AIDS patients. It is caused by bacteria and protozoa, among which are two of the Coccidia, *Cryptosporidium* and *Isospora belli.* Both are animal parasites that are not known to cause infections in humans under normal conditions but have emerged as common pathogens in the AIDS epidemic. In the population at risk for AIDS, the incidence of infection with these coccidian protozoa varies greatly with location, which indicates marked differences in environmental infestation. The incidence of cryptosporidiosis is 3.3% in AIDS patients in the United States, but may be as high as 46% in Haiti. One study found that isosporiasis, which has an incidence of only 0.2% in the United States, occurred in 15% of a series of 131 Haitian AIDS patients.[1] In a study from Zaire, *I. belli* was the cause of diarrhea in 19% of 46 patients with a tentative diagnosis of AIDS.[2] These high incidence figures are related to the tropical climate and to the poor sanitary conditions prevailing in these regions, where fecal contamination of food and water and close contact with potentially infected chickens and dogs are common.[1] In addition, isosporiasis, like amebiasis and giardiasis, may be sexually transmitted within the homosexual population.[3]

In normal hosts, isosporiasis occurs as a self-limited episode of acute diarrhea with fever, malaise, and abdominal pain.[4,5] It has also been identified in children with immuno deficiencies, in whom it is characterized by chronicity, resistance to treatment, and frequent relapse.[6] AIDS patients suffer from profuse, chronic watery diarrhea, with as many as 16 bowel movements a day. The onset is acute, with fever, night sweats, chills, and abdominal cramps, and sometimes with nausea and vomiting as well.[1,4] Diarrhea becomes chronic and leads to malabsorption and severe weight loss.[1,7] In one study of 15 patients with isosporiasis as the only coccidial infection, all 15 lost at least 10% of their weight during the first two months before diagnosis.[1] In the revised definition of AIDS drawn up by the Centers for Disease Control, isosporiasis with diarrhea persisting for more than one month is included as an indicator disease.[8]

The infected hosts continually pass infective isospora oocysts in their stools. Unfortunately, however, these may be missed in the absence of suitable techniques for concentration and staining or of experience in recognizing the oocysts.[4] *I. belli* often resides in the small intestine, and occasionally in the duodenum; therefore, sigmoidoscopy may not recover these oocysts effectively.[4,7] For this reason, duodenal aspirates or small-bowel biopsies have been recommended for patients with chronic diarrhea in whom no other pathogens can be found.[4,5] The oocysts are identified in saline wet mounts or on slides stained with a modified Kinyoun acid-fast stain (**Fig. I.6.5;** see Fig. II.5.38).[3] They appear as large, bright-red, oval cysts on a green background. The oocysts of *I. belli* can be differentiated from those

of *Cryptosporidium, Eimeria,* and *Sarcocystis* (related genera of gastrointestinal coccidial parasites) on the basis of shape, size, and number of sporozoites. *Isospora* oocysts are oval, are about 20 to 30 μm by 10 to 19 μm, and contain two sporozoites, whereas *Cryptosporidium* oocysts are round, are 4 to 6 μm in diameter, and contain four sporozoites.[1]

In a recently published case of isosporiasis in an AIDS patient, the parasite demonstrated an unusual potential for extraintestinal invasion and dissemination. At the autopsy of a 38-year-old homosexual man with CMV pneumonia, *I. belli* was identified in the mucosa and lamina propria of the small and large intestine, as well as in mesenteric and tracheobronchial lymph nodes.[9] Elongated, banana-shaped merozoites of *I. belli* were present within the cytoplasm of histiocytes, and formation of granulomalike aggregates of histiocytes was occasionally apparent. The organisms were 10 to 30 μm long and were made up of a thick PAS-positive sheath, a central nucleus, and a clear paranuclear area.[9] The unusual extension of *Isospora* to extraintestinal organs in this patient follows the pattern of aggressive dissemination exhibited by other infectious agents in AIDS patients.

Effective treatment is available against *Isospora*, which responds quickly to trimethoprim-sulfamethoxazole. Though cures have been obtained, the rate of recurrence remains high.[1,5]

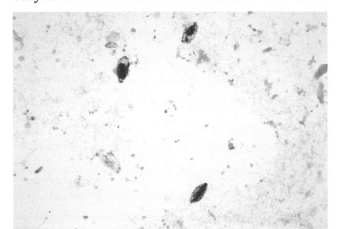

Fig. I.6.5 *Isospora belli;* large, oval, acid-fast–stained oocysts containing two sporozoites.   (Kinyoun's stain, ×400)

ISOSPORIASIS

Isospora belli, coccidian parasite of animals in tropical areas

Large, oval, acid-fast oocysts containing two sporozoites

Contaminant of small and large intestine in immunodeficient hosts

Severe, chronic watery diarrhea with malabsorption and weight loss

Occasional invasion of intestinal wall and dissemination to lymph nodes

REFERENCES

1. DeHovitz JA, Pape JW, Boncy M, et al: Clinical manifestations and therapy of *Isospora belli* infection in patients with the acquired immunodeficiency syndrome. *N Engl J Med* 1986; 315:87–90.
2. Henry MC, De Clercq D, Lokombe B, et al: Parasitological observations of chronic diarrhoea in suspected AIDS adult patients in Kinshasa (Zaire). *Trans R Soc Trop Med Hyg* 1986; 80:309–310.
3. Ma P, Kaufman D, Montana J: *Isospora belli* diarrheal infection in homosexual men. *AIDS Res* 1984; 1:327–338.
4. Kobayashi LM, Kort MP, Berlin OGW, et al: *Isospora* infection in a homosexual man. *Diagn Microbiol Infect Dis* 1985; 3:363–366.
5. Modigliani R, Bories C, Le Charpentier Y, et al: Diarrhoea and malabsorption in acquired immune deficiency syndrome: A study of four cases with special emphasis on opportunistic protozoan infestations. *Gut* 1985; 26:179–187.
6. Arnaud-Battandier F: Cryptosporidiosis, isosporiasis, lambliasis in immunologic deficiencies. *Arch Fr Pediatr* 1985; 42:959–963.
7. Bengoa JM, Widgren S: Gastrointestinal manifestations of acquired immunodeficiency syndrome: Case studies of 14 patients. *Schweiz Med Wochenschr* 1986; 116:1358–1366.
8. Centers for Disease Control: Revision of the CDC surveillance: Case definition for AIDS. *MMWR* 1987; 36:55.
9. Restrepo C, Macher AM, Radany EH: Disseminated extraintestinal isosporiasis in a patient with acquired immune deficiency syndrome. *Am J Clin Pathol* 1987; 87:536–542.

Neoplasias Associated with AIDS

NEOPLASIAS ASSOCIATED WITH AIDS

The increased incidence of neoplasia in the population groups at high risk for AIDS has been noted since the first reports from the Centers for Disease Control in 1981, and has been confirmed repeatedly ever since.[1-4] Kaposi's sarcoma, non-Hodgkin's lymphoma, squamous cell carcinoma of the oropharynx, and cloacogenic carcinoma of the rectum have a significantly higher incidence in homosexual men and intravenous drug users than in the general population.[4-12] It now appears that the immunodeficiency resulting from the initial infection with a human lymphotropic retrovirus provides the opportunity for a second infection, not only with some of a number of opportunistic microorganisms that induce severe systemic diseases, but also with oncogenic viruses that may induce specific types of neoplasms.[3,13]

The relationship between immunodeficiency and neoplasia had been recognized more than a decade before the present AIDS epidemic.[14,15] The risk of developing a malignant tumor for patients with genetic immunodeficiencies is 4%, which is more than 10,000 times the incidence recorded in the general age-matched population.[14,16] In immunosuppressed renal transplant recipients the incidence of neoplasia is 6%; as of May 1983, a total of 1,767 tumors had developed in 1,661 patients according to the transplantation register.[16,17] Of all the tumors developing in immunodeficient individuals, by far the most common are those of the lymphoid system. Non-Hodgkin's lymphomas account for 3% to 4% of all tumors in the general population, but 26% of tumors arising in recipients of renal transplants and 71% of tumors arising in recipients of cardiac transplants.[17] The lymphomas seen in immunodeficient patients are not only more common but also different from those in immunocompetent patients with respect to location, histology, natural history, and response to treatment.[1,18]

Kaposi's sarcoma, a neoplasm with an incidence of only 0.02% in the general population, occurs in 4.9% of transplant patients. It is the malignancy most commonly associated with AIDS, affecting 36% of homosexual men with AIDS.[4] In the course of this tumor, so clearly associated with the status of immune deficiency, additional tumors may develop in as many as 37% of patients, and of these, lymphoid tumors are 20 times more common than other tumors.[19] These and other statistics strongly indicate that lymphoid tumors, more than any other malignancies, are related to various states of immunodeficiency.

On a theoretical level, the high incidence of lymphomas with special biologic features in AIDS patients provides clues to the pathogenesis of neoplasms in general. Normally, cellular immunity controls the cells that express viral and other foreign antigens. When, under the conditions of immune deficiency, cellular immunity fails, unrestricted growth of cells infected by oncogenic viruses becomes possible. Viruses with oncogenic potential are ubiquitous in the general population. Like many other microorganisms, they may become opportunistic in immunodeficient hosts, causing unusual and severe diseases in these individuals.[13] The direct relationship between a viral infection, immunodeficiency, and induction of tumors that has been demonstrated for the first time in the AIDS patients may explain certain mechanisms of human carcinogenesis that to this point have not been well understood.

NEOPLASIAS ASSOCIATED WITH AIDS

High risk of neoplasia in individuals with AIDS

Aggressive behavior of tumors

Tendency to early invasion and dissemination

Occurrence in organs not commonly observed to be involved

Resistance to treatment

Early relapse

Kaposi's sarcoma most common neoplasm in AIDS

Non-Hodgkin's lymphomas (high-grade lesions) second most common neoplasia

REFERENCES

1. Centers for Disease Control: Kaposi's sarcoma and *Pneumocystis* pneumonia among homosexual men: New York City and California. *MMWR* 1981; 25:305–308.
2. Centers for Disease Control: Epidemiologic aspects of the current outbreak of Kaposi's sarcoma and opportunistic infections. *N Engl J Med* 1982; 306:248.
3. Ioachim HL: Acquired immune deficiency disease after three years: The unsolved riddle, editorial. *Lab Invest* 1984; 51:1–6.
4. Selwyn PA: AIDS: What is now known: III. Clinical aspects. *Hosp Pract*, 1986; 21:119–153.
5. Centers for Disease Control: Diffuse, undifferentiated non-Hodgkin's lymphoma among homosexual males: United States. *MMWR* 1982; 31:277.
6. Cooper HS, Patchefsky AJ, Marks G: Cloacogenic carcinoma of the anorectum in homosexual men: An observation of four cases. *Dis Colon Rectum* 1979; 22:557–558.
7. Friedman-Kien AE, Laubenstein LJ, Rubinstein P, et al: Disseminated Kaposi's sarcoma in homosexual men. *Ann Intern Med* 1982; 96:693–700.
8. Ioachim HL, Cooper MC, Hellman GC: Lymphomas in men at high risk for acquired immune deficiency syndrome (AIDS). *Cancer* 1985; 56:2831–2842.
9. Levine AM, Meyer PR, Begandy MK, et al: Development of B-cell lymphoma in homosexual men. *Ann Intern Med* 1984; 100:7–13.
10. Lozada F, Silverman S, Conent M: New outbreak of oral tumors: Malignancies and infectious disease strike young male homosexuals. *Can Dent Assoc J* 1982; 19:39–42.
11. Urmacher C, Myskowski P, Ochoa M, et al: Outbreak of Kaposi's sarcoma with cytomegalovirus infection in young homosexual men. *Am J Med* 1982; 72:569–575.
12. Ziegler JL, and others: Non-Hodgkin's lymphoma in 90 homosexual men: Relationship to generalized lymphadenopathy and acquired immunodeficiency syndrome (AIDS). *N Engl J Med* 1984; 311:565–571.
13. Ioachim HL: Neoplasms associated with immune deficiencies. *Pathol Annu* 1987; 2:147–182.
14. Gatti RA, Good RA: Occurrence of malignancy in immunodeficiency diseases: A literature review. *Cancer* 1971; 28:89–98.
15. Penn I, Hammond A, Brett Scheider L, et al: Malignant lymphomas in transplantation patients. *Transpl Proc* 1969; 1:106.
16. Hanto WH, Frizzera G, Purtillo DT, et al: Clinical spectrum of lymphoproliferative disorders in renal transplant recipients and evidence for the role of Epstein-Barr virus. *Cancer Res* 1981; 41:4253–4261.
17. Penn I: Lymphomas complicating transplantation patients. *Transpl Proc* 1983; 15:2790–2797.
18. Ioachim HL, Cooper MC: Lymphomas of AIDS. *Lancet* 1986; 1:96.
19. Safai B, Mike V, Giraldo G, et al: Association of Kaposi's sarcoma with second primary malignancies: Possible etiopathogenic implications. *Cancer* 1980; 45:1472–1479.

KAPOSI'S SARCOMA

In the more than 100 years from its initial description in 1872 to the report that associated it with the AIDS epidemic in 1981, Kaposi's sarcoma (KS) attracted only limited attention.[1] It was considered a rare tumor, with an incidence of 0.02 to 0.06 per 100,000 cases in the United States and western Europe, though endemic areas were known to exist in equatorial Africa, where KS accounts for 9% of all cancers.[2-4] Certain ethnic backgrounds, particularly Jewish and Italian, have been associated with the classic form of Kaposi's sarcoma; however, the disease does not appear to be genetically transmitted, and familial cases have rarely been documented.[2] Male predominance is characteristic; the male/female ratio ranges from 3/1 in a series of 90 patients seen over 20 years in New York to 15/1 in one group of Africans studied.[2-4] In the classic form, KS lesions usually involve the skin, more often peripherally, on the lower extremities. Involvement of lymph nodes and internal organs is infrequent; it is more likely to occur in African cases, particularly in children.[5] The course of the disease is generally slow and indolent: the average survival time in one American series was eight to 13 years.[2]

That Kaposi's sarcoma has also been reported to occur in recipients of organ transplants and other patients receiving immunosuppressive therapy indicates its close association with conditions of immunoderegulation.[6,7] About 0.4% of all patients undergoing renal transplantation acquire KS within an average of 16 months. This incidence is 150 to 200 times greater than would be expected in the general population.[6] Regression of KS has been recorded in two patients after immunosuppressive treatment was discontinued.[8] A further indication of the significance of a background of immunodeficiency in KS is the uniquely high incidence (37%) of additional malignant tumors in patients with this disease. Lymphoid tumors are seen 20 times more often in such patients than in the general population.[9]

The new Kaposi's sarcoma seen today is also linked with immunodeficient states. It is the second most common manifestation of AIDS and has been included in the definition of the syndrome from the beginning.[1] The incidence of KS in AIDS patients in various series ranges from 21% to 40%, though some authors who have reviewed special groups of individuals at risk report considerably higher figures.[10-13] Homosexual men with AIDS make up the largest population affected by KS. The incidence of the disease is 36% in this population, according to the CDC figures of 1985, whereas its incidence in intravenous drug users is only 4.3%.[13] It is noteworthy that recent trends show that the incidence of KS in AIDS patients is declining, whereas that of pneumocystosis in the same population continues to increase. Before 1984, KS was present in 21% of AIDS cases and pneumocystosis in 35%. In 1985, however, the incidence of KS decreased to 13% of all new cases of AIDS, and that of pneumocystosis increased to 47%.[13]

Investigations into the etiology of KS that predate the present AIDS epidemic indicated that there is a relationship with CMV infection. Virus particles of herpes type have been seen in tissue cultures of KS, and DNA sequences from CMV, as well as CMV-related antigens, have been identified in KS biopsy specimens.[14] In view of these findings, it may be significant that there has been a decrease in the incidence of CMV infections in homosexual men during the past few years that is

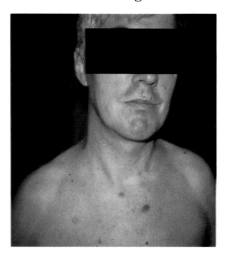

Fig. I.7.1 Numerous patches, plaques, and nodules of Kaposi's sarcoma on face and chest of 35-year-old homosexual man.

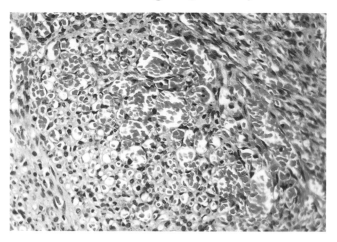

Fig. I.7.2 Kaposi's sarcoma replacing lymph node parenchyma. Spindle-shaped Kaposi's sarcoma cells form bundles and erythrocyte-containing capillaries.
(trichrome Masson stain, ×250)

concurrent with the decrease in the incidence of KS in the same population.[13]

Kaposi's sarcoma involves the skin, the mucosal surfaces, the lymph nodes, and the internal organs. The skin lesions are more numerous and noticeable and are the most frequent presenting complaint. The lesions range in size from 1 to 2 mm to 2 to 3 cm, and in color from pink-red to purple-blue.[5] In form, they can be macules, papules, slightly elevated plaques, or prominent nodules. They can be single or numerous, and they can be widely spread over a single area or over the entire body.[5] Often, they are symmetrical and bilateral and take on a linear shape, following the skin creases.[15] The lesions are classified into three types, patch, plaque, and nodule, which some authors consider to represent stages of progression (**Fig. I.7.1;** see Figs. II.1.14, 17, 18).[15] Patches are early lesions that are small, ovoid, pink-red, and flat. They may become elevated and indurated papules, and eventually they may darken in color and increase in size to become prominent nodules. With time, especially in dark-skinned individuals, the lesions become hyperpigmented. Occasionally, some lesions may flatten and regress spontaneously.[16]

The locations of KS lesions are more varied and widespread in AIDS patients than in patients with the classic form of disease, in whom they tend to arise mainly on the legs and feet (see Figs. II.1.17,18). On the face, the favored sites are the tip of the nose, the medial third of the eyelids (see Figs. II.10.1–3), the area behind the ears, and the earlobes.[15,16] The trunk, the penis (see Fig. II.7.5), and the dorsum of the feet are also common locations. In its new epidemic form, KS also involves mucosal surfaces, especially those of the gastrointestinal tract, lymph nodes, and viscera. At autopsy, almost any internal organ may show Kaposi's sarcoma, with the exception of the brain and the gonads, the involvement of which has not been documented.[4] Visceral lesions are usually perivascular and multifocal. Early lesions in the mouth appear as macules or papules on the mucosa of the hard palate just above the level of the second molar (see Figs. II.5.8,9).[16] On the gum, nodular lesions simulate epulis.[16] Similar red-purple patches and plaques may develop on the tonsils (see Fig. II.5.10), pharynx, esophagus, stomach, intestine (see Figs. II.5.32–35), colon, rectum, and anus. The lungs may also be involved, in which case symptomatic pulmonary disease with dyspnea, hemoptysis, and pleural effusions may result (see Figs. II.4.57–60).

On histologic examination, all types of KS, both sporadic and epidemic, regardless of location, are generally similar (**Fig. I.7.2;** see Figs. II.1.15, 16, 19–21; II.2.48–50; II.5.33–35).[17] They consist of exuberant proliferations of neoplastic spindle-shaped cells arranged in bundles or whorls, with capillarylike slits and clefts that contain a variable amount of red blood cells, a large part of which are extravasated. The nuclei are large but not markedly pleomorphic. Mitoses are usually present. The proliferation of neoplastic blood vessels is accompanied by infiltrates, sometimes abundant, of plasma cells, lymphocytes, and hemosiderin-laden macrophages. An inflammatory form of KS in which the large amount of inflammatory cells obscures the proliferation of neoplastic cells has also been described.[11] The neoplastic cells of KS originate in the endothelial cells of lymphatic or blood vessels, as indicated by their staining with antibody to factor VIII and the immunoperoxidase procedure (**Fig. I.7.3;** see Fig. II.2.51). Early patch lesions in skin, mucosae, or small, transbronchial biopsies are sometimes difficult to recognize; they appear as a lacework of irregularly shaped, thin-walled capillary vessels. Older lesions comprise more inflammatory cells, deposits of hemosiderin, and collagen. In the skin, patchy lesions involve only the superficial dermis

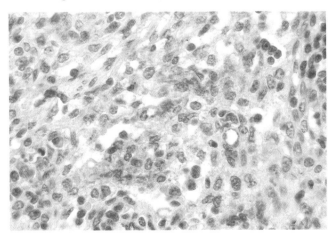

Fig. I.7.3 Spindle-shaped Kaposi's sarcoma cells forming bundles and capillaries show brown granular intracytoplasmic staining with anti–factor VIII antibody.
(perox-antiperox, anti–factor VIII stain, ×400)

and are contiguous with preexisting vessels, sometimes coming to resemble pyogenic granuloma. Plaque and nodular lesions involve the entire dermis and may be confused with dermatofibrosarcoma and hemangiosarcoma.

In the lung, tracheobronchial patches and plaques similar to those in the gastrointestinal tract may be seen, as may purplish, congested nodular infiltrates, usually peribronchial or perivascular, with a lymphatic distribution.[12,18,19] The neoplastic vascular proliferations distend the interalveolar septae without entirely destroying the walls of the collapsed alveolar spaces (see Figs. II.4.58–60). Inflammatory cells, particularly plasma cells, accompany the neoplastic proliferation. Opportunistic infections, such as *Pneumocystis carinii* pneumonia may be associated with pulmonary Kaposi's sarcoma.[12] The lymph nodes are frequently involved in African children with the endemic form of KS and in AIDS patients. Their involvement does not represent metastatic disease, because lymph nodes are sometimes affected in the absence of any other localizations.

In the lymph nodes, the foci of KS appear to arise de novo in multiple locations, and not necessarily in the marginal sinuses as metastatic tumors do (see Figs. II.2.48–51).[15] The T-cell regions of lymph nodes and spleen are primarily involved, as a study of 52 cases has shown.[11] Vascular proliferation in the lymph nodes, as in other organs, varies from focal areas that are difficult to differentiate from the abundant vascular proliferations resembling Castleman's disease that are common in the late stages of HIV lymphadenitides to large replacement of lymphoid nodal tissues.[20,21]

Localized Kaposi's sarcoma is sensitive to radiotherapy, and disseminated disease can be efficiently treated with combination chemotherapy. The prognosis remains poor, however, owing to the background of immunodeficiency. The overall mortality from KS is approximately 41%. About 60% of patients are alive at one year after diagnosis, but the average survival is only 18 months.[22] Death in most patients is caused by associated severe opportunistic infections.[5]

KAPOSI'S SARCOMA

Neoplastic vascular proliferation

Endothelial cells with factor VIII markers

Association with cytomegalovirus

In immunocompetent patients (classic form)

Sporadic in those of Mediterranean ancestry

Endemic in equatorial Africa

Elderly individuals

Skin of legs

Circumscribed lesions

Low aggressiveness

In immunodeficient patients (AIDS form)

No ethnic or age predilection

Predominant in homosexual men

Widespread lesions of skin

Involvement of gastrointestinal tract

Involvement of lymph nodes, lungs

Multicentric

Highly aggressive

Associated with opportunistic infections

REFERENCES

1. Centers for Disease Control: Kaposi's sarcoma and pneumocystis pneumonia among homosexual men—New York City and California. *MMWR* 1981; 25:305–308.

2. DiGiovanna JJ, Safai B: Kaposi's sarcoma: Retrospective study of 90 cases with particular emphasis on the familial occurrence, ethnic background and other diseases. *Am J Med* 1981; 71:779–783.

3. Rothman S: Remarks on sex, age and racial distribution of Kaposi's sarcoma and on possible pathogenetic factors. *Acta Unio Int Cancer* 1962; 18:326–329.

4. Templeton AC: Kaposi's sarcoma. *Pathol Annu* 1981; 16:315–336.

5. Friedman-Kien AE, Laubenstein LJ, Rubinstein P, et al: Disseminated Kaposi's sarcoma in homosexual men. *Ann Intern Med* 1982; 96:693–700.

6. Harwood AR: Kaposi's sarcoma in renal transplant patients, in Friedman-Kien AE, Laubenstein LJ (eds): *AIDS: The Epidemic of Kaposi's Sarcoma and Opportunistic Infections.* New York, Masson, 1984, pp 41–45.

7. Penn I: Kaposi's sarcoma in organ transplant recipients: Report of 20 cases. *Transplantation* 1979; 27:8–11.

8. Myers BD, Kessler E, Levi J, et al: Kaposi's sarcoma in kidney transplant recipients. *Arch Intern Med* 1974; 133:307–311.

9. Urmacher C, Myskowski P, Ochoa M, et al: Outbreak of Kaposi's sarcoma with cytomegalovirus infection in young homosexual men. *Am J Med* 1982; 72:569–575.

10. Centers for Disease Control: Epidemiologic aspects of the current outbreak of Kaposi's sarcoma and opportunistic infections. *N Engl J Med* 1982; 306:248–252.

11. Moskowitz LB, Hensley GT, Gould EW, et al: Frequency and anatomic distribution of lymphadenopathic Kaposi's sarcoma in the acquired immunodeficiency syndrome: An autopsy series. *Hum Pathol* 1985; 16:447–456.

12. Ognibene FP, Steis RG, Macher AB, et al: Kaposi's sarcoma causing pulmonary infiltrates and respiratory failure in the acquired immunodeficiency syndrome. *Ann Intern Med* 1985; 102:471–475.

13. Selwyn PA: AIDS: What is now known: III. Clinical aspects. *Hosp Pract* 1986; 21:119–153.

14. Giraldo G, Beth E, Huang ES: Kaposi's sarcoma and its relationship to cytomegalovirus (CMV): III. CMV, DNA and CMV early antigens in Kaposi's sarcoma. *Int J Cancer* 1980; 26:23–29.

15. Friedman-Kien AE, Ostreicher R: Overview of classical and epidemic Kaposi's sarcoma, in Friedman-Kien AE, Laubenstein LJ (eds): *AIDS: The Epidemic of Kaposi's Sarcoma and Opportunistic Infections.* New York, Masson, 1984; pp 23–25.

16. Farthing CF, Brown SE, Staughton RCD, et al: Kaposi's sarcoma, in *A Colour Atlas of AIDS.* London, Wolfe, Medical Pub, 1986; pp 25–37.

17. Gottlieb GJ, Ackerman AB: Kaposi's sarcoma: An extensively disseminated form in young homosexual men. *Hum Pathol* 1982; 3:882–892.

18. Nash G, Fligiel S: Kaposi's sarcoma presenting as pulmonary disease in the acquired immunodeficiency syndrome: Diagnosis by lung biopsy. *Human Pathol* 1984; 15:999–1001.

19. Purdy LJ, Colby TV, Yousem SA, et al: Pulmonary Kaposi's sarcoma: Premortem histologic diagnosis. *Am J Surg Pathol* 1986; 10:301–311.

20. Ioachim HL, Lerner CW, Tapper ML: The lymphoid lesions associated with the acquired immunodeficiency syndrome. *Am J Surg Pathol* 1983; 7:543–553.

21. Rywlin AM, Rosen L, Cabello B: Coexistence of Castleman's disease. *Am J Dermatopathol* 1983; 5:277–281.

22. Safai B, Johnson KE, Myskowski PL, et al: The natural history of Kaposi's sarcoma in the acquired immunodeficiency syndrome. *Ann Intern Med* 1985; 103:744–750.

HODGKIN'S LYMPHOMA

The incidence of Hodgkin's lymphoma in persons with primary immunodeficiencies, particularly ataxia telangiectasia, is markedly increased over that recorded in age-matched immunocompetent individuals.[1] This increase parallels that of lymphomas in general, which are frequently associated with both congenital and acquired immune deficiencies.[2] In patients with AIDS, however, the expected increase in the incidence of Hodgkin's lymphomas has not been observed.[3] Whereas Hodgkin's lymphoma is the dominant type of lymphoma in the young adult population at large, at an incidence of 3.5 to 5 cases per 100,000 population per year, non-Hodgkin's lymphomas are far more common in homosexual males and others at high risk for AIDS.[4-6] This is reflected in the relatively few reports on Hodgkin's lymphoma in AIDS published so far.[3,5,7,8] Some investigators believe that the unexpectedly low incidence of Hodgkin's lymphoma in AIDS is no more than a statistical coincidence[3]; however, others point out that the clinicopathologic features of Hodgkin's lymphoma are altered in AIDS patients and that there appear to be distinct relations between these two states of immunodeficiency.[4,5,7,8]

The course of Hodgkin's lymphoma is far more aggressive in patients with AIDS, who are more likely to present in advanced stages of the disease. In three studies of a total of 21 patients, 75% to 92% were in stage III or IV at presentation.[3,7,8] Involvement of bone marrow in the absence of other locations, (see Fig. II.2.8), a unique mode of presentation, was noted in four studies.[3,5,7,8] Cutaneous Hodgkin's lymphoma, which is rarely seen in conventional cases, was also reported in AIDS patients, but mediastinal and hilar lymph node involvement, a common occurrence in the general population, was rarely seen in AIDS patients.[7] On histologic examination, the majority of cases in all series were classified as mixed cellularity, thus lesions of a high grade (see Figs. II.2.8,52,53). The course of Hodgkin's disease in AIDS, reflecting the higher grade and stage at diagnosis as well as the background of immunodeficiency, is more aggressive than in comparable non-AIDS patients. Rapid progression and extensive involvement of internal organs, coupled with resistance to treatment and short survival, have been the general experience.[3,5,7,8]

HODGKIN'S LYMPHOMA IN AIDS

Low incidence

Less common than non-Hodgkin's lymphoma

Advanced stage at presentation

Early bone-marrow involvement

High-grade histologic types

Aggressive behavior

Resistant to treatment

REFERENCES

1. Frizzera, G, Rosai J, Dehner LP, et al: Lymphoreticular disorders in primary immunodeficiencies. *Cancer* 1980; 46:692–699.
2. Ioachim HL: Neoplasms associated with immune deficiencies. *Pathol Annu* 1987; 2:147–182.
3. Kaplan LD, Abrams DI, Volberding PA: Clinical course and epidemiology of Hodgkin's disease (HD) in homosexual men in San Francisco (SF). Presented at the Third International Conference on AIDS, Washington DC, June 1–5, 1987.
4. Ioachim HL, Cooper MC: Lymphomas of AIDS. *Lancet* 1986; 1:96–97.
5. Ioachim HL, Cooper MC, Hellman GC: Lymphomas in men at high risk for acquired immune deficiency syndrome (AIDS). *Cancer* 1985; 56:2831–2842.
6. Young JL Jr, Percy C, Asire AJ, et al: Cancer incidence and mortality in the United States. *Natl Cancer Inst Monogr* 1981; 57:72–84.
7. Schoeppel SL, Hoppe RT, Dorfman RF, et al: Hodgkin's disease in homosexual men with generalized lymphadenopathy. *Ann Intern Med* 1985; 102:68–70.
8. Unger PD, Strauchen JA: Hodgkin's disease in AIDS complex patients. *Cancer* 1986; 58:821–825.

NON-HODGKIN'S LYMPHOMA

In 1982, less than one year after having issued the account on the first cases of AIDS, the Centers for Disease Control reported the occurrence of four cases of non-Hodgkin's lymphomas among homosexual men.[1,2] Over the five years since then, the incidence of malignant lymphoma in individuals with HIV infection has rapidly increased, as is documented by a series of reports in the medical literature, as well as by the inclusion of non-Hodgkin's lymphoma in the CDC definition of AIDS.[3,5–11]

Non-Hodgkin's lymphomas associated with AIDS have a number of clinicopathologic features that are similar to those of lymphomas occurring in congenital immune deficiencies and in immunosuppressed organ transplant recipients, but are different from those of lymphomas occurring in the general population.[8,12,13] The distinctive features of the lymphomas associated with AIDS are apparent in the series of cases published so far and have been emphasized in previously published studies.[7,8,12,13] Among these is the reversal of the ratio of non-Hodgkin's to Hodgkin's lymphomas in the population at risk for AIDS. Whereas Hodgkin's lymphoma is prevalent in young adults of the general population, non-Hodgkin's lymphoma is by far the most common form of lymphoma in the age-matched individuals with AIDS.[6-10] In our series of 72 lymphomas in patients with HIV infection, 66 had non-Hodgkin's lymphoma, and only six had Hodgkin's lymphoma.[7]

Another characteristic feature of lymphomas in AIDS patients is their far greater distribution in extranodal locations while in the adult population at large, lymphomas more commonly originate in lymph nodes.[5,6,8,14] In particular, the gastrointestinal tract (see Figs. II.5.12, 13, 40, 41, 50, 51 and Figs. II.9.46–57) and the brain have emerged as the predominant sites for non-Hodgkin's lymphomas associated with AIDS. In the same series of 72 cases of non-Hodgkin's lymphoma in AIDS patients, there were eight primary lymphomas of the brain. A recently recognized special localization of AIDS-associated non-Hodgkin's lymphomas is in the terminal rectum and anus.[15-17] Four cases have been reported of homosexual men who presented with anorectal symptoms and originally underwent surgery for anorectal fistulas or tumor masses (see Figs. II.5.54–57).[16] All four had large

tumor masses confined within the rectum; when staged, three patients had no other organ involvement, and the fourth only had lymphoma in an axillary lymph node.

Involvement of the CNS appears to be another characteristic feature of lymphoma in AIDS. Although in the general population no more than 2% of non-Hodgkin's lymphomas involve the brain primarily, and even secondary involvement is comparatively rare, a series of 90 cases of AIDS-associated lymphomas showed a 42% involvement of the CNS; our series of 72 cases showed CNS involvement in 11% (see Figs. II.9.46–60).[6,7] These high incidences of CNS lymphomas in AIDS are significantly similar to that reported in renal transplant recipients, which were 49% and 50% in two published series.[18,19]

The lymphomas in AIDS patients studied so far have been highly aggressive and have uniformly involved multiple organs. In the autopsies performed, extensive tumor involvement was present, and massive invasion of organs otherwise not commonly affected—such as the heart (see Figs.

Fig. I.7.4A Non-Hodgkin's lymphoma of diffuse, large-cell, immunoblastic type, primary in the small intestine of 33-year-old homosexual man. Starry-sky pattern, large, round nuclei with single prominent nucleolus and frequent mitoses.

(HPS stain, ×400)

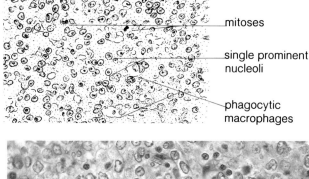

mitoses

single prominent nucleoli

phagocytic macrophages

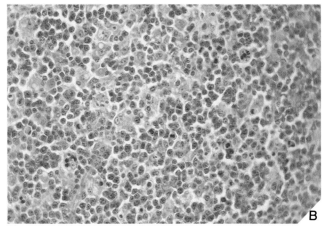

B Non-Hodgkin's lymphoma of diffuse, large-cell type with plasmacytoid features, primary in cecum of 31-year-old man with HIV infection. (HPS stain, ×250)

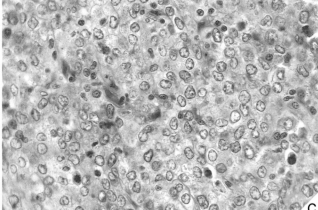

C Non-Hodgkin's lymphoma of diffuse, large, non-cleaved-cell type, primary in axillary lymph nodes of 46-year-old drug addict. Uniform large round nuclei with multiple small nucleoli and numerous mitoses. (HPS stain, ×400)

II.3.4–7), stomach, kidneys (see Fig. II.6.9), testes, urinary bladder, skin (see Figs. II.1.22–24), and eyes (see Figs. II.10.31–32)—were noted. On histologic examination, the non-Hodgkin's lymphomas, though not entirely uniform, generally appear to belong to high-grade categories; they are almost always diffuse, large, noncleaved cell types (**Figs. I.7.4–5.**) A majority in most reports were diagnosed as being of undifferentiated Burkitt's or Burkitt's-like cell type (**Fig. I.7.5**).[6,7,9] Chromosomal studies performed in some cases showed a predominance of t(8:14) translocation, which is characteristic of Burkitt's lymphomas.[9] The phenotype was monoclonal B-cell (**Fig. I.7.6;** see Fig. II.9.60) or non-B non-T-cell in virtually all cases published in the literature so far: to date, only one case of T-cell lymphoma has been reported.[14] Nonneoplastic lymphadenopathies showing the typical AIDS-related morphologic changes precede the lymphomas in most cases (see Figs. II.2.54–55).[7,20,21]

One retrospective study found that lymph nodes in patients with persistent generalized lymphadenopathy who were biopsied before the occurrence of lymphoma were in 80% of cases of the B (II) or C (III) histologic type, which are characterized by the presence of atrophic, involuted follicles, diffuse fibrosis, and extensive proliferation of blood vessels.[20] The observation of focal areas of lymphoma or Kaposi's sarcoma, coexistent in some lymph nodes with residual lesions of HIV lymphadenopathy, clearly establishes the sequence in which the inflammatory and the neoplastic lesions occur in AIDS.[7,20] The relationship with HIV infection is also indicated by the presence of circulating anti-HIV antibodies and the reversed helper/suppressor (T_4/T_8) T-cell ratios in all patients tested in a number of studies.[5,6,7,9,10] The potential of reactive lymph nodes in individuals at high risk for AIDS to undergo neoplastic changes justifies biopsy and, if the changes persist, rebiopsy of enlarged lymph nodes.

Reflecting the immature tumor cell types and the defective immune response, the course of lymphomas in AIDS-related patients has been highly malignant; in one series, the only survivors were those diagnosed within the previous six months. Despite a variety of chemotherapy regimens and a generally positive initial response, almost all patients have relapsed.[5,7] Those with a prior diagnosis of AIDS could not tolerate the necessary aggressive chemotherapy and achieved median survivals of only 2.9 months.[10] Because of the poor results obtained in their treatment, AIDS-related lymphomas should be considered a separate group and should not be included in general clinical or chemotherapy studies.[8]

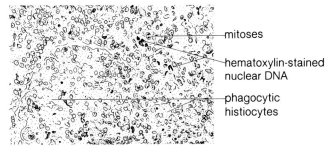

Fig. I.7.5 Non-Hodgkin's lymphoma of diffuse, undifferentiated Burkitt's-cell type, primary in rectum of 39-year-old homosexual man. Starry-sky pattern, round nuclei with fine nucleoli, numerous mitoses, and hematoxylin staining of nuclear DNA released by necrotic cells. (HPS stain, ×250)

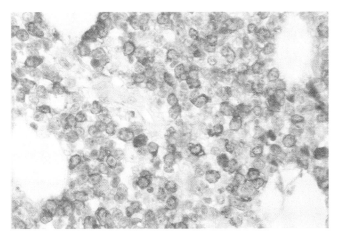

Fig. I.7.6 Non-Hodgkin's lymphoma of diffuse, non-cleaved-cell type, in retroperitoneum and omentum of 33-year-old homosexual man. Anti-κ monoclonal immunoperoxidase staining in almost all lymphoma cells. (PAS stain, ×400)

NON-HODGKIN'S LYMPHOMAS IN AIDS

Incidence increased

Lymphadenopathies often preceding

Non-Hodgkin's lymphoma/Hodgkin's lymphoma ratio increased

Nodal lymphoma/extranodal lymphoma ratio decreased

Frequent gastrointestinal involvement

Frequent CNS involvement

Heterogeneous cells of origin,

High-grade histologic types

B-cell phenotype

Positive for HIV antibodies

Positive for EBV antibodies

Highly aggressive

Initial therapeutic response

Frequent relapse

Short survival

REFERENCES

1. Centers for Disease Control: Kaposi's sarcoma and *Pneumocystis* pneumonia among homosexual men: New York City and California. *MMWR* 1981; 31:249.

2. Centers for Disease Control: Diffuse, undifferentiated non-Hodgkin's lymphoma among homosexual males: United States. *MMWR* 1982; 31:277.

3. Doll DC, List AF: Burkitt's lymphoma in a homosexual. *Lancet* 1982; 1026–1027.

4. Snider WD, Simpson DM, Aronyk KE, et al: Primary lymphoma of the nervous system associated with acquired immune-deficiency syndrome. *N Engl J Med* 1983; 308:45.

5. Levine AM, Meyer PR, Begandy MK, et al: Development of B-cell lymphoma in homosexual men. *Ann Intern Med* 1984; 100:7–13.

6. Ziegler JL, and others: Non-Hodgkin's lymphoma in 90 homosexual men: Relationship to generalized lymphadenopathy and acquired immunodeficiency syndrome (AIDS). *N Engl J Med* 1984; 311:565–571.

7. Ioachim HL, Cooper MC, Hellman GC: Lymphomas in men at high risk for acquired immune deficiency syndrome (AIDS). *Cancer* 1985; 56:2831–2842.

8. Ioachim HL, Cooper MC: Lymphomas of AIDS. *Lancet* 1986; 1:96–97.

9. Kalter SP, Riggs SA, Cabanillas F, et al: Aggressive non-Hodgkin's lymphomas in immunocompromised homosexual males. *Blood* 1985; 66:655–659.

10. Kaplan DL, Volberding PA, Abrams DI: Update on AIDS-associated non-Hodgkin's lymphoma (NHL) in San Francisco. Presented at the Third International Conference on AIDS, Washington, DC, June 1–5, 1987.

11. Centers for Disease Control: Revision of the case definition of acquired immunodeficiency syndrome for national reporting: United States. *MMWR* 1985; 34:373–375.

12. Ioachim HL: Acquired immune deficiency disease after three years: The unsolved riddle, editorial. *Lab Invest* 1984; 51:1–6.

13. Ioachim HL: Neoplasms associated with immune deficiencies. *Pathol Annu* 1987; 2:147–182.

14. Nasr SA, Brynes RK, Garrison CP, et al: Peripheral T-cell lymphoma in a patient with AIDS. *Cancer* 1988; 61:947–951.

15. Burkes RL, Meyer PR, Gill PS, et al: Rectal lymphoma in homosexual men. *Arch Intern Med* 1986; 146:913–915.

16. Ioachim HL, Weinstein MA, Robbins RD, et al: Primary anorectal lymphoma: A new manifestation of the acquired immune deficiency syndrome (AIDS). *Cancer*, 1987; 60:1449–1453.

17. Lee Moon H, Waxman M, Gillooley JF: Primary malignant lymphoma of the anorectum in homosexual men. *Dis Col Rect* 1986; 29:413–416.

18. Hanto DW, Frizzera G, Purtilo DT, et al: Clinical spectrum of lymphoproliferative disorders in renal transplant recipients and evidence for the role of Epstein-Barr virus. *Cancer Res* 1981; 41:4253–4261.

19. Louie S, Schwartz RS: Immunodeficiency and the pathogenesis of lymphoma and leukemia. *Semin Hematol* 1978; 15:117–118.

20. Ioachim HL, Roy M, Cronin W: Histologic patterns of lymphadenopathies in AIDS: Correlation with progress of disease. Presented at the Third International Conference on AIDS, Washington, DC, June 1–5, 1987.

21. Ioachim HL, Ryan JR, Blaugrund SM: Parotid gland lymph nodes: The site of lymphadenopathies and lymphomas associated with the human immunodeficiency virus (HIV) infection. *Arch Pathol Lab Med* (in press).

ANOGENITAL CARCINOMAS

The anogenital region includes the anus, the perianal skin, and external genitalia. In women, the external genitalia comprise the labia majora and minora, the mons pubis, and the vaginal introitus; in men, the penis and the scrotum.[1] Because carcinomas of the anogenital region are infrequent in the general population, the epidemiologic data available are limited. It is estimated that of the 910,000 new cases of cancer that occur annually in the United States, only about 0.5% are located in the anogenital region.[2] In recipients of renal transplants, however, in whom the incidence of neoplasia in general is markedly increased, carcinomas of the anogenital region are more frequent than expected. In a series of 2,150 patients who acquired various tumors after renal transplantation, 2.8% of the tumors were anogenital carcinomas. Similar increases in frequency were recorded in a study from Sweden, in which three cancers of the vulva and anus were observed among 934 renal transplant patients, an incidence that is 100 times the 0.03 expected for these immunosuppressed patients.[3]

The anogenital region is potentially subject to multicentric tumors or multiple primary malignant tumors.[1] Thus, a carcinoma of one organ in this region may indicate that there is a second synchronous or metachronous tumor in the same or another organ. A field effect for the neoplasms of the lower genital and anal area has been noted by several authors.[1,4,5] A study of multiple primary neoplasms of the anogenital region reviewed 15 cases of patients with three or more such tumors.[1] Eight of the patients had synchronous carcinomas (four in situ and four invasive), and seven had sequential multiple primary tumors, all involving the vulva, cervix, vagina, and anus in various combinations.

The explanation for the predisposition to multiple tumors in the anogenital region is the common embryologic origin of the organs in this area. The anal canal develops from the connection of the caudal expansion of the hind gut and the ectodermal depression formed by an anal tubercle.[5] The two rudimentary tubular organs are separated by the cloacal membrane, which eventually disappears, leaving in its place the transitional zone connecting the rectum and the anus. The transitional epithelium lining this area of anal mucosa may give rise to carcinomas that are different from both the adenocarcinomas of the rectum and the squamous-cell or basal-cell carcinomas of the anus. These tumors, designated as transitional, cloacogenic, or basaloid carcinomas of the anus, have distinctive histologic and behavioral features.[4-6] The same embryonic cloacogenic membrane is also the origin of the uterine cervix, vagina, and vulvar region. Women with squamous-cell carcinoma of the cervix are known to have an increased incidence of anal carcinoma, a finding that reflects the common origin of these organs and the field effect that potential carcinogenic agents may induce in this area.[1,4,5]

Carcinomas of the female lower genital organs, particularly of the uterine cervix, have been linked to the activity of human papilloma viruses (HPV) and herpes simplex virus type 2 (HSV-2), either alone or in association. Early sexual intercourse and multiple partners are associated with genital condylomas, dysplasias, and carcinomas.[4] Homosexual men, who are sexually promiscuous, are at high risk for various traumatic lesions, such as anal fistulas and fissures, rectal ulcers, perirectal abscesses, and a variety of infectious complications, including gonorrhea, syphilis, hepatitis, amebiasis and giardiasis.[7,8] Infections with HPV and HSV-2 are particularly common, typically resulting in anal condylomas and ulcers (see Figs. II. 5.58–64).[7] As previously noted for promiscuous women, promiscuity in homosexual men is also associated with dysplasia and carcinomas of the anogenital region.[4]

In individuals at risk for AIDS, condylomas, and carcinomas in situ manifested as Bowen's disease of the anus, are frequently seen. Occasionally, the two lesions are present side by side in the anal mucosa. Condylomas of all three types (planum, acuminatum, and endophytic) can occur in the anogenital area in both males and females (see Figs. II.5.62–64; II.6.11,12; II.7.2,3). On histologic examination, they are characterized, as in other locations, by the presence of koilocytotic atypia involving the upper third of the anal, genital, or cutaneous epithelia. Bowen's disease is characterized by a bandlike hyperplasia of squamous epithelium accompanied by cell disorientation and lack of cellular maturation (see Figs. II.5.65,66). There is marked cytoplasmic basophilia, nuclear pleomorphism (including bizarre and giant nuclei), and typical and atypical mitoses. The subjacent stroma, which is not invaded by tumor, is infiltrated by lymphocytes and plasma cells. Lesions that resemble Bowen's disease histologically but have a benign clinical course are Bowenoid dysplasias of the vulva and anus and Bowenoid papulosis of the penis.[9,10] Compared with the lesions of Bowen's disease, which is a form of carcinoma in situ, the dysplastic changes of Bowenoid lesions show more cellular uniformity and absence of pilosebaceous involvement.[9]

Invasive carcinoma of the anorectum has also been reported to occur in homosexual men.[4] Four cases have been described in men with a long history of receptive homosexual activity.[4] In all these cases, the tumors occurred in the transitional anorectal zone and were of the cloacogenic carcinoma type. On histologic examination, they showed features of transitional-cell carcinoma, with cells containing more uniform, ovoid nuclei, or of basaloid carcinoma, with cells containing smaller, less uniform, more basophilic nuclei.[5] Often, the cloacogenic tumors comprised varying admixtures of all these cell types. The patients had an average age of 42 years, which is younger than the usual age of persons with anorectal carcinomas. The cloacogenic carcinomas in these patients were aggressive, showing a propensity for local invasion and remote metastases.[4,5] Embryonal carcinoma of the testis has been observed in two homosexual men who had no risk factors for this form of cancer but were suffering from cellular immune deficiency and lymphadenopathy.[11]

Squamous-cell carcinoma associated with human papilloma viruses and condylomatous lesions arising in immunodeficient hosts have also been reported to occur in other organs. Accordingly, a squamous-cell carcinoma of the tongue in one young man who had undergone renal transplantation showed adjacent condylomatous lesions, and ultrastructural examination revealed virus particles of papova morphology.[12] Skin cancers, particularly on sun-exposed skin, are 7.1 times more frequent in renal transplant recipients; of these patients squamous-cell carcinoma showed an increase of 36.4 times.[13] Whereas in the general population, where basal-cell carcinomas outnumber squamous-cell carcinoma 4 to 1, in these immunosuppressed individuals squamous-cell carcinomas are much more frequent. Like other tumors, squamous-cell carcinomas are also more aggressive in immunodeficient hosts.[14]

ANOGENITAL CARCINOMAS

Anogenital organs have common origin in cloacogenic membrane

Tendency to multiple tumors in anogenital region

Anogenital carcinomas infrequent in general population

Anogenital carcinomas, 100 times more common in immunodeficient individuals

Associated with promiscuous sexual activity

Associated with anogenital condylomata

Associated with HPV and HSV-2 local infections

Bowen's disease, cloacogenic carcinoma, and basaloid carcinoma more frequent

Squamous-cell carcinoma of other organs also more common in immunodeficient individuals

REFERENCES

1. Choo Y-C, Morley GW: Multiple primary neoplasms of the anogenital region. *Obstet Gynecol* 1980; 56:365–369.
2. Penn I: Cancers of the anogenital region in renal transplant recipients: Analysis of 65 cases. *Cancer* 1986; 58:611–616.
3. Blohmé I, Brynger H: Malignant disease in renal transplant patients. *Transplantation* 1985; 39:23–25.
4. Cooper HS, Patchefsky AS, Marks G: Cloacogenic carcinoma of the anorectum in homosexual men: An observation of four cases. *Dis Col Rect* 1979; 22:557–558.
5. Levin SE, Cooperman H, Freilich M, et al: Transitional cloacogenic carcinoma of the anus. *Dis Col Rect* 1977; 20:17–23.
6. Grinvalski HT, Helwig EB: Carcinoma of the anorectal junction: I. Histological considerations. *Cancer* 1956; 9:480.
7. Owen WF: Sexually transmitted diseases and traumatic problems in homosexual men. *Ann Intern Med* 1980; 92:805–808.
8. Sohn N, Robilotti JG: The gay bowel syndrome: A review of colonic and rectal conditions in 200 male homosexuals. *Am J Gastroenterol* 1977; 67:478–484.
9. Ulbright TM, Stehman FB, Roth LM: Bowenoid papulosis of the vulva. *Cancer* 1982; 50:2910–2919.
10. Wade TR, Kopf AW, Ackerman AB: Bowenoid papulosis of the penis. *Cancer* 1978; 42:1890–1903.
11. Logothetis CJ, Newell GR, Samuels ML: Testicular cancer in homosexual men with cellular immune deficiency: Report of two cases. *J Urol* 1985; 133:484–486.
12. Gisser S: Papovavirus and squamous cell carcinoma. *Hum Pathol* 1981; 12:190–193.
13. Hoxtell EO, Mandel JS, Murray SS, et al: Incidence of skin carcinoma following renal transplantation. *Arch Dermatol* 1977; 113:436–438.
14. Maize JC: Skin cancer in immunosuppressed patients, editorial, *JAMA* 1977; 237:1857–1858.

Ophthalmic Disorders Associated with AIDS

OPHTHALMIC INVOLVEMENT

Ocular symptoms and signs are present in 50% of all patients with AIDS, and 75% of autopsies of AIDS patients reveal ophthalmic involvement.[1] The lesions reported to occur in patients with AIDS are cotton wool spots, CMV retinitis, Kaposi's sarcoma of the conjunctiva and eyelids, mycobacteriosis of the choroid, *Toxoplasma* retinitis, and cranial nerve paralysis.[1-4] In a study of ophthalmic abnormalities in 40 patients with AIDS, the most common findings were CMV retinitis (10 patients), retinal cotton wool spots (11), conjunctival Kaposi's sarcoma (two), and abnormal neuro-ophthalmic motility (three).[1] Postmortem examination of the eyes of 20 of these patients demonstrated pathologic retinal findings in at least one eye in 13 of them.[1]

Cytomegalovirus retinitis can occur in medically immunosuppressed patients, and it is the major cause of visual loss in AIDS patients.[1,5-7] The retinal lesions are white and granular, frequently associated with areas of hemorrhage and necrosis that spread in a centrifugal manner (see Figs. II.10.7–13).[5,7] There is a moderate inflammatory infiltrate with lymphocytes and macrophages. Progression over three to six months produces visual field defects and scotomas, with severe loss of vision shortly before death.[1] Retinal necrosis and disorganization of the underlying pigmented epithelium, accompanied by loss of retinal elements, are followed by atrophy and scarring with pigment dispersion and occasional focal calcifications.[1,6,7]

In one study, electron microscopic examination showed immature and mature virus particles in the nucleus and cytoplasm of involved cells (see Fig.II.10.11).[6] Immunohistochemical staining revealed the presence of CMV antigens in all layers of the retina at the borders of the lesions and in isolated perivascular cells from normal-appearing areas of the retina (see Fig.II.10.12). In situ hybridization using a complementary DNA probe of human CMV confirmed the location of the virus in the retinal cells, adjacent to areas of necrosis, as was previously seen by means of immunohistochemical methods.[6]

Early areas of CMV infection are usually located in the posterior pole, though occasionally the disease may begin at the periphery. Retinal involvement usually follows the vascular distribution, producing large areas of necrosis or smaller perivascular infiltrates.[7]

Lesions typically begin in one eye and start to affect the second eye two to three months later.[1] In a study of 10 cases of CMV retinitis, all of the patients had viremia at the time of examination. Previously, CMV retinitis has been reported to occur with increased frequency in immunosuppressed individuals.[5] In AIDS patients, it appears to occur late in the course of the disease, through hematogenous dissemination of CMV to the retina.

It is noteworthy that in a series of AIDS patients composed primarily of heterosexual drug abusers, CMV retinitis occurred in the only homosexual patient. This finding is perhaps to be expected, given the low incidence of CMV infection in non-homosexual patients with AIDS and the high incidence of CMV infection in the homosexual population and of CMV retinitis in homosexuals with AIDS.[4]

Herpes zoster ophthalmicus is characterized by a vesiculobullous rash in the distribution of the ophthalmic branch of the trigeminal nerve. It may be accompanied by blepharitis, conjunctivitis, keratitis, and uveitis (see Figs. II.10.19–24).[7] Herpes simplex virus infection of the eye, involving all the retinal layers, has also been reported (see Figs. II.10.14–18).

Retinal cotton wool spots are observed in more than 50% of AIDS patients who come for ocular examination; they are the most common ophthalmic lesions associated with AIDS.[1,2,4,8] They appear as white, fluffy, opaque retinal foci that are usually multiple and bilateral. Histologically (see Figs. II.10.5,6), they correspond to cytoid bodies and are the result of microinfarctions in the nerve fiber layer.[8] Retinal cotton wool spots are also known to occur in diabetes, hypertension, and anemia—conditions generally associated with retinal microvascular abnormalities leading to ischemia.[2,4,8] Unlike CMV lesions, they are not associated with hemorrhages and progression, and no visual loss can be attributed to their presence.[1,8] In cases in which the eyes were examined post-mortem, no microorganisms could be identified.[1] Thus, though cotton wool spots do not induce major injury by themselves, they should alert the clinician to the possibility of AIDS when they are found in an asymptomatic individual belonging to a high-risk group.[4]

Involvement of the CNS in AIDS patients may give rise to cranial nerve palsies that result in extraocular motility deficits, visual field defects, pupillary abnormalities, and papilledema.[7] Sometimes, subsequent study can relate these cranial nerve palsies to cryptococcal meningitis, herpes zoster, and cerebral non-Hodgkin's lymphoma (see Figs. II.10.31–33).[1] Granulomas with *Mycobacterium avium-intracellulare* can be seen on the choroid.[2] Toxoplasmic retinochoroiditis (see Figs. II.10.25–27), may be the initial manifestation of AIDS. Permanent loss of vision may develop if the lesion is located in the macula or optic nerve.[7] Kaposi's sarcoma can involve ocular and adnexal structures; in one study, it was present in 24% of patients with ophthalmic manifestations of AIDS.[2] If it is located on the palpebral or bulbar conjunctiva, it enlarges very slowly and does not result in loss of vision.[1] The cutaneous aspects of the eyelids are common sites for Kaposi's sarcoma. Usually it is located in the medial third of the lower lid (see Figs. II.10.1–3).

OPHTHALMIC INVOLVEMENT

Present clinically in 50% of AIDS patients and at autopsy in 75%

Cotton wool spots most common finding; not associated with visual loss

Multiple, white, opaque foci, corresponding to cytoid bodies, result from microinfarctions in the nerve fiber layer

CMV retinitis most common cause of visual loss in AIDS

Foci of hemorrhage and necrosis with mild inflammation, scarring, and atrophy following vascular distribution

Herpes zoster lesions in the distribution of the trigeminal nerve and herpes simplex lesions in the retinal layers

Toxoplasmic retinochoroiditis with possible permanent loss of vision

Cranial nerve palsies, subsequent to meningeal or cerebral infections and lymphomas

Kaposi's sarcoma of conjunctiva and eyelids

REFERENCES

1. Palestine AG, Rodrigues MM, Macher AM, et al: Ophthalmic involvement in acquired immunodeficiency syndrome. *Ophthalmology* 1984; 91:1092–1099.
2. Holland GN, Pepose JS, Pettit TH, et al: Acquired immune deficiency syndrome: Ocular manifestations. *Ophthalmology* 1983; 90:859–873.
3. Macher AM, Palestine A, Masur H, et al: Multicentric Kaposi's sarcoma of the conjunctiva in a male homosexual with the acquired immune deficiency syndrome. *Ophthalmology* 1983; 90:879–884.
4. Rosenberg PR, Uliss AE, Friedland GH, et al: Acquired immunodeficiency syndrome: Ophthalmic manifestations in ambulatory patients. *Ophthalmology* 1983; 90:874–878.
5. Egbert PR, Pollard RB, Gallagher JG, et al: Cytomegalovirus retinitis in immunosuppressed hosts. *Ann Intern Med* 1980; 93:664–670.
6. Pepose JS, Newman C, Bach MC, et al: Pathologic features of cytomegalovirus retinopathy after treatment with the antiviral agent ganciclovir. *Ophthalmology* 1987; 94:414–424.
7. Schuman JS, Orellana J, Friedman AH, et al: Acquired immunodeficiency syndrome (AIDS). *Survey Ophthalmol* 1987; 31:384–410.
8. Rodrigues MM, Palestine A, Nussenblatt R, et al: Unilateral cytomegalovirus retinochoroiditis and bilateral cytoid bodies in a bisexual man with the acquired immunodeficiency syndrome. *Ophthalmology* 1983; 90:1577–1582.

Cutaneous Disorders Associated with AIDS

CUTANEOUS DISORDERS

A number of skin conditions noted in the general population occur with increased frequency in persons at high risk for AIDS. Like many other diseases, these skin disorders tend to be atypical, more severe, more disseminated, and more resistant to treatment when associated with AIDS.[1] Skin disorders frequently recognized in AIDS patients include infections induced by a variety of agents and neoplasias. The most common of these are molluscum contagiosum, herpes simplex, herpes zoster, dermatophytic infections, candidiasis, impetigo, folliculitis, seborrheic dermatitis, verrucae, and Kaposi's sarcoma.[2]

CUTANEOUS DISORDERS

Infections and neoplasias

Increased incidence in AIDS

More atypical, more severe, more disseminated

More resistant to treatment

Occasionally preceding ARC or AIDS

Severe forms indicative of poor prognosis of AIDS

REFERENCES

1. Hatcher VA: Mucocutaneous infections in acquired immune deficiency syndrome, in Friedman-Kien AE, Laubenstein LJ (eds): *AIDS: The Epidemic of Kaposi's Sarcoma and Opportunistic Infections.* New York, Masson, 1984, pp 245–252.

2. Mathes BM, Douglass MC: Seborrheic dermatitis in patients with acquired immunodeficiency syndrome. *J Am Acad Dermatol* 1985; 13:947–951.

SEBORRHEIC DERMATITIS

Seborrheic dermatitis is a benign skin eruption characterized by erythematous patches and plaques covered with small, yellowish, greasy scales and areas of crusting (see Fig. II.1.1).[1] It has a predilection for the scalp, the cheeks, the ears, and the seborrheic areas of the face, including the eyebrows, the nasolabial surfaces, and the beard.[2] Involvement of the malar area often results in a butterfly rash resembling that of lupus.[3] It may also be found in other hairbearing areas, such as the axillae, groin, and chest, though this is less common. Scarring does not occur.

The histologic lesions consist of extensive parakeratosis with exudation of serum and infiltration by neutrophils, lymphocytes, and plasma cells.[1] Follicular plugging and psoriasiform epidermal hyperplasia are observed. The underlying dermis shows vascular congestion and moderate perivascular lymphocytic infiltration.[3]

Seborrheic dermatitis is known to occur in association with various neurologic conditions, particularly Parkinson's disease, cerebrovascular accidents, CNS trauma, and facial nerve palsy.[2] It is more extended and more severe in AIDS patients than in healthy individuals. In one study, the incidence of seborrheic dermatitis was 83% among patients with AIDS and 42% among patients with ARC, but only 1% to 3% in normal control individuals.[2] The severity of seborrheic dermatitis seemed to correlate with the degree of the patients' immunodeficiency, and therefore may have some prognostic significance.

The occurrence of severe seborrheic dermatitis in apparently healthy homosexual men and intravenous drug abusers may be indicative of impending AIDS.[1,2] The cause of seborrheic dermatitis is unknown. One suggested explanation is that the decrease in the number of Langerhans cells known to occur in AIDS alters the immune reactions of the skin, thus favoring the development of dermatitis and other cutaneous infections.[1]

SEBORRHEIC DERMATITIS

Benign skin eruption predominant on hair-bearing areas

Erythematous patches covered with greasy scales and crusts

Parakeratosis, exudation, and inflammatory cellular infiltrates

Cause unknown; associated with neurological conditions

High incidence in individuals with AIDS and ARC

Severe seborrheic dermatitis indicative of poor prognosis of AIDS

REFERENCES

1. Soeprono FF, Schinella RA, Cockerell CJ, et al: Seborrheic-like dermatitis of acquired immunodeficiency syndrome. *J Am Acad Dermatol* 1986; 14:242–248.
2. Mathes BM, Douglass MC: Seborrheic dermatitis in patients with acquired immunodeficiency syndrome. *J Am Acad Dermatol* 1985; 13:947–951.
3. Eisenstat BA, Wormser GP: Seborrheic dermatitis and butterfly rash in AIDS. *N Engl J Med* 1984; 311:189.

MOLLUSCUM CONTAGIOSUM

Molluscum contagiosum is a common viral-induced cutaneous disease that affects children and adults worldwide. The lesions are skin-colored or pearly-white papules 2 to 5 mm in diameter that are dome-shaped and umbilicated and contain a waxy substance that can be expressed from their cores (see Fig. II.1.11).[1] The papules appear singly or in clusters and may either remain unnoticed or disseminate, sometimes into the hundreds. In children, the lesions appear on the face, hands, forearms, and legs. They persist for variable amounts of time and often regress spontaneously. In adults, molluscum contagiosum is generally sexually transmitted, and the lesions in both men and women are typically confined to the genital organs and the adjacent areas.[2] In a study of molluscum contagiosum in an outpatient clinic at a general hospital, young, sexually active men and women aged 17 to 26 years (mean, 20 years) were the only individuals affected.[2]

The etiologic agent, molluscum contagiosum virus, belongs to the family of poxviruses, which also includes the small pox (variola), vaccinia, and cowpox viruses. Poxviruses are DNA viruses and are the largest of animal viruses; they can be seen with phase optics or even in stained preparations under the light microscope. The molluscum body is a large inclusion body composed of numerous virions present within the cytoplasm of infected cells. The viral particles, also called elementary bodies, are round or brick-shaped and have a complex structure consisting of an internal mass (the nucleoid) surrounded by two membrane layers.[3] Clusters of DNA viral particles embedded in a protein matrix form the molluscum bodies, which infect the cells by contiguity.

In the skin, the lesion is confined to the epidermis, where infected keratinocytes are markedly enlarged and contain the molluscum bodies (**Fig. I.9.1;** see Figs.II.1.12,13). These increase in size up to 35 μm and fill the cytoplasm, compressing the nuclei, which appear pyknotic and crescent-shaped at the periphery of the cell.[1,4] The enlarged keratinocytes form large lobules that protrude into the dermis and form a central cystic area where the infected cells are desquamated. The basement membrane remains intact, and the basal cells increase in volume as they become infected and move toward the surface. The content of the cyst is eventually extruded, leaving behind an empty crater in the center of the papule. The lesions show no parakeratosis and no significant dermal inflammatory reaction.[1] In normal immunocompetent persons, the lesions involute spontaneously after several months, leaving no traces unless secondary infection occurred.

Diagnosis is made by biopsy or by crushing the content of a papule on a slide and staining with Gram or Giemsa stains, which reveal the large, diagnostic molluscum bodies.[2] The treatment of choice is cryotherapy or curettage of the papules in order to eradicate the molluscum bodies and prevent the spread of the infection.[1]

In normal individuals, recurrences are rare after adequate therapy. Molluscum contagiosum with large numbers of papules has been reported in pregnant women, individuals with congenital immune deficiencies, and patients undergoing immunosuppressive treatment with prednisone or methotrexate.[2,5] Recently, molluscum contagiosum has been reported in AIDS patients. These cases were remarkable for the large number, unusual distribution, and rapid recurrence of lesions, despite adequate treatment,[5] which indicate that molluscum may be yet another cutaneous lesion that is dependent on the deficient cellular immunity induced by AIDS.

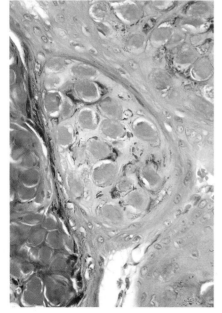

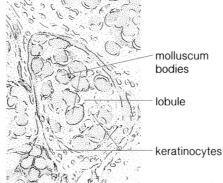

molluscum bodies

lobule

keratinocytes

Fig. I.9.1 Molluscum bodies within elarged keratinocytes of epidermis. Disticnt lobules formed by the involved cells. (HPS stain, ×400)

MOLLUSCUM CONTAGIOSUM

Virus-induced cutaneous disease

Worldwide distribution

Large DNA poxviruses forming molluscum bodies in cytoplasm of infected cells

Confined to epidermis by infection of keratinocytes and formation of papules

In children, self-healing lesions on face and extremities

In adults, sexually transmitted and genital distribution

In AIDS patients, numerous lesions, unusual distribution, rapid recurrence

REFERENCES

1. Remigio PA: Molluscum contagiosum, in Sun T (ed): *Sexually Related Infectious Diseases.* New York, Field, Rich & Assoc, 1986, pp 135–141.
2. Wilkin JK: Molluscum contagiosum venereum in a women's outpatient clinic: A venereally transmitted disease. *Am J Obstet Gynecol* 1977; 128:531–535.
3. Dulbecco R, Ginsberg HS: Poxviruses, in Davis BD, Dulbecco R, Eisen HN (eds): *Microbiology.* New York, Harper & Row, 1973, pp 1258–1277.
4. Kwittken J: Molluscum contagiosum: Some new histologic observations. *Mt Sinai J Med* 1980; 47:583–588.
5. Lombardo P: Molluscum contagiosum and the acquired immune-deficiency syndrome. *Arch Dermatol* 1985; 121:834–835.

AIDS in Children

AIDS IN CHILDREN

Cases of infants with cellular immune deficiency and various opportunistic infections have been reported in increasing numbers during the past few years, indicating that the AIDS epidemic has now extended to children.[1-5] In the first reports, the infants were predominantly of Haitian origin; however, the majority of the later cases have occurred in children of mothers with known risk factors for AIDS, such as intravenous drug abuse, prostitution, or sexual contact with bisexual men at risk for AIDS.[1,4,5]

The affected infants fail to thrive and suffer from recurrent febrile episodes, anemia, hepatosplenomegaly, and diarrhea. They may also have persistent oral infection with *Candida albicans*, cutaneous rashes, and severe neurologic impairment. A variety of opportunistic infections similar to those seen in adult patients with AIDS have been observed in children, including *Pneumocystis* pneumonia, CMV and HSV infections, mycobacteriosis, and candidiasis and cases of Kaposi's sarcoma in children have even been reported.[4,5] Bacterial infections, particularly with gram-negative organisms, are common and are frequently the cause of death in children; this is rarely the case in adult AIDS patients.[4,5] The persistent generalized lymphadenopathies of the adult pre-AIDS phase are not seen in children. Severe immune alterations, mainly affecting cellular immunity, are the common background in pediatric AIDS. These include substantial reductions of T lymphocytes, with inverted helper/suppressor T-cell ratios; reduced lymphocyte response to mitogens; marked hypergammaglobulinemia; and circulating antigen-antibody complexes.[4,5] The thymus may show the development of lymphoid follicles in the medulla, infiltration by plasma cells, and progressive atrophy.[6]

The most common and characteristic manifestation of AIDS in infants and children, however, is the involvement of lungs and brain by the initial infection with HIV. Lymphocytic interstitial pneumonitis (LIP) is more common in children than in adults, and it may occur in the absence of other infections.[1,4,5,7] On radiologic examination (see Figs. II.4.4,5), the lesions appear as diffuse, bilateral reticulonodular densities; the diagnosis is usually confirmed by open-lung biopsy. On microscopic examination (see Figs. II.4.6–9), the lung sections show diffuse and nodular infiltration of interalveolar septa and peribronchiolar areas by accumulations of small mature lymphocytes, sometimes including germinal centers and scattered plasma cells.[4,5,8] The lymphocytes are of polyclonal B-cell type (without nuclear atypia), and have relatively infrequent mitoses.[9] In studies aimed at identifying the etiologic agent in LIP, EBV DNA was detected in eight of ten lung biopsy specimens from children with LIP and in none of the lung specimens from the patients infected with CMV, *Pneumocystis*, or *Mycobacterium*.[1] The children with LIP also had elevated serum antibody titers to EBV. In other studies, HIV RNA was identified in lymphocytes of LIP patients by in situ hybridization techniques, which suggests that HIV might be implicated in the etiology of LIP, either directly or, perhaps, through activation of EBV.[1,7,9]

A syndrome of progressive neurologic deterioration similar to the subacute encephalitis of adult AIDS has also been observed in affected children.[3] The clinical manifestations include failure of neurologic and intellectual development, hyperreflexia, spastic quadriparesis, microcephaly (in infants), and cortical atrophy on CT scans.[3,10,11] Progressive encephalopathy, often manifested by dementia, typically ends in death in two to 16 months, as one study of 11 children, aged four months to 11 years, with this syndrome indicated.[10] On gross examination, the brains are atrophic; weight is markedly diminished, and ventricles and sulci are enlarged.

On microscopic examination, the major findings are loss of myelin, glial microglial nodules, blood-vessel calcifications, perivascular inflammatory infiltrates, and multinucleated giant cells.[10,11] The white matter is diminished in the cerebral hemispheres and cerebellum, and there is little stainable myelin. Blood vessels—mostly small ones, and usually in the basal ganglia—show deposition of calcium in or next to their walls. In addition, more abundant calcification is seen in large vessels of the putamen.[10] The cellular infiltrates are focal and frequently perivascular, composed of glial and microglial cells, along with lymphocytes and monocytes in many instances and even with plasma cells on occasion. In one study, multinucleated giant cells associated with the cellular infiltrates were seen in eight of 11 cases.[10] Two types of giant cells were described. In one type, the cells have a cluster of overlapping nuclei and minimal cytoplasm, resembling those seen in the lymphadenopathies of HIV infection in adults; in the other type, the giant cells resemble Langhans or Touton cells, with abundant acidophilic cytoplasm and peripherally arranged nuclei. The presence of transitional forms may indicate that these two types represent progressive stages, and the foamy cytoplasm in some of these cells may indicate that they derive from macrophages or histiocytes.[10] In the same study, viral particles morphologically consistent with HIV were seen around mitochondria in the central region of giant cells, in the cytoplasm of astrocytes, and in extracellular clusters adjacent to the cell membranes of giant cells.[10]

The progressive encephalopathy noted in children with AIDS is morphologically similar to the subacute encephalitis noted in adult AIDS patients with dementia. As pointed out by the authors of one comprehensive study, these neuropathologic findings are different from those of any encephalopathy previously seen in humans, including those observed in immunocompromised patients.[10] This unique morphologic appearance and the presence of HIV particles in the affected tissues strongly suggest a causative role for HIV in the induction of encephalitis by direct infection of the brain.

AIDS IN CHILDREN

Infants and children whose mothers are at high risk for AIDS

Failure to thrive

Recurrent febrile episodes

Anemia

Rashes

Diarrhea

Opportunistic infections

Gram-negative bacterial sepsis

Severe cellular immune deficiency

Lymphocytic interstitial pneumonitis (LIP), more common in children than in adults

HIV RNA detectable in lymphocytes of LIP patients

Progressive encephalopathy with failure of neurologic development, spastic paresis, and dementia

Cortical atrophy

Loss of myelin

Vascular calcifications

Cellular infiltrates with multinucleated giant cells

HIV-like virus particles within and around giant cells

REFERENCES

1. Andiman WA, Eastman R, Martin K, et al: Opportunistic lymphoproliferations associated with Epstein-Barr viral DNA in infants and children with AIDS. *Lancet* 1985; 2:1390–1393.
2. Centers for Disease Control: Revision of case definition of AIDS for national reporting—United States. *MMWR* 1985; 34:373–375.
3. Epstein LG, Sharer LR, Joshi VV, et al: Progressive encephalopathy in children with AIDS. *Ann Neurol* 1985; 17:488–496.
4. Oleske J, Minnefor A, Cooper R Jr, et al: Immune deficiency syndrome in children. *JAMA* 1983; 249:2345–2349.
5. Scott GB, Buck BE, Leterman JG, et al: Acquired immunodeficiency syndrome in infants. *N Engl J Med* 1984; 310:76–81.
6. Joshi VV, Oleske JM: Pathologic appraisal of the thymus gland in AIDS in children. *Arch Pathol Lab Med* 1985; 109:142–146.
7. Chayt KJ, Harper ME, Marselle LM, et al: Detection of HTLV-III RNA in lungs of patients with AIDS and pulmonary involvement. *JAMA* 1986; 256:2356–2359.
8. Joshi VV, Oleske JM: Pulmonary lesions in children with AIDS: A reappraisal based on data in additional cases and follow-up study of previously reported cases. *Hum Pathol* 1986; 17:641–642.
9. Joshi VV, Kaufmann S, Oleske JM, et al: Polyclonal polymorphic B-cell lymphoproliferative disorder with prominent pulmonary involvement in children with acquired immune deficiency syndrome. *Cancer* 1987; 59:1455–1462.
10. Sharer LR, Epstein LG, Cho E-S: Pathologic features of AIDS encephalopathy in children: Evidence of LAV/HTLV-III infection of brain. *Hum Pathol* 1986; 17:271–284.
11. Shaw GM, Harper ME, Hahn BH, et al: HTLV-III infection in brains of children and adults with AIDS encephalopathy. *Science* 1985; 227:177–182.

Atlas of AIDS Pathology

section
TWO

Skin

SEBORRHEIC DERMATITIS

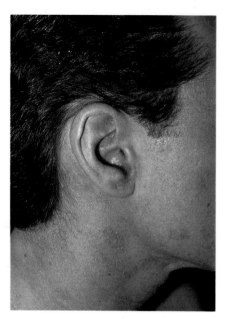

Fig. II.1.1 Erythematous scaling plaques on the neck and face in a young homosexual man.

CUTANEOUS HERPES SIMPLEX

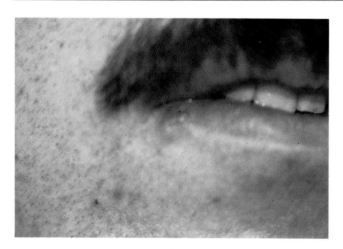

Fig. II.1.2 Herpetic vesicles on indurated red skin adjacent to the vermilion border of the lip

Biopsy, skin of forearm, in 34-year-old homosexual man with HIV infection.

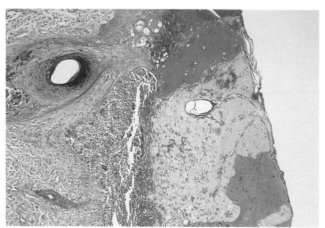

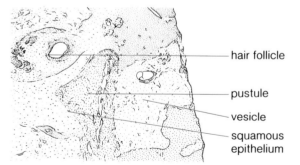

Fig. II.1.3 Epidermis with squamous epithelium, hair follicle, fluid-filled herpetic vesicle, and formation of pustule at the base.   HPS stain, × 100

hair follicle

pustule

vesicle

squamous epithelium

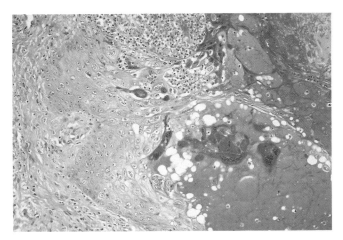

Fig. II.1.4 Same section as in Fig. II.1.3. Squamous epithelium with vesicle and accumulation of polymorphonuclear leukocytes forming pustule. HSV inclusion bodies in the peripheral area.   HPS stain, ×200

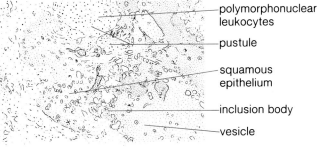
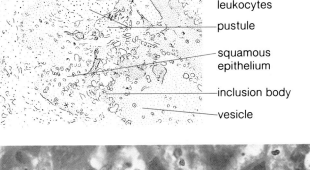

— polymorphonuclear leukocytes

— pustule

— squamous epithelium

— inclusion body

— vesicle

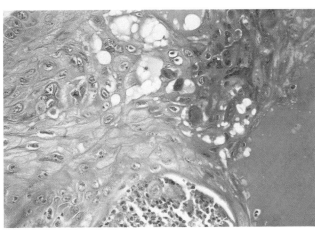

Fig. II.1.5 Same section as in Fig. II.1.3. Squamous epithelium with ballooning degeneration of keratinocytes, polymorphonuclear leukocytes forming pustule, and HSV inclusion bodies.   HPS stain, ×400

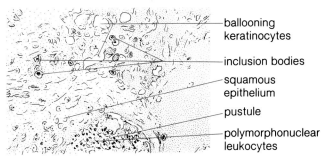

— ballooning keratinocytes

— inclusion bodies

— squamous epithelium

— pustule

— polymorphonuclear leukocytes

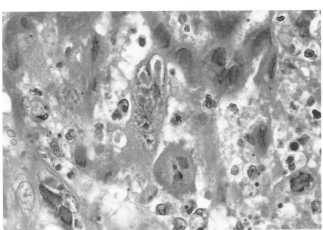

Fig. II.1.6 Same section as in Fig. II.1.3. Lilac-stained, ground-glass HSV early inclusions filling the nuclei and multinucleated giant cells with eosinophilic haloed intranuclear inclusion bodies.   HPS stain, ×1,000

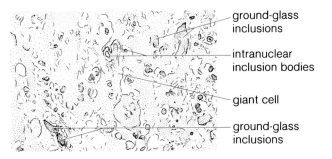

— ground-glass inclusions

— intranuclear inclusion bodies

— giant cell

— ground-glass inclusions

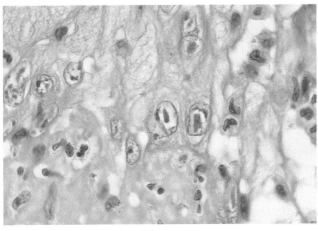

Fig. II.1.7 Same section as in Fig. II.1.3. Ballooning degeneration of squamous cells; intranuclear, haloed HSV inclusion bodies with the nuclei molded around the vacuoles.   HPS stain, ×1,000

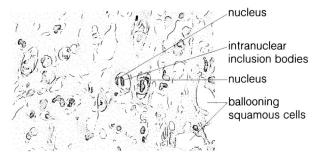

— nucleus

— intranuclear inclusion bodies

— nucleus

— ballooning squamous cells

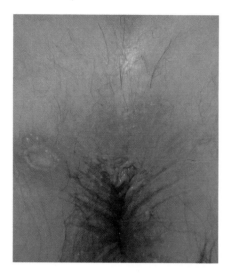

Fig. II.1.8
Perianal herpes
with cluster of
vesicles and ulcer.

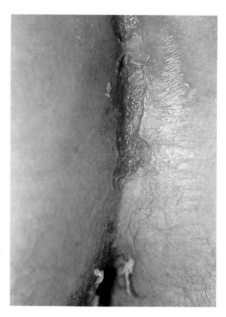

Fig. II.1.9
Ulcerated
confluent herpetic
lesions in perianal
skin

CUTANEOUS HERPES ZOSTER

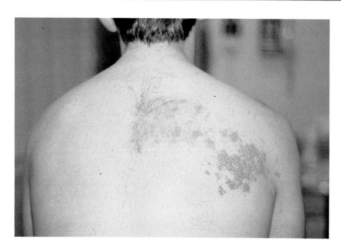

Fig. II.1.10 Clusters of herpes zoster vesicles, partially
healing, in a dermatome distribution on the skin of the back of
a 28-year-old homosexual man.

MOLLUSCUM CONTAGIOSUM

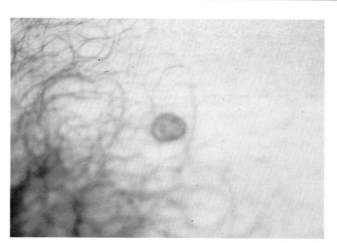

Fig. II.1.11 White, waxy, dome-shaped papule on abdominal
skin of 26-year-old HIV-positive homosexual man.

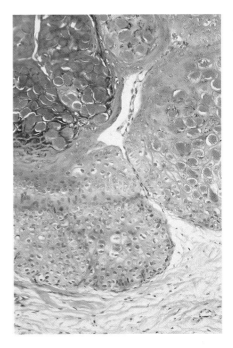

Fig. II.1.12 Skin biopsy specimen showing lobules composed of enlarged keratinocytes containing molluscum bodies and penetrating into the dermis.
HPS stain, ×200

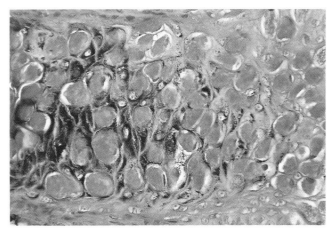

Fig. II.1.13 Same section as in Fig. II.1.12. Enlarged keratinocytes in squamous epithelium, containing molluscum bodies and peripheralized nuclei. HPS stain, ×400

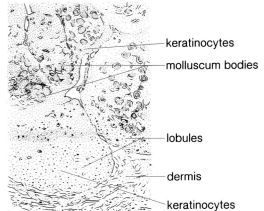

keratinocytes

molluscum bodies

lobules

dermis

keratinocytes

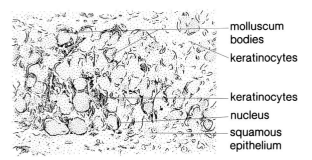

molluscum bodies

keratinocytes

keratinocytes

nucleus

squamous epithelium

KAPOSI'S SARCOMA: SKIN OF FACE

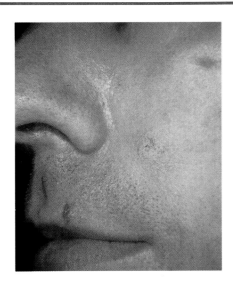

Fig. II.1.14 Kaposi's sarcoma on the skin of the face in a 28-year-old homosexual man. Nodule on the upper lip and plaque on the cheek.

A pink-red patch on the cheek of a 24-year-old man.

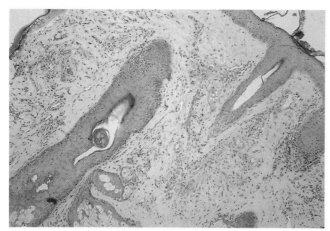

Fig. II.1.15 Clusters of fine capillaries and spindle-shaped cells in upper dermis.   HPS stain, ×100

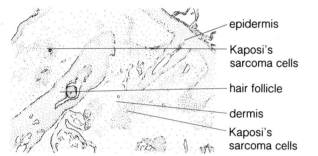

- epidermis
- Kaposi's sarcoma cells
- hair follicle
- dermis
- Kaposi's sarcoma cells

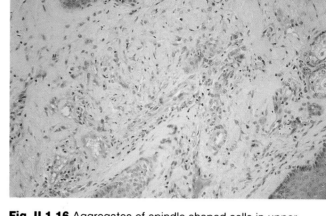

Fig. II.1.16 Aggregates of spindle-shaped cells in upper dermis form bundles or fine vascular slits and clefts. A sprinkling of lymphocytes and plasma cells accompanies this early lesion.   HPS stain, ×200

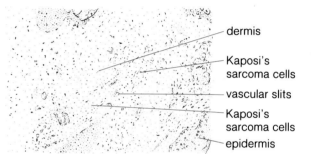

- dermis
- Kaposi's sarcoma cells
- vascular slits
- Kaposi's sarcoma cells
- epidermis

KAPOSI'S SARCOMA: SKIN OF ARMS AND LEGS

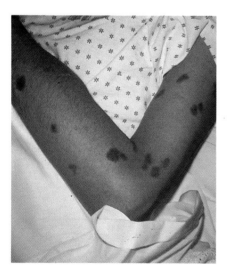

Fig. II.1.17 Kaposi's sarcoma on the skin of the arm in a 32-year-old homosexual man. Multiple, large, irregularly shaped plaques.

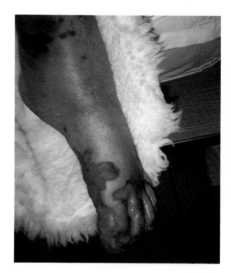

Fig. II.1.18 Kaposi's sarcoma on the skin of the leg and foot in a 34-year-old homosexual man. Large, confluent, partially ulcerated plaques and nodules.

Numerous dark-red patches and plaques are observed on the arms, chest, and back of a 33-year-old homosexual man.

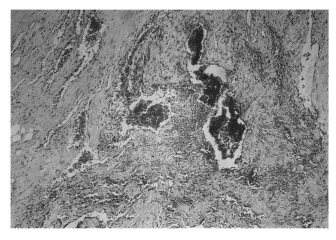

Fig. II.1.19 Dark-red plaque on skin of back, with multiple newly formed, irregularly shaped, congested vascular spaces.
HPS stain, ×100

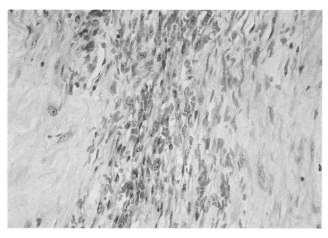

Fig. II.1.20 Red patch on the skin of the arm, with bundles of spindle-shaped cells with atypical nuclei forming slits and clefts containing erythrocytes.
HPS stain, ×400

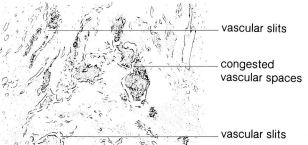

vascular slits

congested vascular spaces

vascular slits

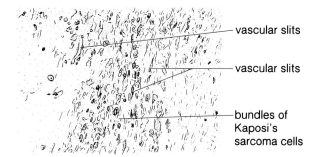

vascular slits

vascular slits

bundles of Kaposi's sarcoma cells

Fig. II.1.21 Dark-red plaque on the skin of the back, with rudimentary vascular spaces containing erythrocytes. Spindle-shaped cells with atypical nuclei form bundles and line the lumina.
HPS stain, ×400

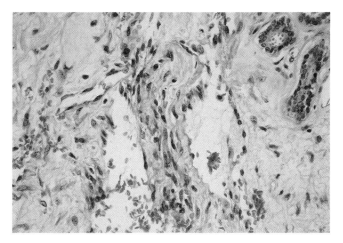

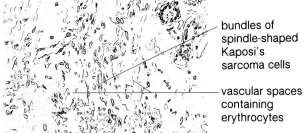

bundles of spindle-shaped Kaposi's sarcoma cells

vascular spaces containing erythrocytes

NON-HODGKIN'S LYMPHOMA OF SKIN

A 39-year-old homosexual man has non-Hodgkin's diffuse, large cleaved-cell lymphoma of the lymph nodes and a cutaneous rash composed of red, irregularly shaped plaques on the back, arms, and legs.

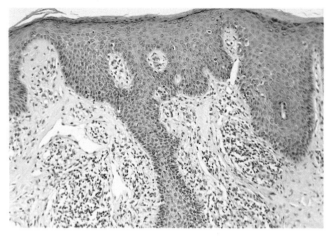

Fig. II.1.22 Skin of back with epidermis uninvolved and perivascular, nodular cellular infiltrates.   HPS stain, ×25

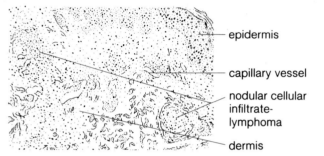

Fig. II.1.23 Perivascular nodular cellular infiltrates in the papillary dermis.   HPS stain, ×100

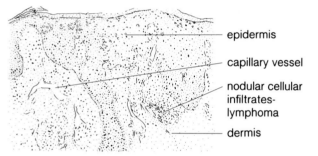

- epidermis
- capillary vessel
- nodular cellular infiltrates-lymphoma
- dermis

- epidermis
- capillary vessel
- nodular cellular infiltrate-lymphoma
- dermis

Fig. II.1.24 Cellular infiltrates, frequently perivascular, composed of small, darkly-stained lymphocytes and large, palely-stained, cleaved lymphoma cells.   HPS stain, ×250

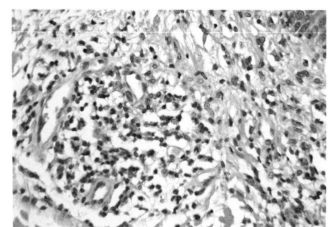

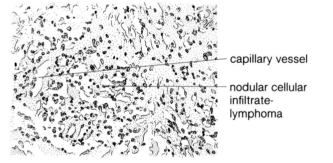

- capillary vessel
- nodular cellular infiltrate-lymphoma

Hemato-lymphopoietic System

BONE MARROW

Bone Marrow in HIV Infection

A 28-year-old homosexual man with low grade fever, fatigue, and moderate weight loss.

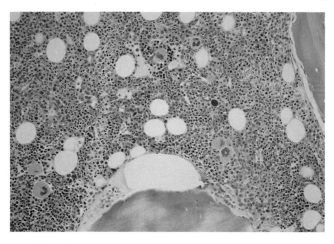

Fig. II.2.1 Hypercellular hematopoietic bone marrow. All hematopoietic series are represented and show cellular maturation. Megakaryocytes are numerous and often aggregated.   HPS stain, ×250

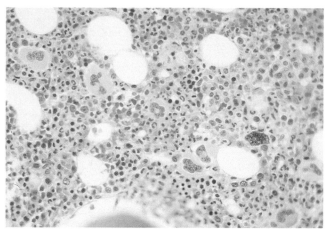

Fig. II.2.2 Hypercellular hematopoietic bone marrow with leukocytosis and megakaryocytosis. Megakaryocytes are frequently clustered and have immature, bizarre nuclei that are often pyknotic and devoid of cytoplasm.   HPS stain, ×400

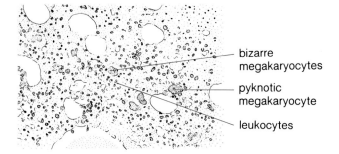

bizarre megakaryocytes

pyknotic megakaryocyte

leukocytes

A 33-year-old homosexual man with low grade fever and lymphadenopathy.

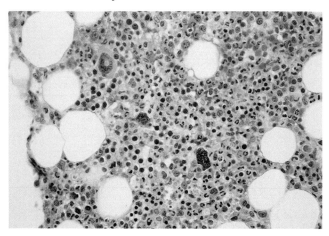

Fig. II.2.3 Hypercellular hematopoietic bone marrow with leukocytosis and megakaryocytosis. Megakaryocytes show immature, bizarre, and pyknotic nuclei that lack cytoplasm.
                          HPS stain, ×400

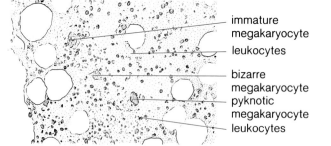

immature megakaryocyte

leukocytes

bizarre megakaryocyte

pyknotic megakaryocyte

leukocytes

Bone-Marrow Granulomas

A 29-year-old homosexual male heroin addict who was healthy prior to this admission developed low-grade fever, fatigue, moderate anemia, and thrombocytopenia.

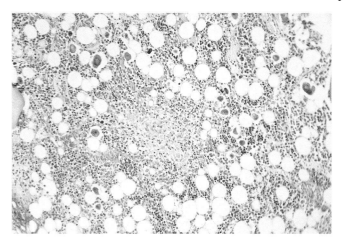

Fig. II.2.4 Hematopoietic bone marrow is mildly hypercellular and shows increased numbers of atypical megakaryocytes, isolated and in clusters, as well as nonnecrotizing granuloma. HPS stain, ×100

Fig. II.2.5 Granuloma in bone marrow is composed of epithelioid cells with peripheral lymphocytes and plasma cells. Necrosis and giant cells are not present. Acid-fast and silver staining reveal no microorganisms. HPS stain, ×250

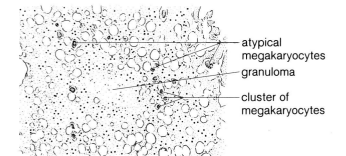

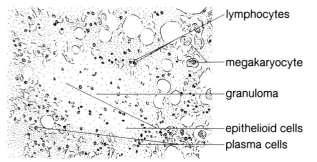

Bone-Marrow Mycobacteriosis

A 36-year-old homosexual man with low grade fever, fatigue, loss of weight, and mild anemia.

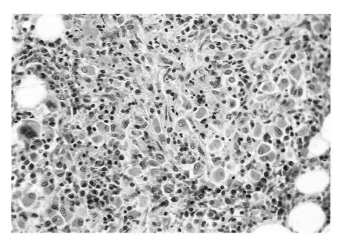

Fig. II.2.6 Bone marrow with granuloma composed of macrophages, peripheral lymphocytes, and plasma cells. Necrosis and giant cells not present. HPS stain, ×250

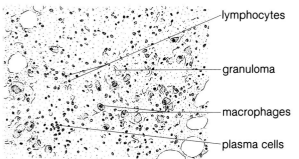

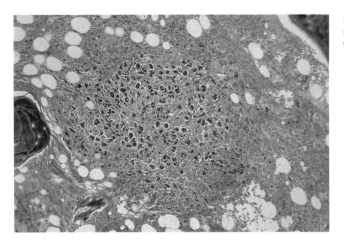

Fig. II.2.7 Same bone-marrow biopsy as in Fig. II.2.6. Silver staining reveals large amounts of bacilli, singly and in clusters, within the macrophages of granuloma. GMS stain, ×100

Hodgkin's Lymphoma in Bone Marrow

A 40-year-old homosexual man has Hodgkin's disease limited to the bone marrow at the time of presentation.

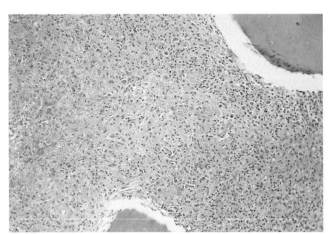

Fig. II.2.8 Mixed cellular infiltrate with lymphocytes, plasma cells, eosinophils, Hodgkin's cells, and a few Reed-Sternberg cells, entirely replaces the hematopoietic and adipose tissues of the bone marrow. HPS stain, ×100

Non-Hodgkin's Lymphoma in Bone Marrow

A 41-year-old homosexual man has non-Hodgkin's lymphoma of the lymphocytic, small-cleaved-cell type, involving lungs, lymph nodes, and bone marrow.

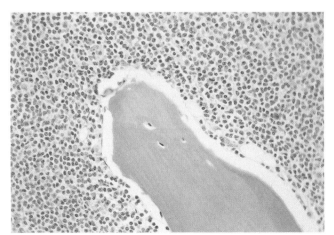

Fig. II.2.9. In the bone marrow, there is total replacement of hematopoietic and adipose tissues by a uniform population of lymphoid cells with small, angular, cleaved nuclei.
HPS stain, ×250

THYMUS

Thymic Dysplasia

A male infant manifests respiratory distress, disseminated CMV infection, and toxoplasmosis. The child's mother is an IV drug addict.

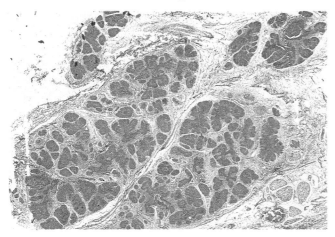

Fig. II.2.10 Thymic lobules with lack of corticomedullary differentiation and loss of Hassall's corpuscles. Microcysts in lobules.   H&E stain, ×10

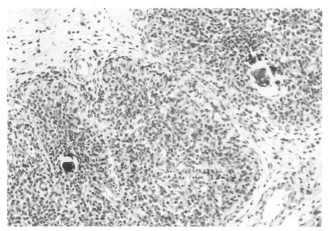

Fig. II.2.11 Thymic lobules with marked lymphocyte depletion and lack of corticomedullary differentiation. Two calcified Hassall's corpuscles.   ˜ H&E stain, ×100

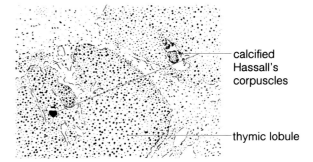

calcified Hassall's corpuscles

thymic lobule

LYMPH NODES

Persistent Generalized Lymphadenopathy

Acute lymphadenitis (type A pattern)
Cervical and axillary lymph nodes of three homosexual patients with HIV infection and lymphadenopathies.

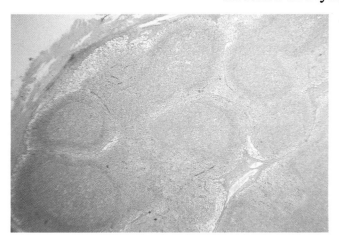

Fig. II.2.12 Axillary lymph node with enlarged coalescing lymphoid follicles containing hyperplastic germinal centers. Sinuses distended.   HPS stain, ×100

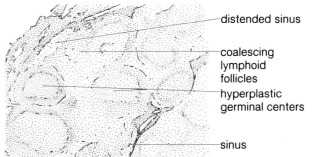

distended sinus

coalescing lymphoid follicles

hyperplastic germinal centers

sinus

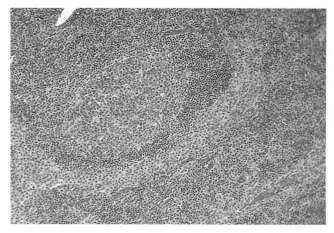

Fig. II.2.13 Cervical lymph node showing enlarged follicle with hyperplastic germinal center and focal invagination of small mantle lymphocytes. Perifollicular area of monocytoid clear cells.   HPS stain, ×100

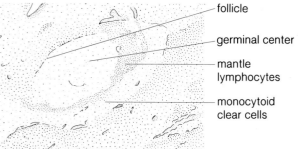

- follicle
- germinal center
- mantle lymphocytes
- monocytoid clear cells

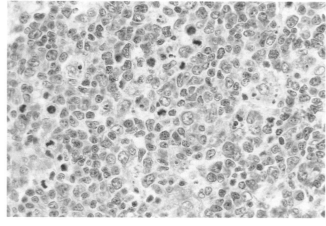

Fig. II.2.14 Same section as in Fig. II.2.13. Germinal center with tingible-body macrophages containing nuclear debris, activated lymphocytes, and frequent mitoses.
                                                   HPS stain, ×400

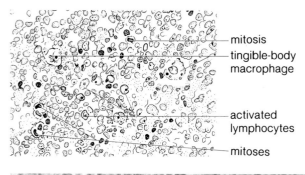

- mitosis
- tingible-body macrophage
- activated lymphocytes
- mitoses

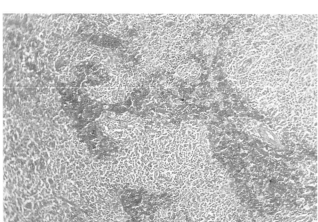

Fig. II.2.15 Axillary lymph node with areas of hemorrhage.
                                                   HPS stain, ×100

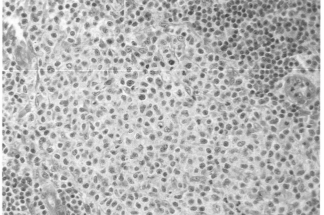

Fig. II.2.16 Cervical lymph node with large aggregate of monocytoid cells. In contrast to the small lymphocytes, these cells have sharp borders, abundant clear cytoplasm, and a central nucleus.   HPS stain, ×250

Fig. II.2.17 Same section as in Fig. II.2.16, showing aggregate of monocytoid cells with interspersed neutrophils around blood vessel. Area of small lymphocytes.
                                                   HPS stain, ×250

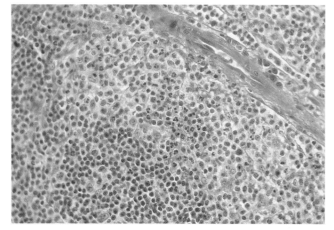

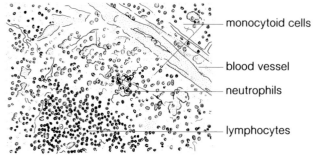

- monocytoid cells
- blood vessel
- neutrophils
- lymphocytes

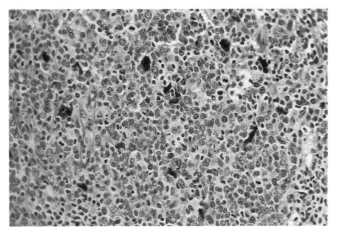

Fig. II.2.18 Axillary lymph node with activated lymphocytes, frequent mitoses, and multiple, randomly distributed multinucleated giant cells. H&E stain, ×250

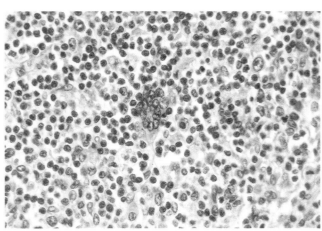

Fig. II.2.19 Multinucleated giant cell with grapelike cluster of nuclei (Warthin-Finkeldey type) in cervical lymph node.
HPS stain, ×400

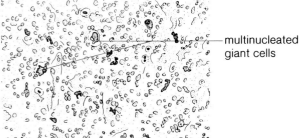

multinucleated giant cells

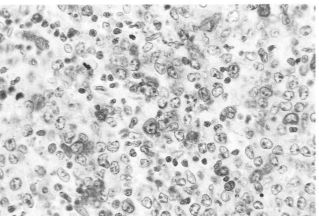

multinucleated giant cell

Fig. II.2.20 Positive staining for λ light-chain immunoglobulin in monocytoid cells, indicating their B-cell origin. (In parallel section, κ light chain-positive cells were also present.
Perox-antiperox stain, ×400

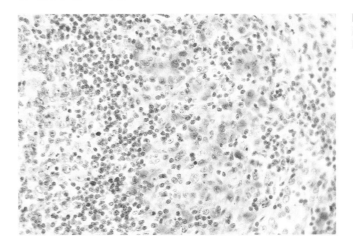

Fig. II.2.21 Langerhans cells stained with anti-S-100 antibody in cortex of axillary lymph node of patient with acute HIV lymphadenopathy. Follicle with hyperplastic germinal center.
Perox-antiperox stain, ×250

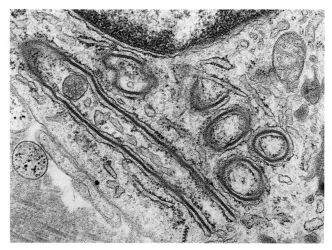

Fig. II.2.22 Test tube or ring-shaped forms in longitudinal or criss-cross section within cytoplasm of interdigitating cell of lymph node. (From Sidhu GS et al: The acquired immunodeficiency syndrome: An ultrastructural study. *Hum Pathol* 1985; 16:380.)   (×44,000)

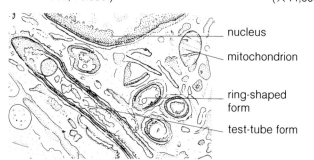

nucleus

mitochondrion

ring-shaped form

test-tube form

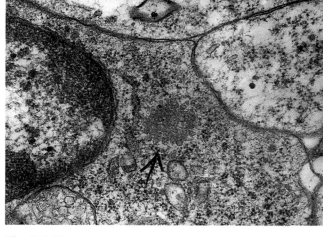

Fig. II.2.23 Vesicular body (rosette) (arrow) in cytoplasm of immunoblast. Cervical lymph node of a homosexual man with persistent generalized lymphadenopathy.   (×36,000)

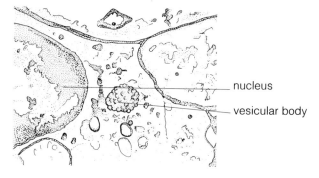

nucleus

vesicular body

HIV in Lymph Nodes

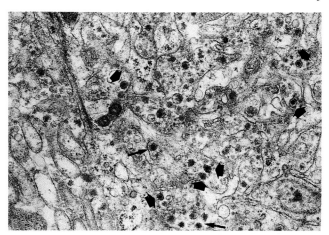

Fig. II.2.24 Numerous HIV particles situated between the altered cytoplasmic extensions of dendritic reticular cells (thick arrows) in affected lymph node. Round forms without defined structure (thin arrows). (From Le Tourneau A et al 1986   (× 32,000)

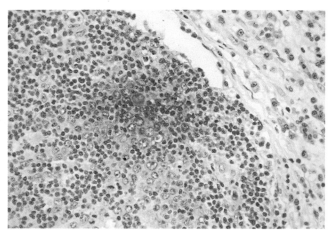

Fig. II.2.25 Focus of activated lymphocytes in lymph node cortex stained positively with anti-P$_{24}$, an HIV component.
                    Perox-antiperox stain, ×250

Subacute lymphadenitis (type B pattern)
Axillary lymph node in a 34-year-old homosexual man with HIV infection and lymphadenopathy.

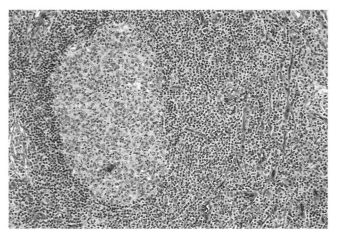

Fig. II.2.26 Persistent hyperplastic germinal center and perifollicular vascular hyperplasia.   HPS stain, ×100

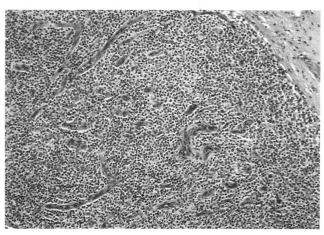

Fig. II.2.27 Effacement of lymphoid follicles and marked vascular proliferation without lymphocyte depletion.

HPS stain, ×100

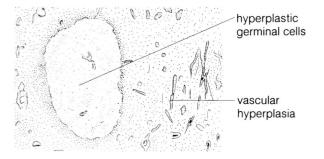

— hyperplastic germinal cells

— vascular hyperplasia

Chronic lymphadenitis (type C pattern)
A cervical lymph node in a 42-year-old homosexual man with HIV infection and lymphadenopathies.

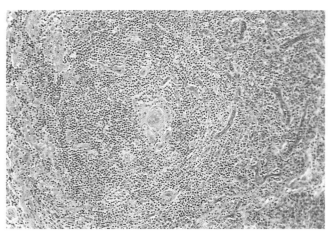

Fig. II.2.28 Atrophic, burnt-out follicle with central arteriole, perivascular hyalinization and marked vascular proliferation.
HPS stain, ×100

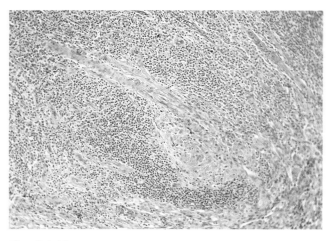

Fig. II.2.29 Atrophic follicle with germinal center replaced by penetrating arteriole (lollipop appearance). Morphology resembling that of Castleman's disease.   HPS stain, ×100

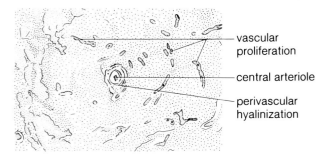

— vascular proliferation

— central arteriole

— perivascular hyalinization

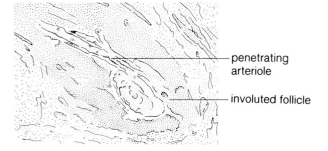

— penetrating arteriole

— involuted follicle

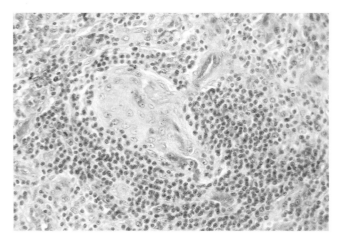

Fig. II.2.30 Burnt-out follicle showing penetrating arteriole, hyalinization, and narrow mantle of small lymphocytes.
HPS stain, ×250

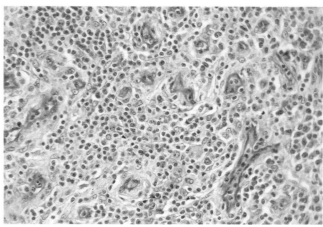

Fig. II.2.31 Extensive vascular proliferation, perivascular fibrosis, and lymphocyte depletion.
HPS stain, ×250

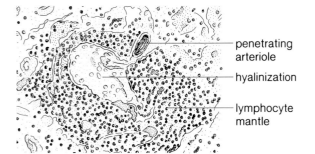

penetrating arteriole

hyalinization

lymphocyte mantle

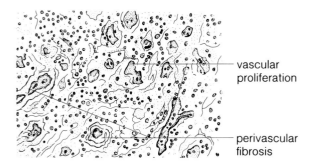

vascular proliferation

perivascular fibrosis

Mycobacteriosis of Lymph Nodes

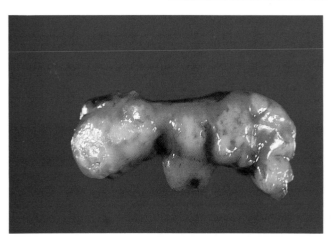

Fig. II.2.32 Cervical lymph node, enlarged and bulging after sectioning. Areas of discoloration and softening but not caseation.

A 34-year-old homosexual man with mycobacteriosis of cervical lymph node. The foamy histiocytes pattern characteristic of MAI lymphadenitis can be seen.

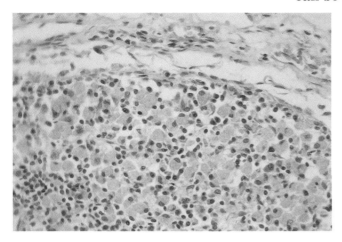

Fig. II.2.33 Capsule, distended marginal sinus, and cortex entirely occupied by large, foamy histiocytes with a few scattered residual lymphocytes.   HPS stain, ×250

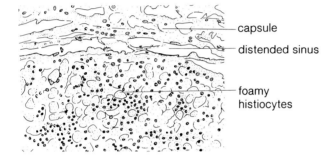

capsule

distended sinus

foamy histiocytes

Fig. II.2.34 Accumulation of histiocytes filled with acid-fast MAI bacilli, separated by uninvolved distended sinuses.   Kinyoun's stain, ×25

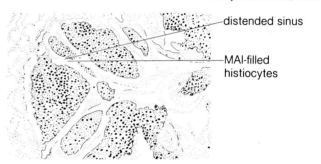

distended sinus

MAI-filled histiocytes

A 39-year-old homosexual man with mycobacteriosis of mediastinal lymph node. The spindle-shaped histiocytes (histoid) pattern found in MAI lymphadenitis is seen.

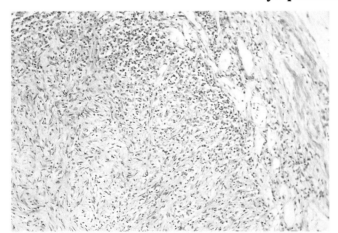

Fig. II.2.35 Mediastinal lymph node in which lymphoid tissue is totally replaced by proliferation of spindle cells forming whorls and bundles in a histoid pattern. Marginal sinus is obliterated; a few residual lymphocytes are seen below the capsule.   HPS stain, ×250

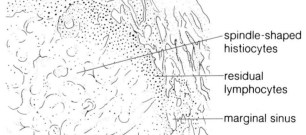

spindle-shaped histiocytes

residual lymphocytes

marginal sinus

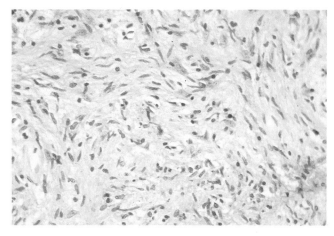

Fig. II.2.36 Histoid pattern in MAI lymphadenitis composed of histiocytes with abundant cytoplasm and spindle-shaped nuclei, along with a sprinkling of lymphocytes.

HPS stain, ×250

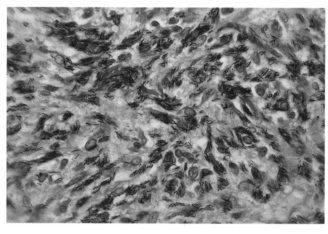

Fig. II.2.37 Acid-fast staining of Fig. II.2.36 shows cytoplasm of histiocytes filled with large amounts of MAI bacilli.

Kinyoun's stain, ×400

Cryptococcal Lymphadenitis

A 37-year-old homosexual man with enlarged cervical lymph node and no other manifestations of HIV infection.

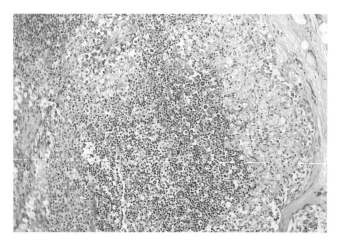

Fig. II.2.38 Lymph node architecture totally effaced. Broad area below the capsule replaced by sheets of foamy histiocytes. HPS stain, ×100

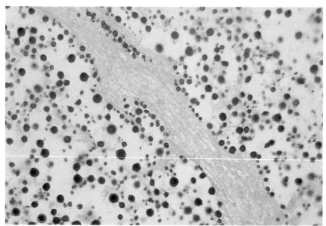

Fig. II.2.39 Section of same lymph node as in Fig. II.2.38, showing numerous silver-stained fungal organisms of varying size. GMS stain, ×250

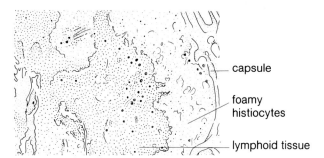

capsule

foamy histiocytes

lymphoid tissue

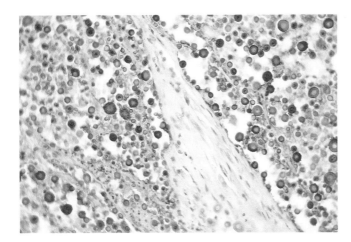

Fig. II.2.40 Section of same lymph node as in Fig. II.2.38, with large amounts of single or budding yeasts that vary in size and have intensely PAS-positive capsules.

PAS stain, ×250

Axillary lymphadenitis in 39-year-old homosexual man with disseminated cryptococcosis.

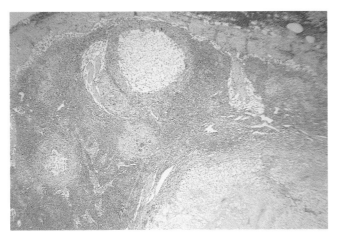

Fig. II.2.41 Enlarged axillary lymph node with subcapsular and medullary cystic formations. HPS stain, ×25

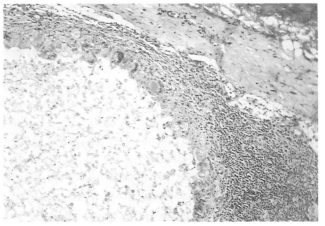

Fig. II.2.42 Same lymph node as in Fig. II.2.41, showing large cyst within nodal cortex, filled with fungi and tissue debris and lined by epithelioid and giant cells. HPS stain, ×100

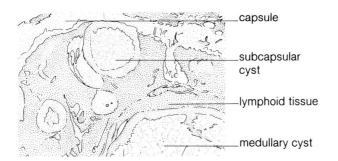

- capsule
- subcapsular cyst
- lymphoid tissue
- medullary cyst

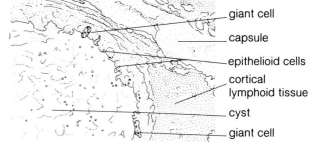

- giant cell
- capsule
- epithelioid cells
- cortical lymphoid tissue
- cyst
- giant cell

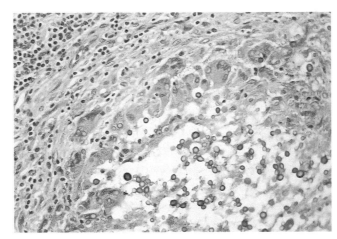

Fig. II.2.43 Cyst in lymph node cortex, lined by epithelioid and giant cells and containing numerous budding cryptococcal yeasts with unstained center and strongly stained mucicarmine-positive capsule. Mucicarmine stain, ×250

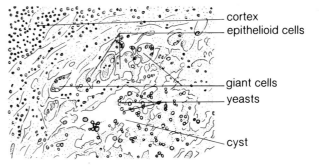

- cortex
- epithelioid cells
- giant cells
- yeasts
- cyst

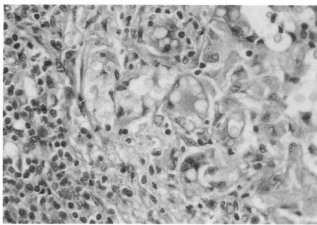

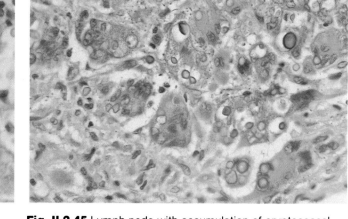

Fig. II.2.44 Cryptococcal cyst in lymph node cortex, containing numerous multinucleated giant cells with engulfed degenerated yeasts. HPS stain, ×250

Fig. II.2.45 Lymph node with accumulation of cryptococcal yeasts: some budding; some single, showing thick mucicarmine-positive capsule; and some degenerated, engulfed within multinucleated giant cells.

Mucicarmine stain, ×250

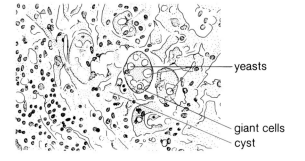

yeasts

giant cells

cyst

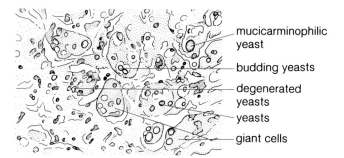

mucicarminophilic yeast

budding yeasts

degenerated yeasts

yeasts

giant cells

Coccidioidomycosis of Lymph Node

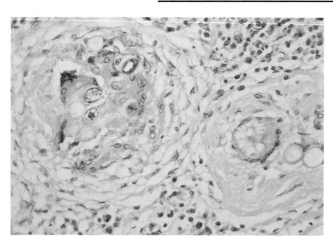

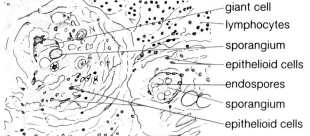

Fig. II.2.46 Mesenteric lymph node in 52-year-old homosexual man with systemic coccidioidomycosis. Partly degenerated, capsulated sporangia, some containing endospores, in the center of granulomas composed of multinucleated giant cells, epithelioid cells, and lymphocytes. HPS stain, ×250

giant cell

lymphocytes

sporangium

epithelioid cells

endospores

sporangium

epithelioid cells

Toxoplasmosis of Lymph Node

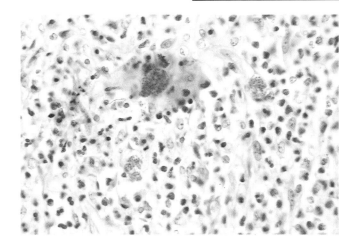

Fig. II.2.47 Cervical lymphadenitis in 41-year-old homosexual man with toxoplasmosis. *Toxoplasma gondii* cyst containing tachyzoites surrounded by multinucleated giant cell and epithelioid cells, singly and in small clusters, in lymph node cortex.   HPS stain, ×400

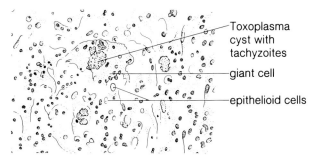

Toxoplasma cyst with tachyzoites

giant cell

epithelioid cells

Kaposi's Sarcoma of Lymph Nodes

A 29-year-old homosexual male has multiple enlarged peripheral lymph nodes. Two axillary lymph nodes are biopsied. One shows the features of acute-phase HIV lymphadenopathy, and the other is almost entirely replaced by Kaposi's sarcoma.

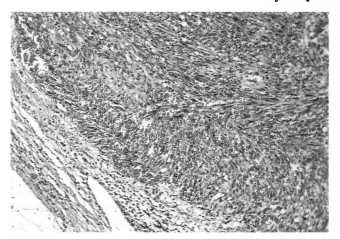

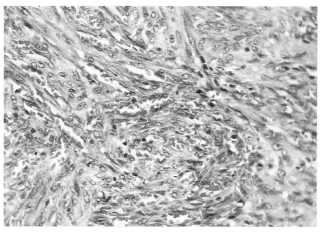

Fig. II.2.48 Lymph node cortex replaced by sheets of capillary vessels and neoplastic endothelial cells. Abundant erythrocytes extravasated and within lumina of newly formed vessels.   Masson stain, ×100

Fig. II.2.49 Spindle-shaped Kaposi's sarcoma cells aggregated in criss-cross bundles and forming erythrocyte-containing vascular clefts.   Masson stain, ×250

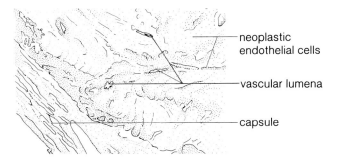

neoplastic endothelial cells

vascular lumena

capsule

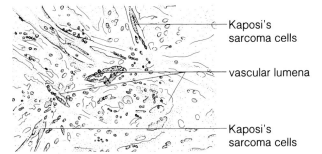

Kaposi's sarcoma cells

vascular lumena

Kaposi's sarcoma cells

A 42-year-old homosexual man has disseminated Kaposi's sarcoma.

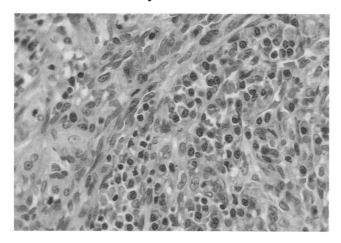

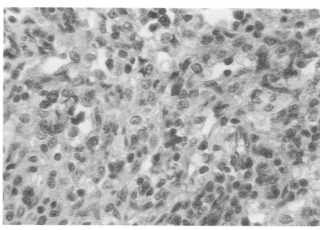

Fig. II.2.50 Peritoneal lymph node with bundles of elongated cells containing spindle-shaped nuclei that form rudimentary vascular lumina. Abundant accumulations of plasma cells and lymphocytes. HPS stain, ×400

Fig. II.2.51 Abdominal lymph node with proliferation of spindle-shaped Kaposi's sarcoma cells lining vascular clefts which stain with factor VIII antibody. Reactive plasma cells and lymphocytes. Perox-antiperox anti–factor VIII stain, ×400

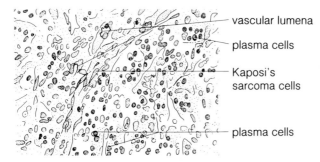

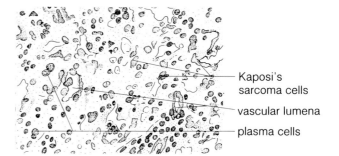

Hodgkin's Lymphoma of Cervical Lymph Node

A 52-year-old homosexual man with positive HIV-antibody test, developed Hodgkin's disease.

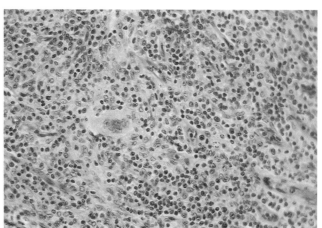

Fig. II.2.52 Cervical lymph node shows Hodgkin's lymphoma (mixed cellularity type) with Reed-Sternberg cell, plasma cells, and marked vascular proliferation of HIV-lymphoadenopathy, chronic phase. HPS stain, ×250

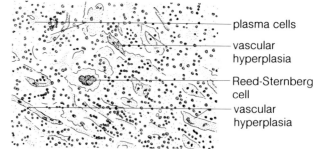

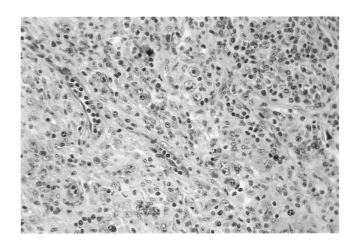

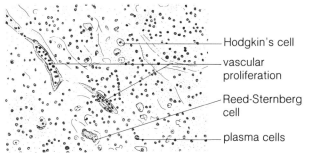

Fig. II.2.53 Same lymph node as in Fig. II.2.52, showing Hodgkin's cells, Reed-Sternberg cells, plasma cells, and marked vascular proliferation of HIV-lymphoadenopathy, chronic phase. HPS stain, ×250

- Hodgkin's cell
- vascular proliferation
- Reed-Sternberg cell
- plasma cells

Non-Hodgkin's Lymphoma of Cervical Lymph Node

An enlarged cervical lymph node in a 38-year-old homosexual man shows coexistent lesions of HIV-related lymphadenopathy and non-Hodgkin's lymphoma.

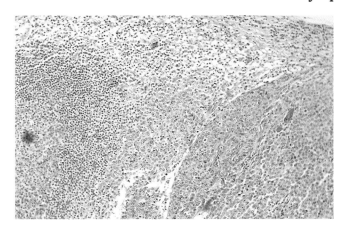

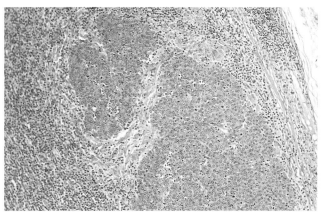

Fig. II.2.54 Enlarged follicle with hyperplastic germinal center next to nodular area of non-Hodgkin's lymphoma in lymph node cortex. HPS stain, ×100

Fig. II.2.55 Confluent nodules of non-Hodgkin's lymphoma (Burkitt's cell type) in lymph node cortex. HPS stain, ×100

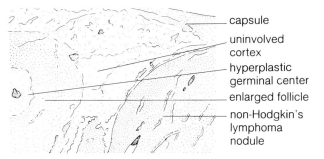

- capsule
- uninvolved cortex
- hyperplastic germinal center
- enlarged follicle
- non-Hodgkin's lymphoma nodule

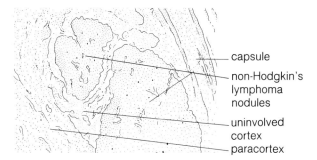

- capsule
- non-Hodgkin's lymphoma nodules
- uninvolved cortex
- paracortex

SPLEEN

Spleen in Idiopathic Thrombocytopenia

A 20-year-old homosexual man who recently traveled to Haiti presents because of repeated bleeding episodes. The platelet count is 8,000 per μL and the spleen weighs 220g.

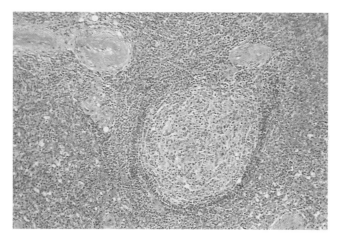

Fig. II.2.56 Lymphoid follicle, moderately enlarged, with layered peripheral area of small lymphocytes. Trizonal follicles are not present. Thick-walled arterioles are noted.

HPS stain, ×200

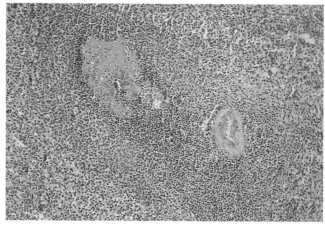

Fig. II.2.57 Ill-defined, irregularly shaped perivascular follicle composed exclusively of small lymphocytes. Deposits of extravascular PAS-positive amorphous material.

PAS stain, ×200

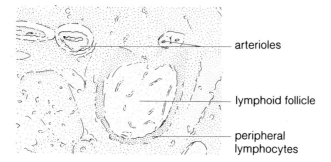

arterioles

lymphoid follicle

peripheral lymphocytes

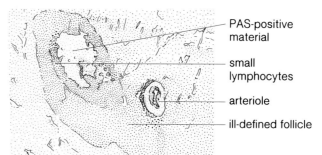

PAS-positive material

small lymphocytes

arteriole

ill-defined follicle

Fig. II.2.58 Markedly thickened, fibrosed arteriole with perivascular follicle composed exclusively of small lymphocytes.

HPS stain, × 400

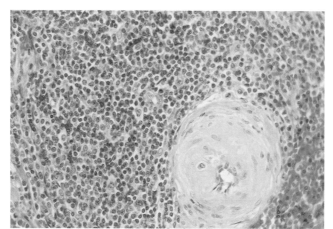

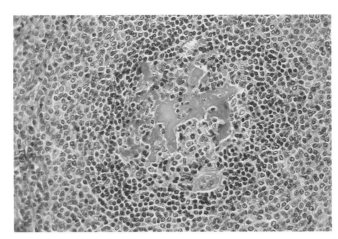

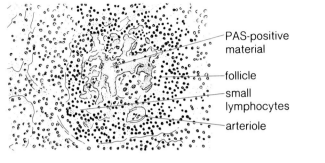

Fig. II.2.59 Deposits of amorphous, PAS-positive material in periarteriolar follicle composed of small lymphocytes.
PAS stain, ×400

- PAS-positive material
- follicle
- small lymphocytes
- arteriole

Tuberculosis of Spleen

A 44-year-old drug abuser developed miliary tuberculosis.

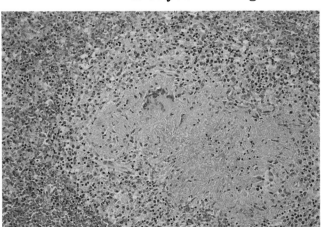

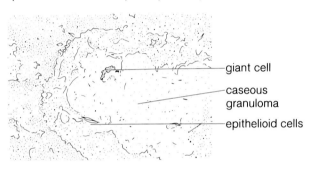

Fig. II.2.60 Caseating granuloma with giant cells and epithelioid cells within splenic parenchyma.   HPS stain, ×200

- giant cell
- caseous granuloma
- epithelioid cells

Mycobacteriosis of Spleen

A 46-year-old man with previously diagnosed mycobacteriosis has a massively enlarged spleen (620g) with a distinct follicular pattern on gross examination.

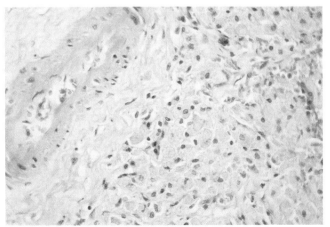

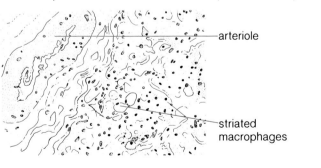

Fig. II.2.61 Accumulation of foamy, striated macrophages around splenic arteriole.   HPS stain, ×250

- arteriole
- striated macrophages

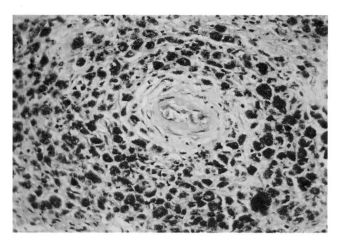

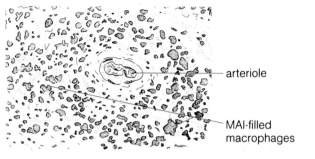

Fig. II.2.62 Huge amounts of acid-fast bacilli (MAI) fill and distend the macrophages that have accumulated exclusively around the splenic arterioles.   Kinyoun's stain, ×250

arteriole

MAI-filled macrophages

Coccidioidomycosis of Spleen

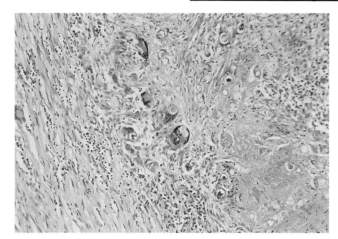

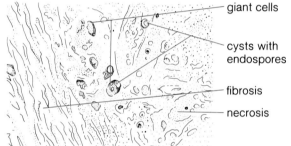

Fig. II.2.63 Granuloma with necrosis, fibrosis, and cysts containing endospores engulfed by giant cells within splenic parenchyma.   HPS stain, ×100

giant cells

cysts with endospores

fibrosis

necrosis

Cardiovascular System

three

CARDIOMYOPATHY

A 48-year-old homosexual man with *Pneumocystis* carinii pneumonia has an enlarged heart at autopsy.

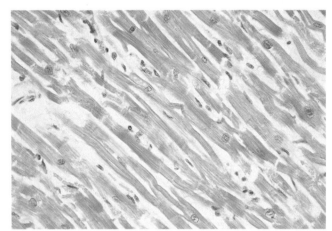

Fig. II.3.1 Myocardium shows numerous foci of myocytic necrosis and chronic inflammation.   HPS stain, ×200

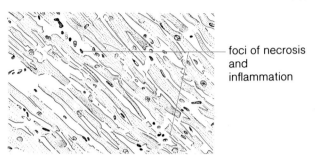

foci of necrosis and inflammation

A 29-year-old homosexual man exhibits acute congestive cardiac failure of no apparent cause. At autopsy, pleural and pericardial effusions and four-chamber cardiac dilatation are noted.

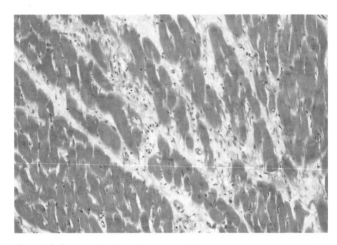

Fig. II.3.2 Multiple foci of myocardial necrosis, inflammation, and fibrosis.   HPS stain, ×200

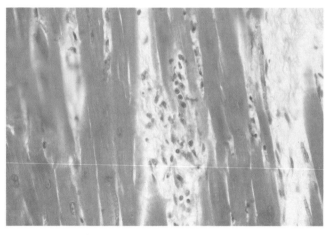

Fig. II.3.3. Same section as in Fig. II.3.2. Necrosis of myocardial fibers with accumulation of lymphocytes and histiocytes.   HPS stain, ×400

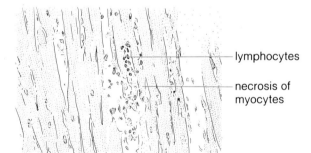

lymphocytes

necrosis of myocytes

LYMPHOMA OF THE HEART

Non-Hodgkin's lymphoma, (large-cell immunoblastic type) in a 42-year-old man involves multiple organs, including the heart, which has tumor nodules in the epicardium of the atria, around the coronary arteries, and deep into the myocardium.

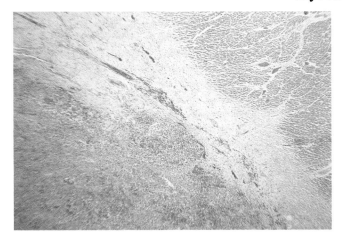

Fig. II.3.4 Mass of lymphoma cells in the epicardium, still separated from myocardium by band of fibrous tissue.

HPS stain, ×25

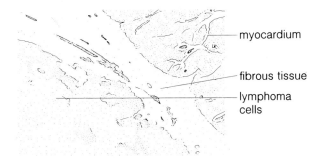

— myocardium

— fibrous tissue

— lymphoma cells

Fig. II.3.5 Lymphoma cells of plasmacytoid type infiltrating the myocardium. Lymphoma cells present within the cytoplasm of invaded myocardial fibers. Inflammatory reaction with lymphocytes accumulating around degenerated myocardial fibers.

HPS stain, ×400

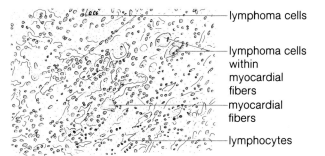

— lymphoma cells

— lymphoma cells within myocardial fibers

— myocardial fibers

— lymphocytes

Non-Hodgkin's lymphoma (large-cell pleomorphic type) of the intestine in a 52-year-old man also involves the right atrium and right ventricle.

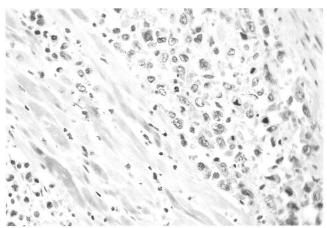

Fig. II.3.6 Lymphoma cells with large, irregularly shaped nuclei and frequent mitoses invade and largely replace the myocardium.

HPS stain, ×100

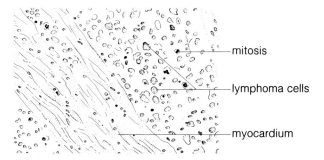

— mitosis

— lymphoma cells

— myocardium

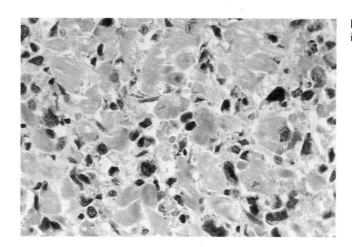

Fig. II.3.7 Myocardial fibers, frequently degenerated, infiltrated by lymphoma cells with bizarre, pleomorphic nuclei. HPS stain, ×400

Respiratory Tract

chapter
four

LYMPHOCYTIC INTERSTITIAL PNEUMONITIS

A 46-year-old homosexual man has fever and tests positive for HIV-antibody.

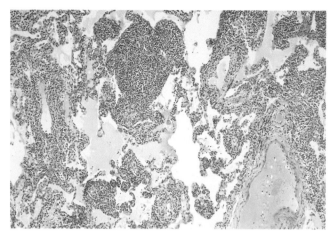

Fig. II.4.1 Cellular infiltrates accumulating around blood vessels, extending along interalveolar septae and forming nodules.
HPS stain, ×100

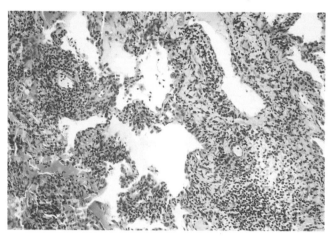

Fig. II.4.2 Monocellular infiltrates around blood vessel and interalveolar septae. Alveolar spaces uninvolved.
HPS stain, ×200

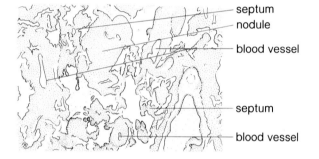

septum
nodule

blood vessel

septum

blood vessel

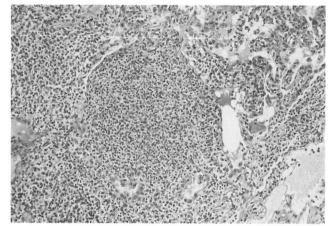

Fig. II.4.3 Interstitial nodule composed primarily of lymphocytes, with occasional macrophages and plasma cells. Compressed alveoli lined by metaplastic alveolar cells.
HPS stain, ×200

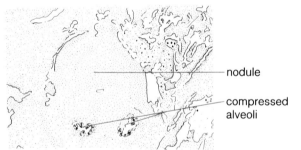

nodule

compressed alveoli

LYMPHOCYTIC INTERSTITIAL PNEUMONITIS IN CHILDREN

Persistent bilateral interstitial pneumonitis with reticulonodular infiltrates developed in a seven-year-old girl. She, her five-month-old brother, and both drug-addicted parents test positive for HIV-antibody.

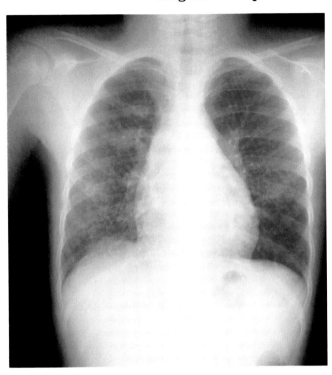

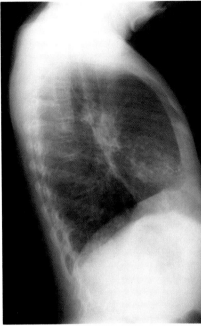

Fig. II.4.5 Same case as in Fig. II.4.4. Lateral view showing interstitial infiltrate with characteristic reticulonodular pattern.

Fig. II.4.4 Bilateral diffuse interstitial nodular infiltrates consistent with LIP. Widened mediastinum indicative of lymphadenopathy.

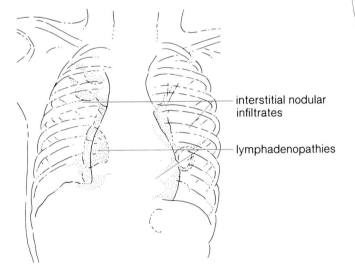

interstitial nodular infiltrates

lymphadenopathies

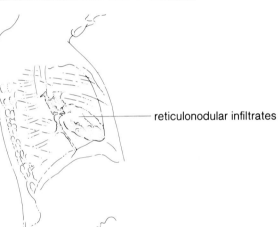

reticulonodular infiltrates

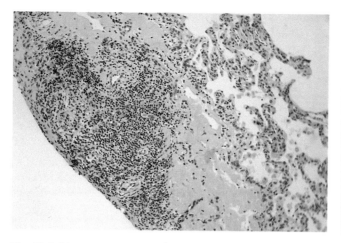

Fig. II.4.6 Lung biopsy with subpleural nodular lymphocytic infiltrate. Alveoli are uninvolved.   HPS stain, ×100

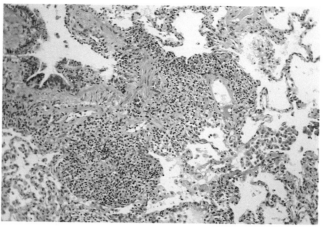

Fig. II.4.7 Interstitial reticulonodular lymphocytic infiltrates. Alveoli and bronchi uninvolved.   HPS stain, ×100

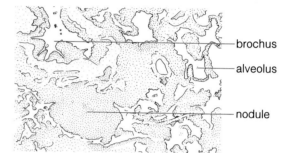

brochus

alveolus

nodule

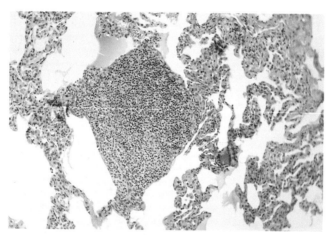

Fig. II.4.8 Sharply demarcated lymphocytic nodule in interalveolar septum. Alveoli and other septae uninvolved.
HPS stain, ×100

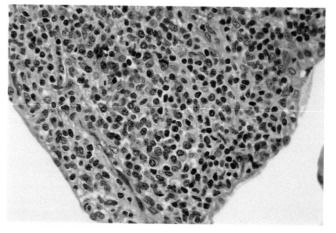

Fig. II.4.9 Cellular nodule composed of lymphocytes and plasma cells within interalveolar septum.

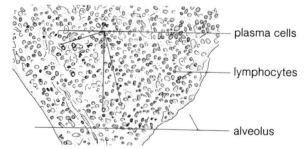

plasma cells

lymphocytes

alveolus

CYTOMEGALOVIRUS PNEUMONITIS

Focal areas of pneumonia are apparent in the lungs of a 36-year-old man who died with disseminated CMV infection.

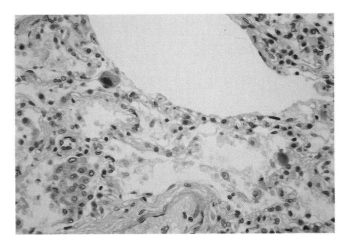

Fig. II.4.10 Alveoli with exudate and desquamated pneumocytes. Lymphocytes and plasma cells in interalveolar septae. Intranuclear and intracytoplasmic CMV inclusions.
HPS stain, ×400

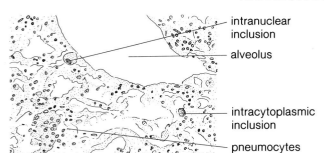

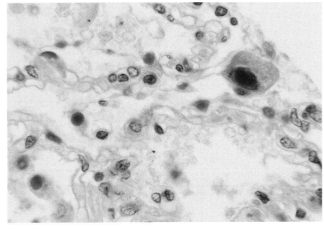

Fig. II.4.11 Macrophage with intranuclear CMV inclusion totally obscuring the nucleus. HPS stain, ×1,000

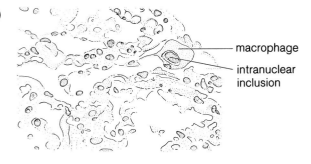

LEGIONELLA PNEUMOPHILIA PNEUMONITIS

Poorly defined, patchy bilateral infiltrates can be seen in the lungs of a 48-year-old homosexual man.

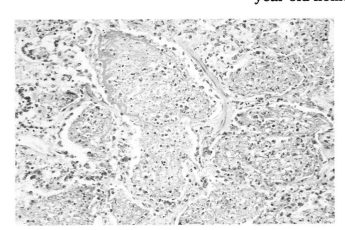

Fig. II.4.12 Alveoli filled with fibrinous exudate containing leukocytes and cellular debris. HPS stain, ×100

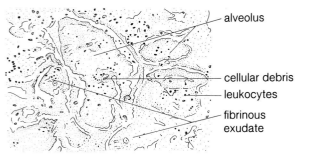

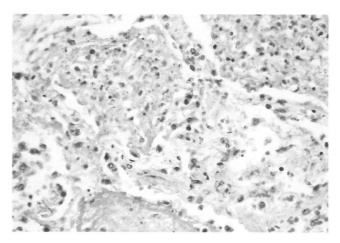

Fig. II.4.13 Alveoli with fibrinous exudate and areas of necrosis, containing macrophages, polymorphonuclear leukocytes, and nuclear debris (leukocytoclasis).
HPS stain, ×400

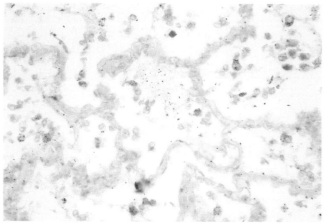

Fig. II.4.14 Short, fine, black-stained bacilli within intra-alveolar fibrinous exudate.   Dieterle silver stain, ×400

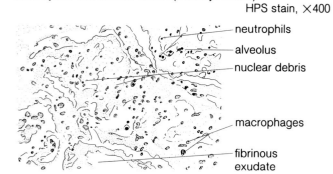

- neutrophils
- alveolus
- nuclear debris
- macrophages
- fibrinous exudate

PULMONARY MYCOBACTERIOSIS

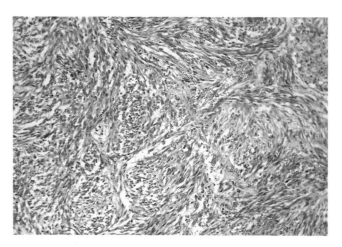

Fig.II.4.15 Pulmonary mycobacteriosis, histoid type. Alveoli are filled with spindle-shaped macrophages arranged in bundles that special staining shows to contain numerous acid-fast bacilli.   HPS stain, ×100

PULMONARY CANDIDIASIS

Autopsy of a 34-year-old homosexual man with AIDS reveals massive pulmonary involvement in disseminated candidiasis.

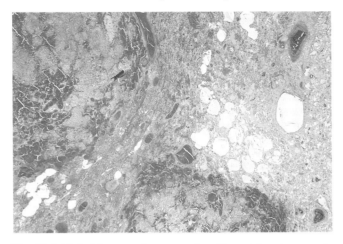

Fig. II.4.16 Solid areas of pneumonia with peripheral areas of hemorrhage and areas of uninvolved alveolar tissues.

HPS stain, ×25

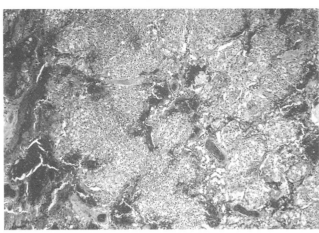

Fig. II.4.17 Alveoli filled with exudate, still separated by septae in some areas but becoming confluent in others. Areas of abundant hemorrhage.

HPS stain, ×100

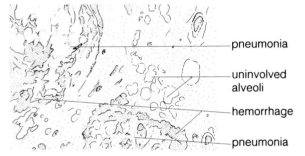

pneumonia

uninvolved alveoli

hemorrhage

pneumonia

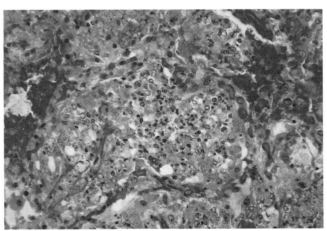

Fig. II.4.18 Alveolus surrounded by hemorrhage and filled with exudate, desquamated alveolar cells, neutrophils, and large amounts of yeasts.

HPS stain, ×400

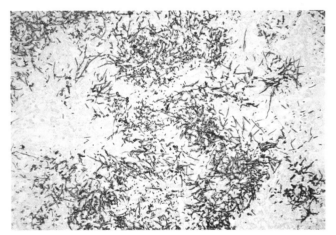

Fig. II.4.19 Abundant mats of pseudohyphae and yeasts (blastospores) within alveolar spaces.

GMS stain, ×100

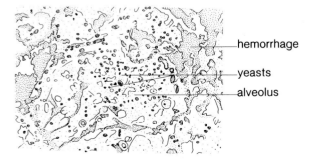

hemorrhage

yeasts

alveolus

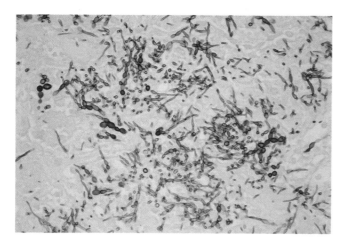

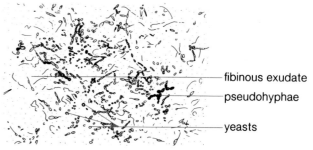

Fig. II.4.20 *Candida albicans* yeasts (blastospores) and pseudohyphae that are formed by juxtaposition of yeasts with points of narrowing without branchings.   GMS stain, ×400

— fibinous exudate

— pseudohyphae

— yeasts

PULMONARY ASPERGILLOSIS

A 43-year-old bisexual man with disseminated Kaposi's sarcoma presents with a large area of consolidation in the right lower lobe of the lung.

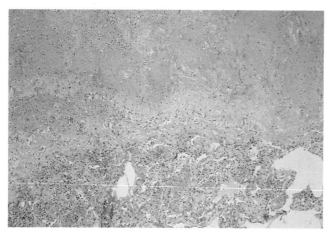

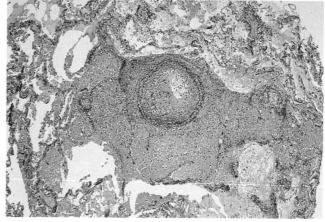

Fig. II.4.21 Large infarcted area with ischemic necrosis of lung tissues. Some alveoli show inflammatory exudate; others are patent.   HPS stain, ×100

Fig. II.4.22 Thrombosed pulmonary arteriole surrounded by infarcted necrotic tissues. No apparent inflammatory reaction in the outside alveoli.   EVG stain, ×100

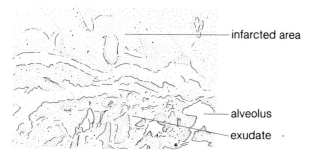

— infarcted area

— alveolus

— exudate

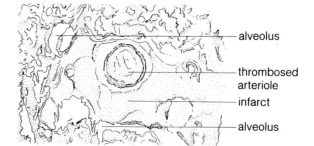

— alveolus

— thrombosed arteriole

— infarct

— alveolus

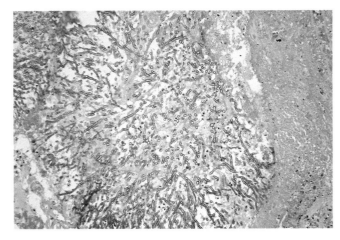

Fig. II.4.23 Large fungal colony composed of branching hyphae surrounded by necrotic, noninflamed pulmonary tissues. HPS stain, ×250

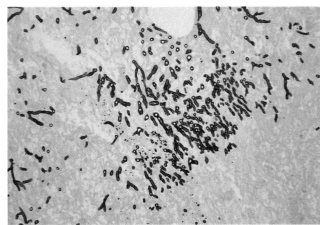

Fig. II.4.24 Characteristic hyphae of *Aspergillus:* uniform in size, with dichotomic branchings advancing in the same direction. Necrotic lung tissue. GMS stain, ×400

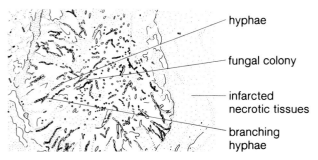

hyphae

fungal colony

infarcted necrotic tissues

branching hyphae

Fig. II.4.25 Colony of *Aspergillus* in the lung of AIDS patient. Characteristic regularly septated hyphae with dichotomic branchings at about 45° advancing in the same direction. HPS stain, ×400

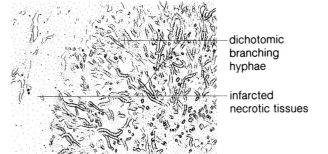

dichotomic branching hyphae

infarcted necrotic tissues

PULMONARY CRYPTOCOCCOSIS

A 48-year-old male drug addict has pulmonary cryptococcosis.

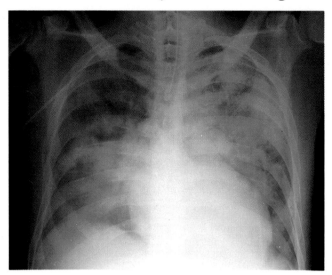

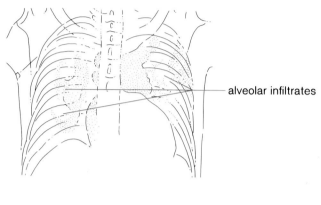

Fig. II.4.26 Multiple bilateral diffuse, confluent alveolar infiltrates have developed rapidly. No significant pleural effusions are apparent.

alveolar infiltrates

Transbronchial biopsy in 36-year-old homosexual man with nodular infiltrates in the right lung. This 0.2 × 0.3 cm fragment of tissue was obtained, from which imprints and sections were prepared.

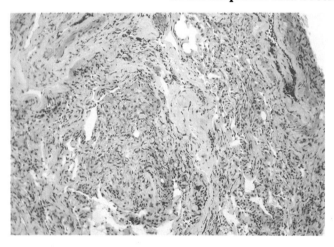

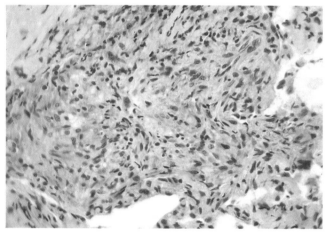

Fɪɢ. II.4.27 Confluent granulomas in interstitial pulmonary tissue, partially occluding alveolar spaces. HPS stain, ×100

Fig. II.4.28 Ill-formed, nonnecrotizing granulomas in peribronchial tissue and interalveolar septae. HPS stain, ×250

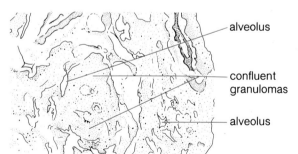

alveolus

confluent granulomas

alveolus

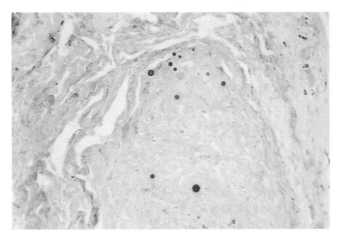

Fig. II.4.29 Confluent mass of granulomas obliterating alveoli, with scattered cryptococcal yeasts of variable size.

GMS stain, ×250

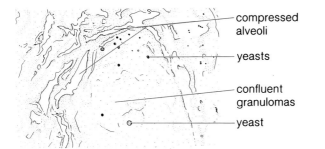

compressed alveoli

yeasts

confluent granulomas

yeast

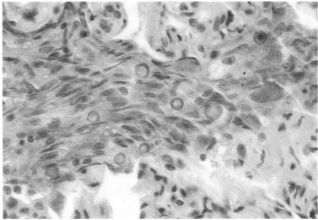

Fig. II.4.30 Thickened interalveolar septum with proliferation of epithelioid cells and fibroblasts. Numerous cryptococcal yeasts, characterized by variable size, unstained center, and strongly staining mucicarminophilic capsule.

Mucicarmine stain, ×400

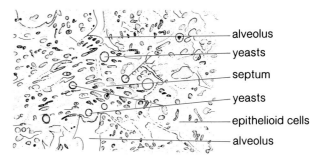

alveolus

yeasts

septum

yeasts

epithelioid cells

alveolus

A 53-year-old homosexual man has pulmonary cryptococcosis.

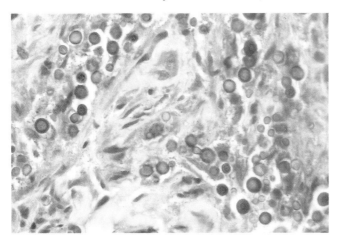

Fig. II.4.31 Numerous round, single and budding, strongly mucicarminophilic yeasts with clear capsules in alveolus and interalveolar septae. Mucicarmine stain, ×100

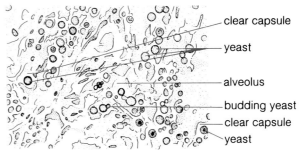

clear capsule

yeast

alveolus

budding yeast

clear capsule

yeast

PULMONARY HISTOPLASMOSIS

Transbronchial biopsy in a 31-year-old homosexual man with fever and bilateral small pulmonary infiltrates.

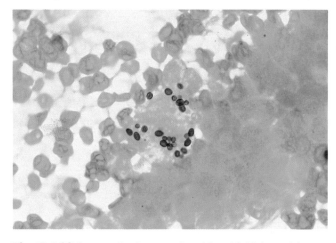

Fig. II.4.32 Smear of pulmonary brushing. Multiple ovoid yeasts with frequent narrow-based budding forms.
GMS stain, ×1,000

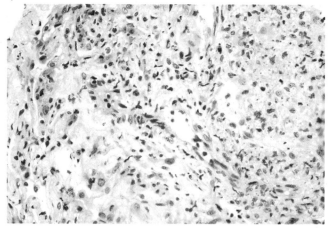

Fig. II.4.33 Pulmonary infiltrate with numerous lymphocytes and macrophages, some with intracellular fine, small organisms that are palely stained.
HPS stain, ×400

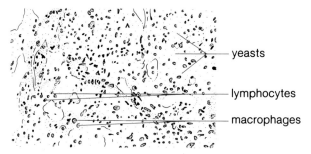

yeasts

lymphocytes

macrophages

Fig. II.4.34 Section of same tissue as in Fig. II.4.33, showing yeasts, including budding forms, either free or within lung macrophages.
GMS stain, ×1,000

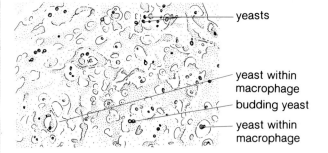

yeasts

yeast within macrophage

budding yeast

yeast within macrophage

PULMONARY COCCIDIOIDOMYCOSIS

A 52-year-old homosexual man has systemic coccidioidomycosis.

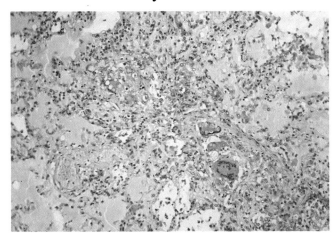

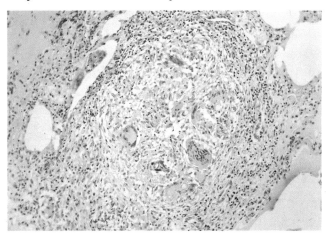

Fig. II.4.35 Area of pulmonary infiltrate showing ill-defined granulomas in interalveolar septae, with epithelioid cells, lymphocytes, and giant cells. Numerous endospores are present within giant cells and scattered throughout the tissues.   HPS stain, ×100

Fig. II.4.36 Sporangia with thick double capsules and degenerated endospores. Endospores released in tissues and phagocytosed by giant cells.   HPS stain, ×250

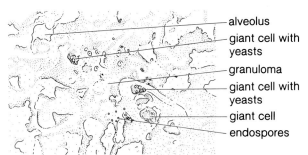

alveolus
giant cell with yeasts
granuloma
giant cell with yeasts
giant cell
endospores

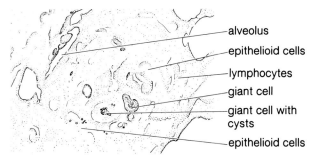

alveolus
epithelioid cells
lymphocytes
giant cell
giant cell with cysts
epithelioid cells

Fig. II.4.37 Sporangium of *Coccidioidomycosis immitis* with thick double capsule and degenerated endospores. Numerous spores released in the tissues.   HPS stain, ×400

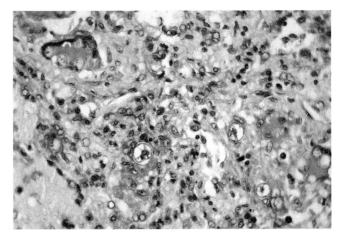

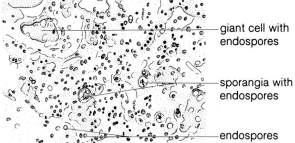

giant cell with endospores

sporangia with endospores

endospores

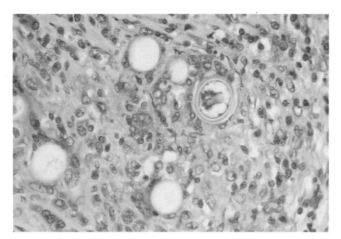

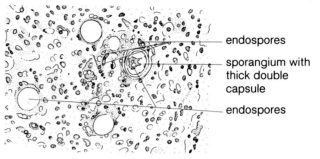

Fig. II.4.38 Lung granuloma composed of multinucleated giant cells, with engulfed cysts, epithelioid cells, and lymphocytes. Compressed alveoli.   HPS stain, ×1000

— endospores

— sporangium with thick double capsule

— endospores

PULMONARY BLASTOMYCOSIS

Blastomycosis is diagnosed in a 48-year-old male IV drug addict from Tennessee who has bilateral pulmonary infiltrates.

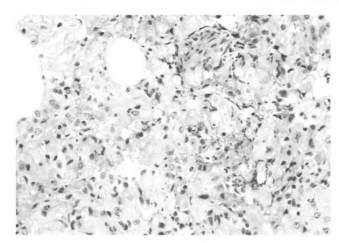

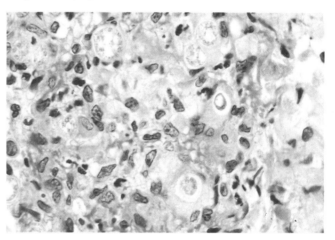

Fig. II.4.39 Coalescing granulomas, composed of macrophages and lymphocytes, accumulated around numerous *Blastomyces* organisms.   HPS stain, ×400

Fig. II.4.40 Same section as in Fig. II.4.39. Pulmonary granuloma with large, multinucleated *Blastomyces* cells. Some are degenerating, either surrounded by or within macrophages and lymphocytes.   HPS stain, ×1,000

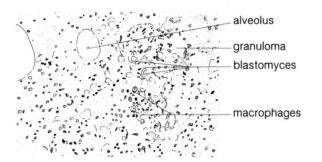

— alveolus

— granuloma

— blastomyces

— macrophages

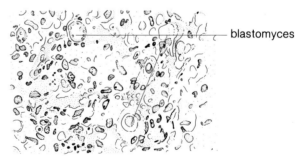

— blastomyces

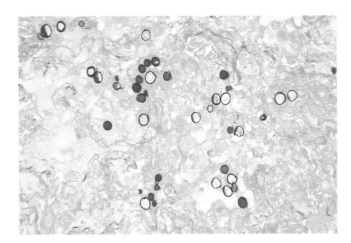

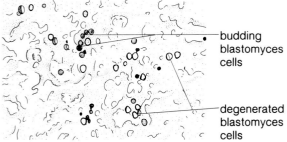

Fig. II.4.41 Same section as in Fig. II.4.39. Numerous large, thick-walled *Blastomyces* cells, some degenerated, single or budding from broad base.   GMS stain, ×400

budding blastomyces cells

degenerated blastomyces cells

PULMONARY MUCORMYCOSIS

A 49-year-old man, a long-term heroin addict, died with multiple bilateral pulmonary infarcts and areas of consolidation.

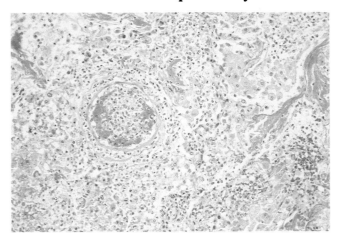

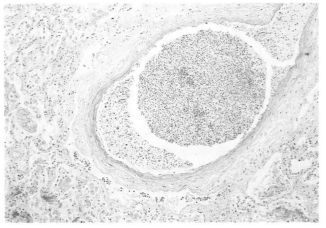

Fig. II.4.42 Pulmonary arteriole occluded by thrombus made up of fibrin and leukocytes. Surrounding tissues are infarcted, with loss of alveolar architecture and infiltration of leukocytes.   HPS stain, ×100

Fig. II.4.43 Pulmonary arteriole obstructed by thrombus of fibrin, fungi, and granulocytes. Surrounding alveoli filled with fibrin, granulocytes, and macrophages.   HPS stain, ×100

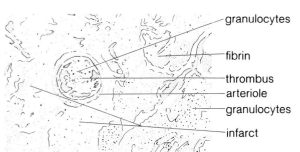

granulocytes

fibrin

thrombus

arteriole

granulocytes

infarct

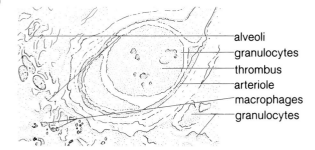

alveoli

granulocytes

thrombus

arteriole

macrophages

granulocytes

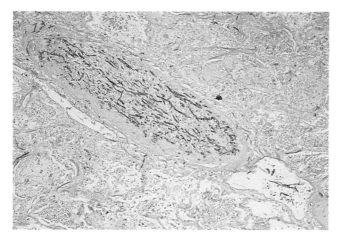

Fig. II.4.44 Pulmonary arteriole completely occluded by thrombus of fibrin and fungi. Surrounding parenchyma is infarcted.   GMS stain, ×100

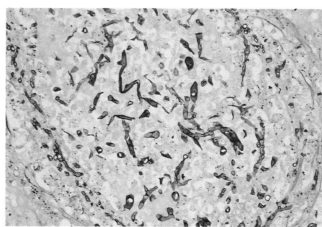

Fig. II.4.45 Same section as in Fig. II.4.44. Intravascular thrombus shows the broad hyphae of *Mucor* with right-angle branchings. Cross-sections of hyphae resemble yeasts.
                                        GMS stain, ×400

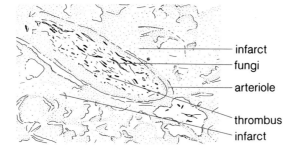

infarct
fungi
arteriole
thrombus
infarct

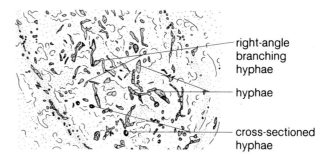

right-angle
branching
hyphae
hyphae
cross-sectioned
hyphae

PNEUMOCYSTIS CARINII PNEUMONIA

A 50-year-old man with multiple cutaneous and mucosal lesions of Kaposi's sarcoma also has *Pneumocystis carinii* pneumonia.

Fig. II.4.46 Extensive bilateral alveolar fluffy infiltrates

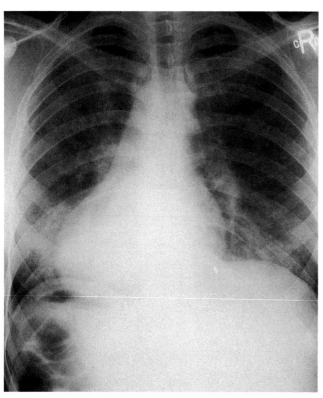

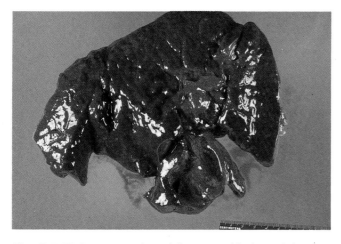

Fig. II.4.47 *Pneumocystis carinii* pneumonitis. Lung is heavy, expanded, and congested.

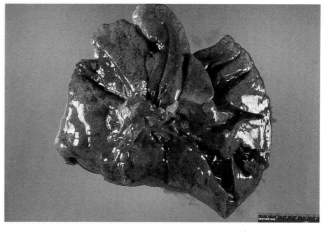

Fig. II.4.48 *Pneumocystis carinii* pneumonitis. Section shows uniform consolidation with loss of alveolar patterns.

Pneumocystis carinii pneumonia in a 34-year-old homosexual man with dry cough, increasing dyspnea, and bilateral reticulonodular infiltrates.

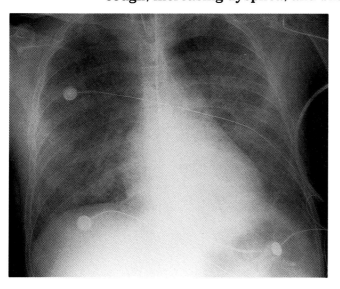

Fig. II.4.49 Bilateral reticulonodular alveolar infiltrates, progressing rapidly in two weeks.

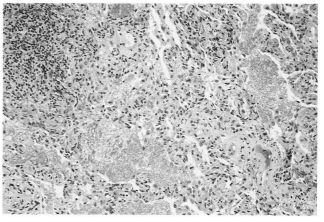

Fig. II.4.50 Consolidation of pulmonary parenchyma with abundant intraalveolar exudate and accumulations of lymphocytes, both diffusely and in nodules.   HPS stain, ×200

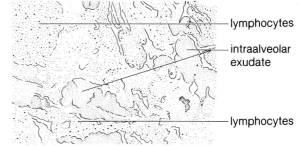

Fig. II.4.51 Alveolus with abundant foamy, fibrinous, acellular exudate. Moderate interstitial infiltrates of lymphocytes and macrophages.   HPS stain, ×400

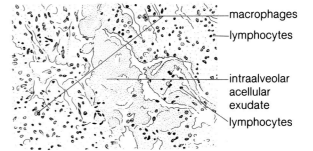

Respiratory Tract **159**

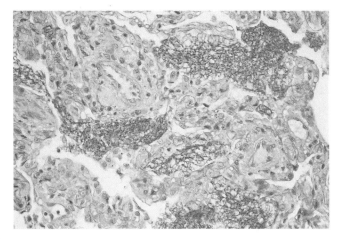

Fig. II.4.52 Characteristic foamy, fibrinous, PAS-positive, poorly cellular exudate filling the alveoli. Thickened interalveolar septae, and lining alveolar cells with cuboidal metaplasia. PAS stain, ×400

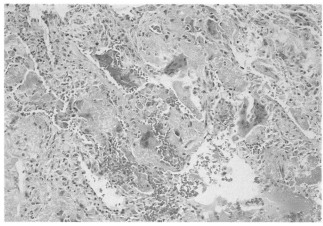

Fig. II.4.53 Foamy exudate and trophozoites in alveoli, with numerous multinucleated giant cells in active phagocytosis. HPS stain, ×200

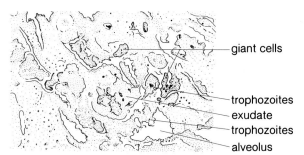

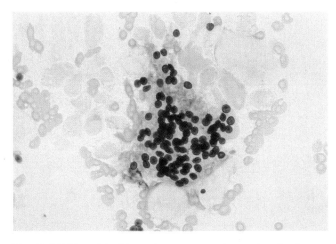

Fig. II.4.54 Imprint of bronchoscopy specimen showing large cluster of characteristic ovoid, nonhomogeneous *Pneumocystis* trophozoites. GMS stain, ×400

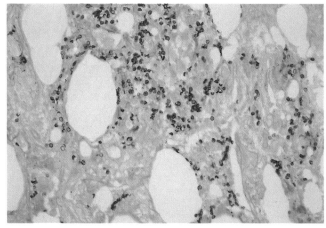

Fig. II.4.55 Section of bronchoscopy specimen showing numerous ovoid and crescent-shaped *Pneumocystis* trophozoites within the alveolar foamy exudate and the interalveolar septae. Some are degenerating. GMS stain, ×400

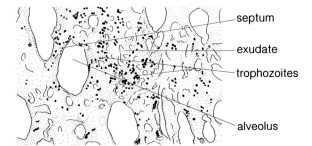

PULMONARY FOREIGN-BODY GRANULOMA

A 40-year-old male IV drug addict has a pulmonary foreign-body granuloma.

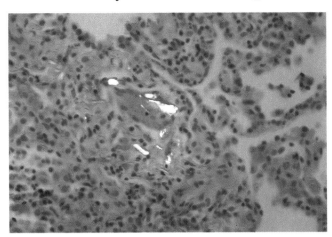

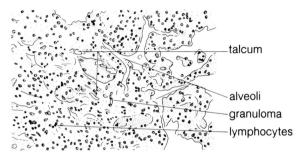

Fig. II.4.56 Ill-defined granuloma, composed of epithelioid cells, lymphocytes, and foreign-body giant cells, compressing adjacent alveoli. Talcum crystals, mostly within giant cells, appear refractile in polarized light.   H&E stain, ×200

PULMONARY KAPOSI'S SARCOMA

A 36-year-old homosexual man has Kaposi's sarcoma of the lung.

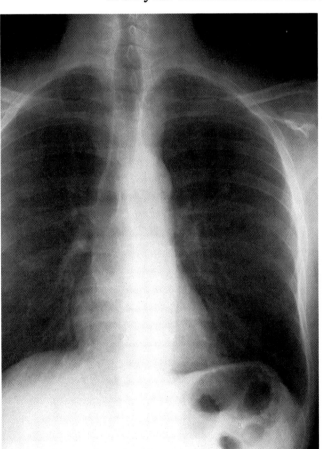

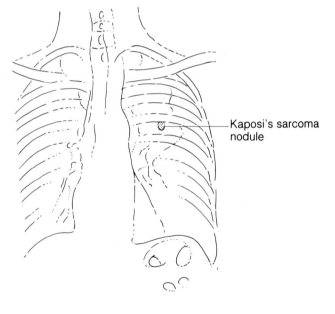

Fig. II.4.57 A round nodule in the left upper lobe has increased slowly in diameter over the past three months.

A 49-year-old homosexual male undergoes surgery for a lung tumor. The tumor consists of a large, solid mass in the right middle lobe measuring 8.5 × 5 × 3.5 cm.

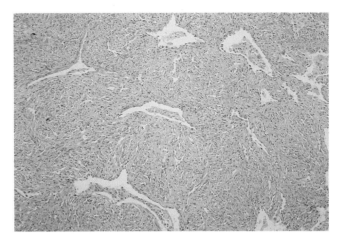

Fig. II.4.58 The tumor cells grow in the interalveolar septae, which are greatly expanded, compressing and obliterating the alveoli. They are spindle-shaped and arranged in bundles and whorls.   HPS stain, ×100

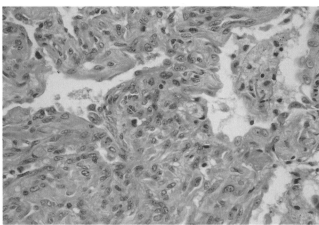

Fig. II.4.59 Kaposi's sarcoma cells with spindle-shaped nuclei occupy the interalveolar spaces, compressing but not destroying the alveoli.   HPS stain, ×400

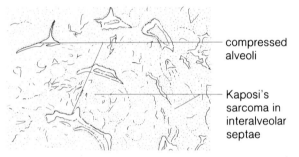

compressed alveoli

Kaposi's sarcoma in interalveolar septae

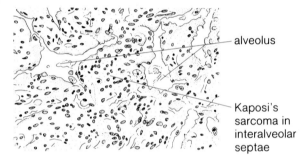

alveolus

Kaposi's sarcoma in interalveolar septae

Fig. II.4.60 Nodule of Kaposi's sarcoma cells, with palisading spindle-shaped nuclei and rare mitoses, pushing into an alveolar space.   HPS stain, ×400

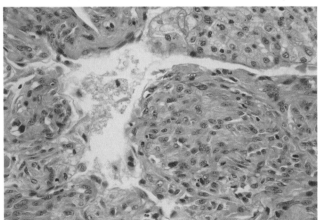

NON-HODGKIN'S LYMPHOMA OF LUNG

A 51-year-old homosexual man has non-Hodgkin's lymphoma, with
mediastinal and retroperitoneal lymph node involvement.

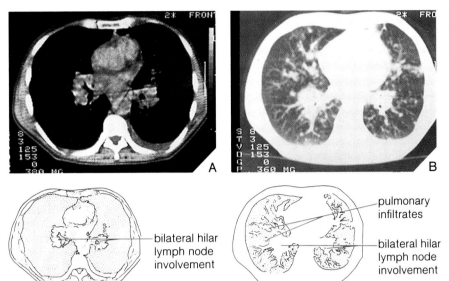

Fig. II.4.61 A. and B. On CT scan, large bilateral hilar adenopathies and interstitial pulmonary infiltrates are apparent.

A 42-year-old homosexual man has pulmonary lymphoma, with involvement
of bone marrow and retroperitoneal lymph nodes.

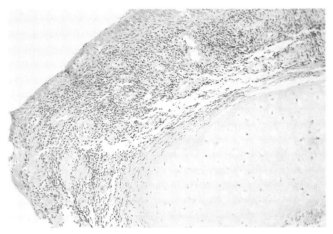

Fig. II.4.62 Bronchial biopsy showing fragment of right lower lobe bronchus with squamous metaplasia of surface epithelium, abundant infiltration of submucosa by lymphoma cells, and uninvolved cartilage of bronchial wall.

HPS stain, ×100

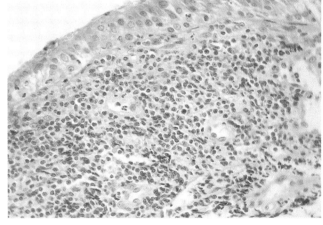

Fig. II.4.63 Surface stratified metaplastic squamous epithelium of bronchus and submucosa, with heavy infiltration by homogeneous population of lymphoma cells.

HPS stain, ×250

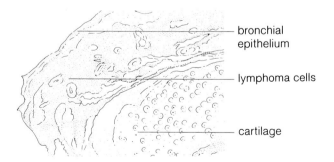

A 46-year-old homosexual man has primary non-Hodgkin's lymphoma of the lung.

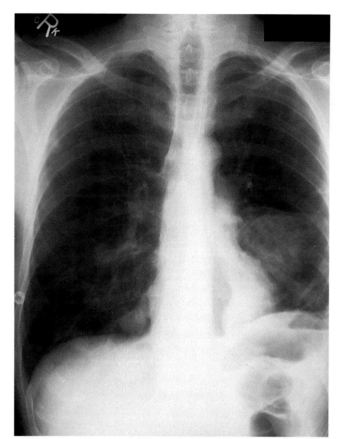

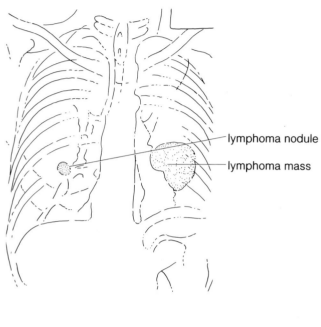

Fig. II.4.64 Large, irregularly shaped mass in left lower lobe and smaller mass in right middle lobe.

lymphoma nodule

lymphoma mass

Fig. II.4.65 Same case as in Fig. II.4.64, lateral view. Large lymphoma mass in left lower lobe of lung.

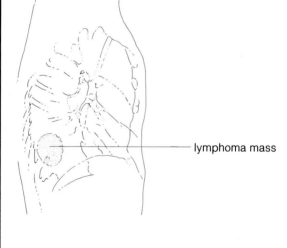

lymphoma mass

A 42-year-old homosexual man with brain lymphoma also has pulmonary lymphoma. A 4 x 3 x 3 cm tumor mass, partially infarcted and necrotic, is found in the left lower lobe of the lung at autopsy.

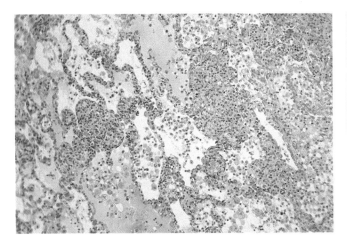

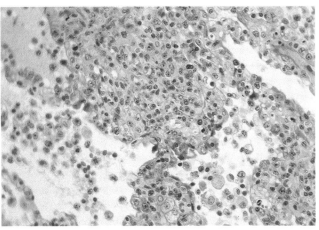

Fig. II.4.66 Lung parenchyma shows patent alveoli containing mostly desquamated alveolar cells and large, nodular, interstitial infiltrates composed of a homogeneous population of lymphoid cells.   HPS stain, ×250

Fig. II.4.67 Alveoli containing desquamated pneumocytes and interstitial nodular infiltrate composed of undifferentiated lymphoma cells with round nuclei, prominent nucleoli, and frequent mitoses. Phenotype was monoclonal IgG κ.

HPS stain, ×250

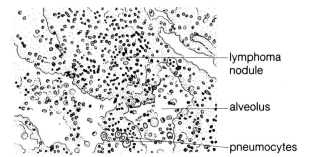

Gastrointestinal Tract and Associated Organs

MOUTH

Hairy Leukoplakia of Tongue

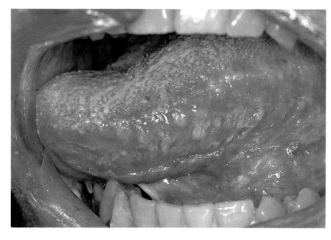

Fig. II.5.1 Hairy leukoplakia in HIV-positive homosexual man. White, confluent, corrugated, excrescences on lateral, dorsal, and ventral aspects of tongue.

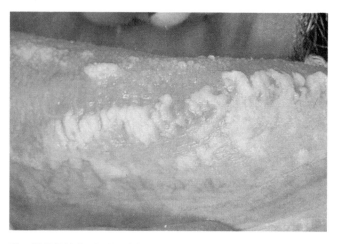

Fig. II.5.2 Hairy leukoplakia. White confluent, raised, adherent keratin plaques on lateral border of tongue.

A white, raised area 1 x 1.4 cm in size, with fine projections, is seen on the dorsal and lateral sides of the tongue in a 28-year-old homosexual man.

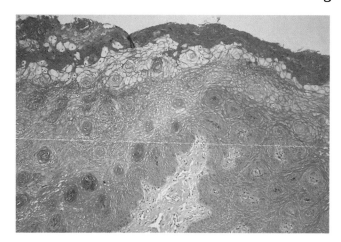

Fig. II.5.3 Flat condyloma of tongue with multiple cross-sectioned papillary projections: keratin layer, vacuolated squamous cells, stratified squamous epithelium, and subepithelial stroma.　　　　HPS stain, ×100

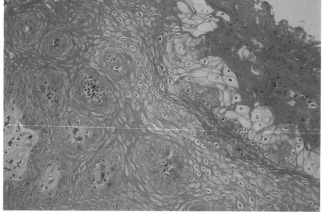

Fig. II.5.4 Cross-sectioned papillary projections with fibrovascular cores, stratified squamous epithelium with koilocytotic atypia, and keratin deposits.　　HPS stain, ×200

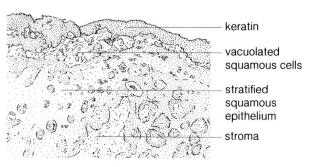

- keratin
- vacuolated squamous cells
- stratified squamous epithelium
- stroma

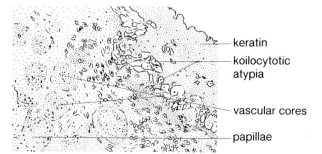

- keratin
- koilocytotic atypia
- vascular cores
- papillae

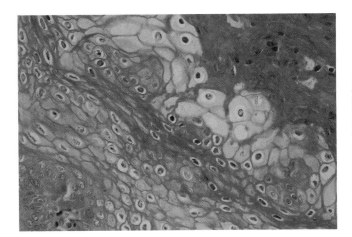

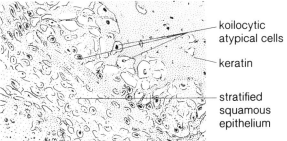

Fig. II.5.5 Stratified squamous epithelium of papilla with koilocytotic atypical cells containing large, pyknotic nuclei within vacuolated cytoplasm. Thick deposits of keratin.

HPS stain, ×400

koilocytic atypical cells

keratin

stratified squamous epithelium

Hairy Leukoplakia of Tongue and Kaposi's Sarcoma of Palate

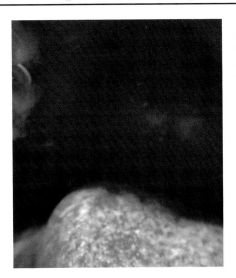

Fig. II.5.6 Protruding white excrescences cover dorsal aspect of tongue in 46-year-old homosexual man. Purplish plaque of Kaposi's sarcoma on the palate.

Candidiasis of Tongue

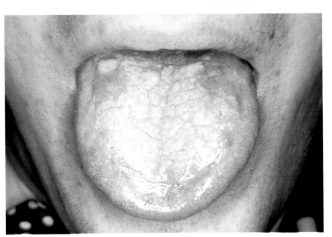

Fig. II.5.7 Tongue covered by thick white coating typical of oral candidiasis.

Kaposi's Sarcoma of Mouth

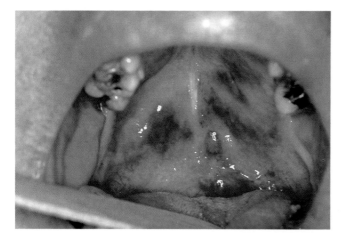

Fig. II.5.8 Raised, dark-red lesions on hard palate at level of second molar tooth.

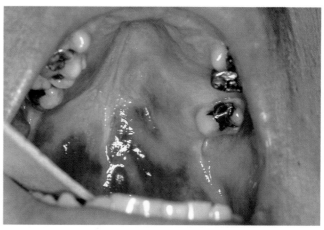

Fig. II.5.9 Multiple red and purplish lesions on hard and soft palate.

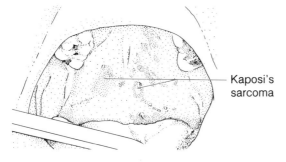

Kaposi's sarcoma

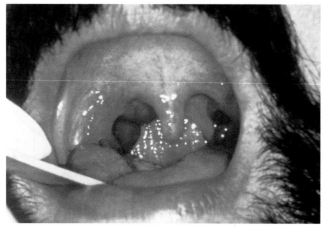

Fig. II.5.10 Nodular lesions on both tonsils.

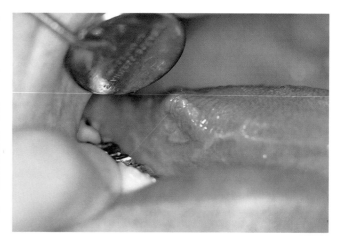

Fig. II.5.11 Protruding, ulcerated Kaposi's sarcoma on lateral border of tongue.

Non-Hodgkin's Lymphoma of Gum

A homosexual 33-year-old man presents to the dentist with a swelling area next to the lower right cuspid.

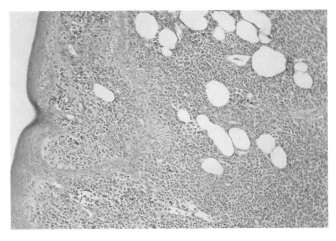

Fig. II.5.12 Masses of lymphoma cells invading fibroadipose tissues below the surface stratified squamous epithelium of oral mucosa.   HPS stain, ×100

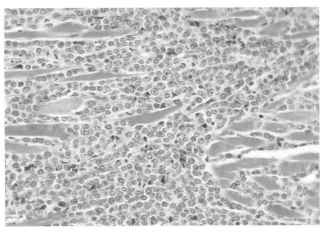

Fig. II.5.13 Lymphoma cells with scarce cytoplasm, round nuclei, conspicuous nucleoli, and frequent mitoses dissociate and replace skeletal muscle fibers of gum.   HPS stain, ×250

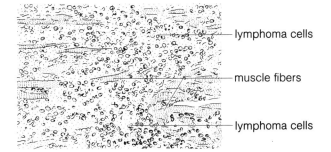

lymphoma cells

muscle fibers

lymphoma cells

SALIVARY GLANDS

Salivary Gland Lymphadenopathy

Tumorlike painless masses in the parotid glands increase slowly in size in HIV-positive homosexual men with no other symptoms.

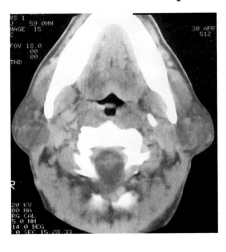

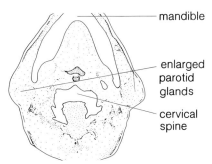

mandible

enlarged parotid glands

cervical spine

Fig. II.5.14 Diffuse symmetric swelling of both parotid glands on contrast-enhanced CT scan.

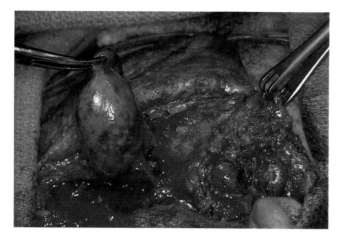

Fig. II.5.15 Right parotid mass, 6 x 4.5 cm in size, entirely removed.

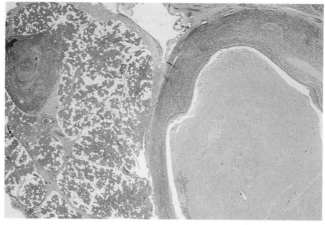

Fig. II.5.16 Parotid gland parenchyma with hyperplastic lymph node and cystically dilated duct surrounded by lymphoid tissue and containing masses of keratin.

HPS stain, ×25

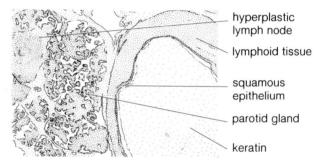

hyperplastic lymph node

lymphoid tissue

squamous epithelium

parotid gland

keratin

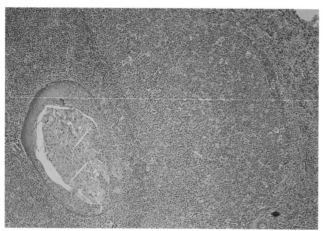

Fig. II.5.17 Intraparotid lymph node with hyperplastic germinal center showing starry-sky pattern indicative of active macrophages. Salivary duct cyst lined by squamous epithelium and filled with keratin.   HPS stain, ×100

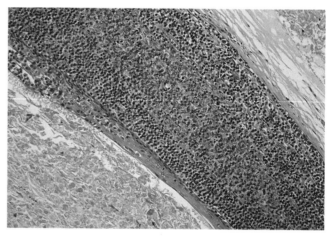

Fig. II.5.18 Large keratin-filled cyst lined by squamous epithelium and surrounded by lymphatic tissue, with large, elongated hyperplastic germinal center.   HPS stain, ×100

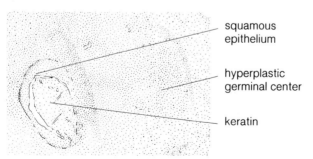

squamous epithelium

hyperplastic germinal center

keratin

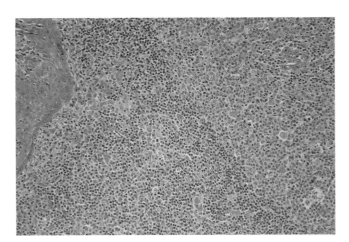

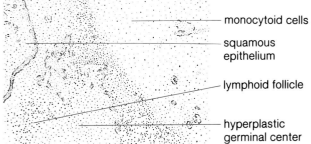

Fig. II.5.19 Intraparotid lymph node with enlarged follicle, hyperplastic germinal center, and area of monocytoid cells. Duct obliterated by squamous metaplasia and hyperplasia.
HPS stain, ×200

- monocytoid cells
- squamous epithelium
- lymphoid follicle
- hyperplastic germinal center

Salivary Gland Lymphoma

Non-Hodgkin's lymphomas in the intraparotid lymph nodes of HIV-positive homosexual men.

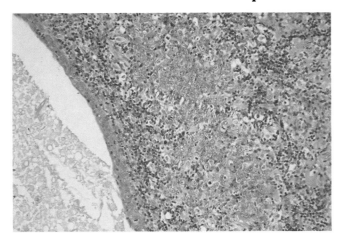

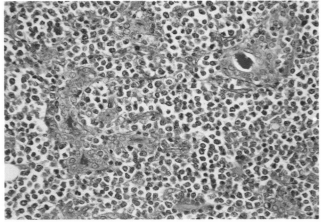

Fig. II.5.20 Non-Hodgkin's lymphoma (undifferentiated Burkitt's type) replacing lymph node parenchyma. Adjacent cystic duct with squamous epithelial lining and keratin content.
HPS stain, ×100

Fig. II.5.21 Non-Hodgkin's lymphoma (large-cell plasmacytoid type) entirely replacing lymph node parenchyma and surrounding residual salivary gland ducts.
PAS stain, ×400

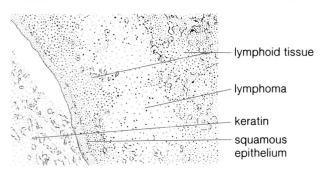

- lymphoid tissue
- lymphoma
- keratin
- squamous epithelium

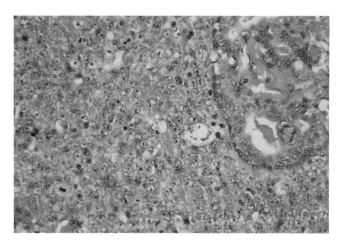

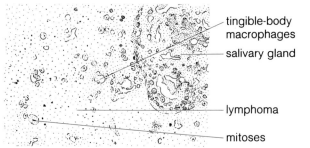

Fig. II.5.22 Non-Hodgkin's lymphoma undifferentiated Burkitt's type with frequent mitoses and scattered tingible-body histiocytes surrounding hyperplastic salivary gland myoepithelial formation.　　　　H&E stain, ×400

tingible-body macrophages

salivary gland

lymphoma

mitoses

ESOPHAGUS

Candida Esophagitis

A 51-year-old homosexual man with *Pneumocystis carinii* pneumonia has *Candida albicans* esophagitis.

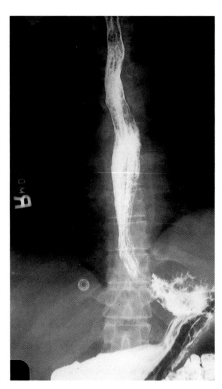

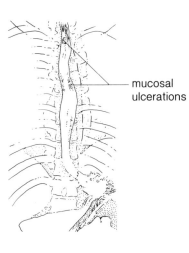

mucosal ulcerations

Fig. II.5.23 Esophageal mucosa is thickened and exhibits a cobblestone pattern. Numerous tiny collections of barium represent mucosal ulcerations. The barium traversed the esophagus slowly, because of motor dysfunction expressed by shallow and inefficient esophageal contractions.

Candida–Cytomegalovirus Esophagitis

A 38-year-old man who tests positive for HIV-antibody presents with extensive esophagitis.

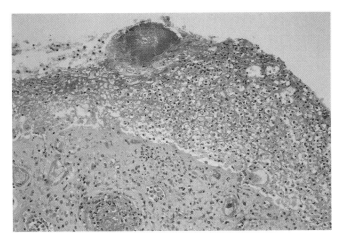

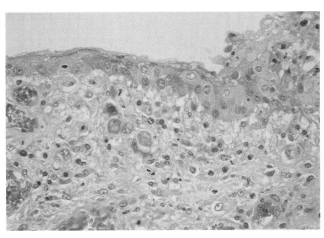

Fig. II.5.24 Esophageal mucosa, ulcerated and covered by tissue debris and colonies of *Candida albicans* pseudohyphae and yeasts. Surface squamous epithelium is acanthotic and vacuolized. CMV inclusion in endothelial cell of blood vessel.
HPS stain, ×200

Fig. II.5.25 Esophageal mucosa with vacuolization and necrosis of surface squamous epithelium. Inflammatory infiltrates, mostly lymphocytes, in subjacent stroma. Histiocyte with cytoplasmic CMV (smudge cell).
HPS stain, ×400

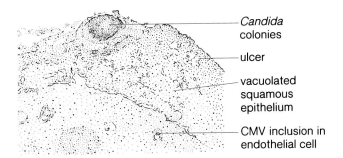

Candida colonies

ulcer

vacuolated squamous epithelium

CMV inclusion in endothelial cell

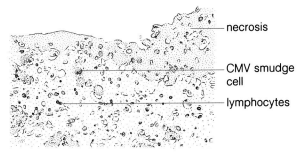

necrosis

CMV smudge cell

lymphocytes

Herpetic Esophagitis

A 36-year-old homosexual man presents with an esophageal ulcer.

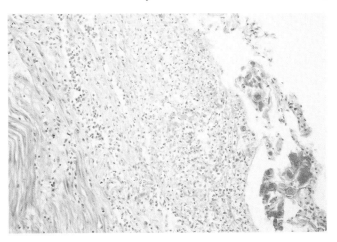

Fig. II.5.26 Esophageal muscular wall, denuded mucosa infiltrated by inflammatory cells, and large ground-glass intranuclear HSV inclusion bodies in squamous epithelial cells on ulcer bed.
HPS stain, ×200

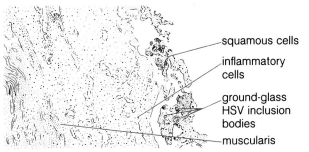

squamous cells

inflammatory cells

ground-glass HSV inclusion bodies

muscularis

Kaposi's Sarcoma of Esophagus

A 41-year-old man with Kaposi's sarcoma of the rectum and skin also has esophageal lesions.

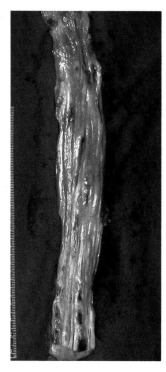

Fig. II.5.27 Deep hemorrhagic ulcerations in distal part of esophagus and areas of pseudomembranes comprising *Candida albicans* yeasts, in proximal part.

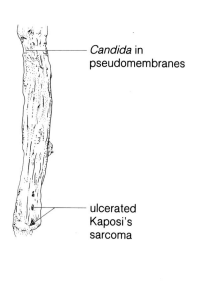

Candida in pseudomembranes

ulcerated Kaposi's sarcoma

STOMACH

Gastric Herpes

A biopsy specimen of the gastric mucosa is obtained from a 36-year-old AIDS patient.

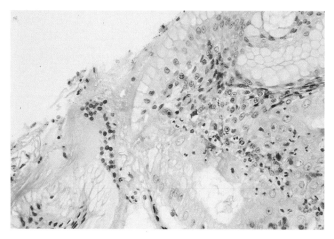

Fig. II.5.28 Gastric antral mucosa with infiltrate made up of polymorphonuclear leukocytes, lymphocytes, and macrophages. Intranuclear inclusion body in histiocyte.
HPS stain, ×400

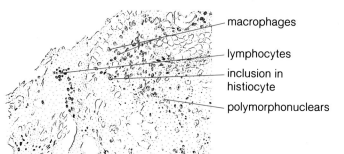

macrophages

lymphocytes

inclusion in histiocyte

polymorphonuclears

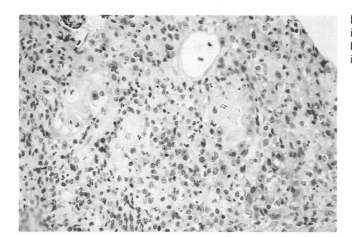

Fig. II.5.29 Gastric mucosa with abundant inflammatory infiltrate made up of polymorphonuclear leukocytes, lymphocytes, and macrophages. Intranuclear inclusion bodies in epithelial cells of glands. HPS stain, ×400

Kaposi's Sarcoma of Stomach

A 33-year-old homosexual man presents with multiple lesions in the stomach, small intestine, colon, rectum, and anus.

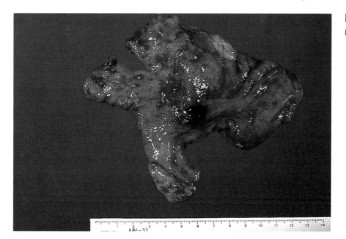

Fig. II.5.30 Raised, dark-red lesion, 1.2 cm in size, on gastric mucosa; large curvature.

Lymphoma of Stomach

A 41-year-old homosexual man has primary gastric non-Hodgkin's lymphoma.

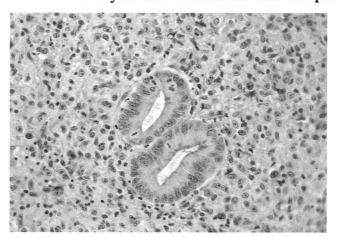

Fig. II.5.31 Two residual glands with well-preserved, mucus-secreting cells with occasional mitoses in mucosa infiltrated by lymphoma cells. Mucicarmine stain, ×250

SMALL INTESTINE

Kaposi's Sarcoma of Duodenum

Multiple purplish, slightly raised, irregularly shaped areas on the gastric and duodenal mucosae are observed and biopsied by endoscopy in a 31-year-old homosexual man.

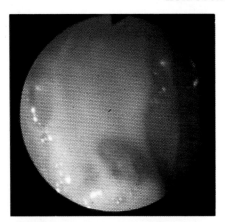

Fig. II.5.32 Purple, ovoid, raised area on the duodenal mucosa, as seen on endoscopy.

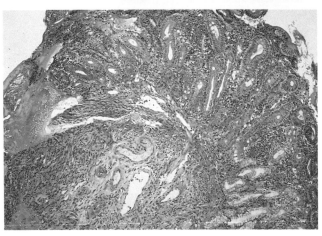

Fig. II.5.33 Duodenal mucosa with glands of normal appearance that are raised by nodular growths located in the submucosa and muscularis mucosae and are composed of spindle-shaped sarcoma cells and numerous vascular spaces. HPS stain, ×100

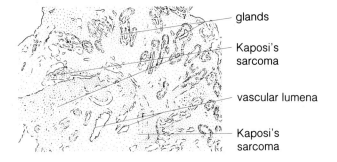

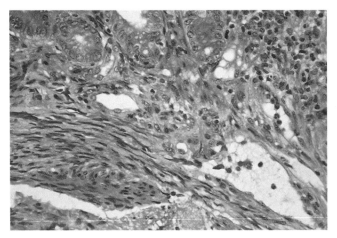

Fig. II.5.34 Duodenal mucosal glands, bundles of Kaposi's sarcoma cells with vascular spaces and mild inflammatory infiltrate. HPS stain, ×400

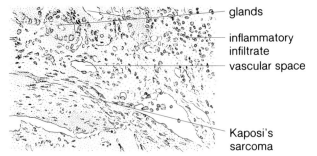

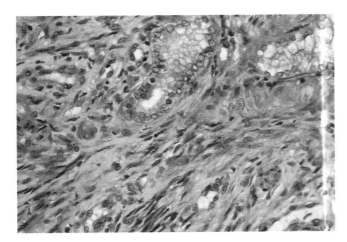

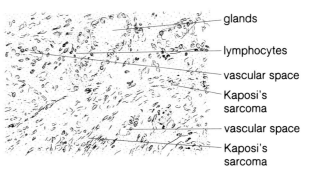

Fig. II.5.35 Duodenal glands, Kaposi's sarcoma cells forming vascular clefts and mild lymphocytic infiltrate.

HPS stain, ×400

- glands
- lymphocytes
- vascular space
- Kaposi's sarcoma
- vascular space
- Kaposi's sarcoma

Mycobacteriosis of Jejunum

A 46-year-old homosexual man with mycobacteriosis involving the spleen, intestine, and lymph nodes.

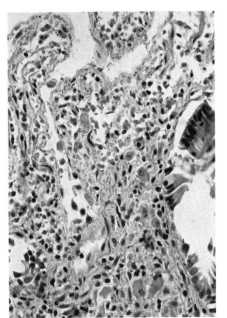

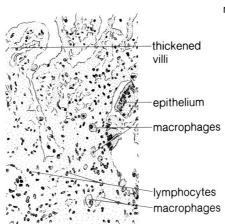

Fig. II.5.36 Thickened intestinal villi with partially preserved surface epithelium are infiltrated by numerous macrophages and lymphocytes.

HPS stain, ×400

- thickened villi
- epithelium
- macrophages
- lymphocytes
- macrophages

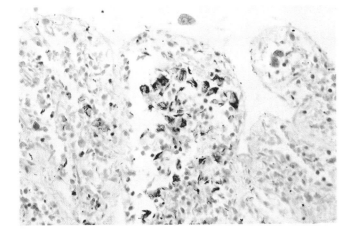

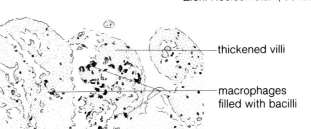

Fig. II.5.37 Thick, short intestinal villi contain numerous macrophages filled with large amounts of acid-fast bacilli.

Ziehl-Neelsen stain, ×400

- thickened villi
- macrophages filled with bacilli

Isosporiasis of Ileum

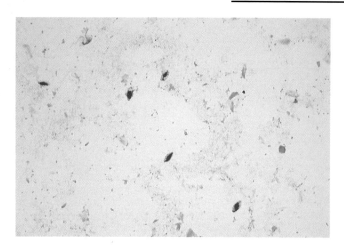

Fig. II.5.38 Multiple acid-fast oocysts of *Isospora belli* with internal sporozoites in small intestine of Haitian man with profuse diarrhea of three months' duration.

Kinyoun's stain, ×200

Lymphoma of Duodenum and Ileum

A 29-year-old homosexual man has primary non-Hodgkin's lymphoma (B-cell Burkitt's-like type) of the duodenum and ileum.

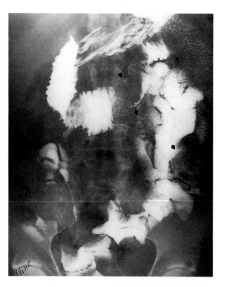

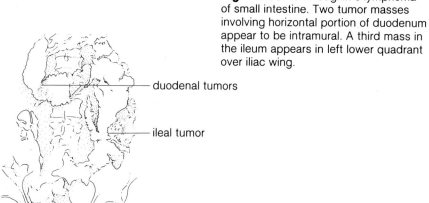

Fig. II.5.39 Non-Hodgkin's lymphoma of small intestine. Two tumor masses involving horizontal portion of duodenum appear to be intramural. A third mass in the ileum appears in left lower quadrant over iliac wing.

— duodenal tumors

— ileal tumor

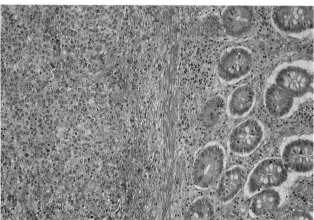

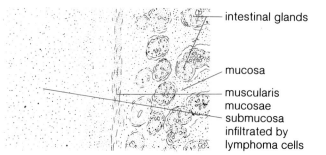

Fig. II.5.40 Masses of lymphoma cells replace submucosa and infiltrate mucosa, sparing muscularis mucosae and glandular epithelium with well-preserved mucus-secreting cells.

HPS stain, ×200

— intestinal glands

— mucosa

— muscularis mucosae
— submucosa infiltrated by lymphoma cells

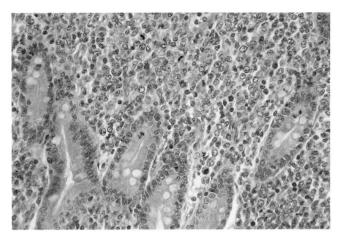

Fig. II.5.41 Same section as in Fig. II.5.40. Sheets of lymphoma cells with numerous mitoses replace mucosa but partially spare epithelium lining intestinal villi. HPS stain, ×400

LARGE INTESTINE

Cytomegalovirus Colitis

Endoscopic biopsies of cecum are performed in a 31-year-old homosexual man with colitis of four months' duration.

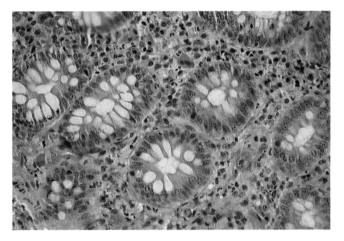

Fig. II.5.42 Mucosa of cecum with diffuse inflammatory infiltrate made up of lymphocytes, plasma cells, and neutrophils in lamina propria. CMV inclusion bodies in stromal and epithelial cells. Colonic crypts maintain normal configuration.   HPS stain, ×400

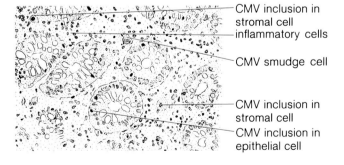

CMV inclusion in stromal cell
inflammatory cells

CMV smudge cell

CMV inclusion in stromal cell
CMV inclusion in epithelial cell

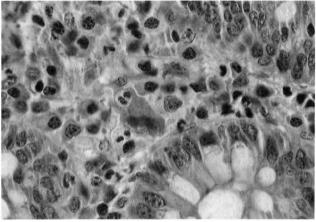

Fig. II.5.43 Mucosa of cecum with large intracytoplasmic CMV inclusions in one histiocyte of lamina propria and epithelial cells of colonic crypt. Lymphocytes, plasma cells, and neutrophils form diffuse inflammatory infiltrate.
HPS stain, ×1,000

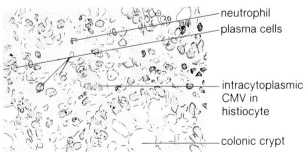

neutrophil
plasma cells

intracytoplasmic CMV in histiocyte

colonic crypt

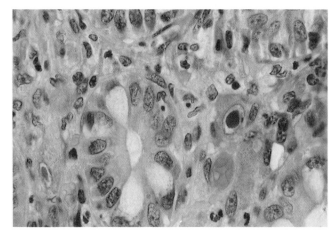

Fig. II.5.44 Large intranuclear CMV inclusions and surrounding clear haloes in histiocytes of inflamed colonic lamina propria, with lymphocytes, plasma cells, and neutrophils. HPS stain, ×100

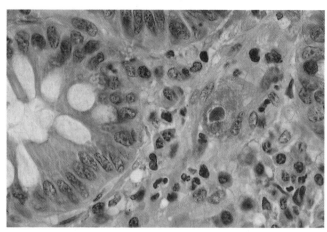

Fig. II.5.45 Large intracytoplasmic CMV inclusions and surrounding clear haloes in histiocytes of inflamed colonic lamina propria with neutrophils, lymphocytes, and plasma cells. HPS stain, ×100

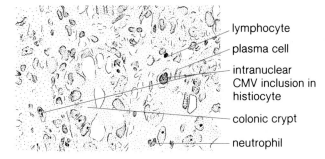

lymphocyte
plasma cell
intranuclear CMV inclusion in histiocyte
colonic crypt
neutrophil

Endoscopic biopsies of sigmoid colon are performed in a 36-year-old homosexual man with colitis of one year's duration.

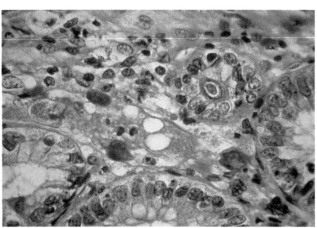

Fig. II.5.46 Numerous smudge intracytoplasmic CMV inclusions in histiocytes of lamina propria and intranuclear inclusions in epithelial cells of colonic crypts. HPS stain, ×1,000

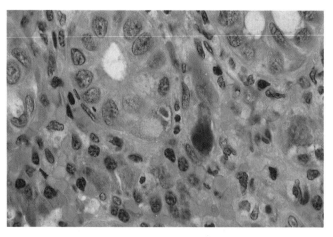

Fig. II.5.47 Large, smudge intracytoplasmic inclusion in a histiocyte of lamina propria and intranuclear inclusion in an epithelial cell of colonic crypt. HPS stain, ×1,000

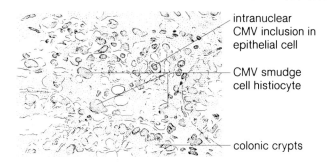

intranuclear CMV inclusion in epithelial cell

CMV smudge cell histiocyte

colonic crypts

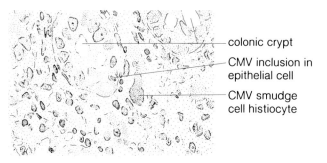

colonic crypt

CMV inclusion in epithelial cell

CMV smudge cell histiocyte

Cryptosporidiosis of Colon

A 26-year-old homosexual man manifests severe, chronic diarrhea, dehydration, malnutrition, and weight loss.

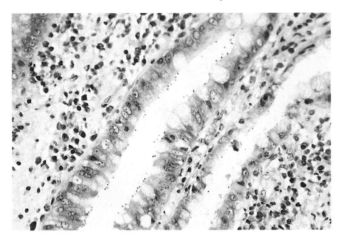

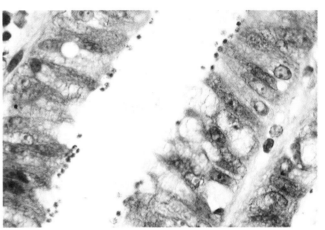

Fig. II.5.48 Biopsy specimen from descending colon showing two crypts lined by mucinous and goblet cells with sporozoites attached to their surfaces. Plasma cells and lymphocytes in lamina propria.   Giemsa stain, ×400

Fig. II.5.49 Same section as in Fig. II.5.48. Colonic crypt with numerous cryptosporidial sporozoites attached to the apical pole of lining goblet cells and absorbing epithelial cells.
Giemsa stain, ×1,000

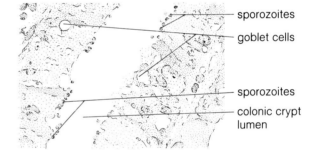

- sporozoites
- goblet cells
- sporozoites
- colonic crypt lumen

Non-Hodgkin's Lymphoma of Colon

A 40-year-old man who tests positive for HIV-antibody has primary non-Hodgkin's lymphoma in the cecum.

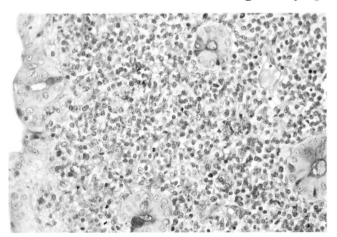

Fig. II.5.50 Mucin-secreting epithelial cells lining surface mucosa and a few preserved glands in a mass of lymphoma cells.   PAS stain, ×200

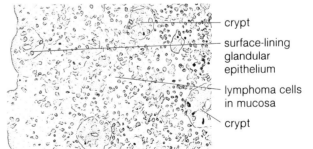

- crypt
- surface-lining glandular epithelium
- lymphoma cells in mucosa
- crypt

A 33-year-old homosexual man has primary non-Hodgkin's lymphoma in the ascending colon.

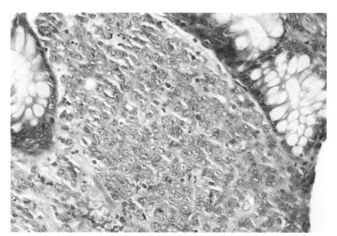

Fig. II.5.51 Masses of large noncleaved lymphoma cells infiltrate mucosa but not colonic crypts lined by goblet cells.
PAS stain, ×250

Kaposi's Sarcoma of Descending Colon

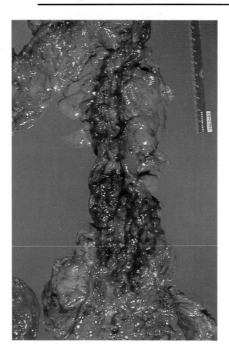

Fig. II.5.52 Multiple confluent purplish, flat, and nodular lesions replacing a large area of colonic mucosa.

RECTUM AND ANUS

Kaposi's Sarcoma of Rectum

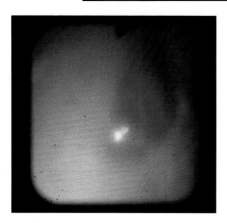

Fig. II.5.53 Round, reddish, protruding nodular lesion on rectal mucosa, as seen on endoscopy.

Non-Hodgkin's Lymphoma of Rectum and Anus

Non-Hodgkin's lymphoma can occur as a primary or major tumor in the lower rectum and anus. A 33-year-old homosexual man who tests positive for HIV-antibody presents with anal fistulas and no other organ involvement. The diagnosis is non-Hodgkin's lymphoma (undifferentiated Burkitt's-cell type).

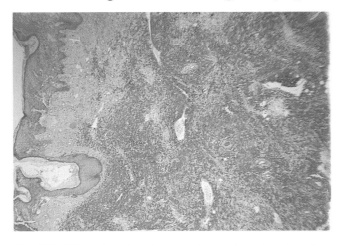

Fig. II.5.54 Sheets of lymphoma cells invade and replace the wall of the anal canal without penetrating into the covering squamous epithelium and its underlying stroma.
HPS stain, ×25

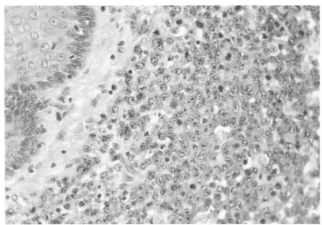

Fig. II.5.55 Same section as in Fig. II.5.54, at higher magnification.
HPS stain, ×250

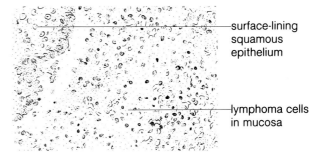

surface-lining squamous epithelium

lymphoma cells in mucosa

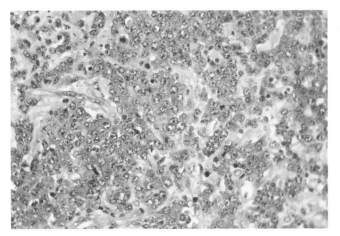

Fig. II.5.56 Sheets of lymphoma cells with large, round nuclei containing conspicuous nucleoli and frequent mitoses. Diagnosis is non-Hodgkin's lymphoma, undifferentiated Burkitt's cell type.
HPS stain, ×250

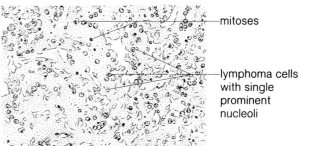

mitoses

lymphoma cells with single prominent nucleoli

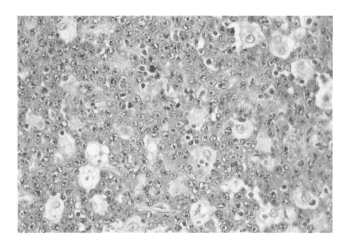

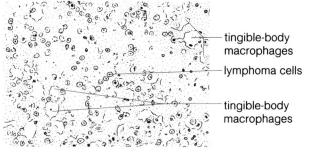

Fig. II.5.57 Same section as Fig. II.5.56. Numerous, evenly scattered tingible-body macrophages with engulfed nuclear debris resulting in starry-sky pattern.   HPS stain, ×250

tingible-body macrophages

lymphoma cells

tingible-body macrophages

Anal Herpes

A 40-year-old homosexual man presents with persistent anal ulcers.

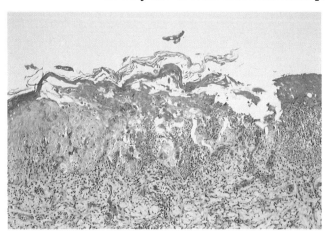

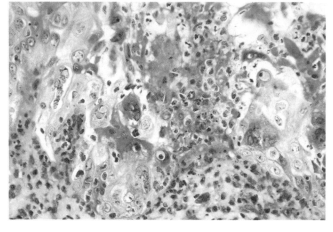

Fig. II.5.58 Intraepithelial vesicle with ulceration. Ballooning squamous cells and abundant leukocytic infiltration in epithelium and dermis, with formation of pustule.
HPS stain, ×200

Fig. II.5.59 Same section as in Fig. II.5.58. Multinucleated giant cells. Ground-glass inclusion bodies within nuclei of squamous cells. Abundant infiltration of polymorphonuclear leukocytes.   HPS stain, ×400

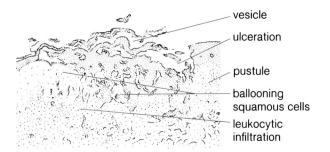

vesicle

ulceration

pustule

ballooning squamous cells

leukocytic infiltration

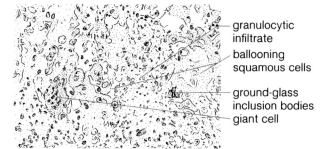

granulocytic infiltrate

ballooning squamous cells

ground-glass inclusion bodies

giant cell

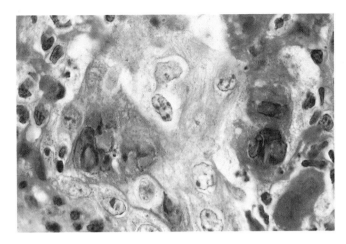

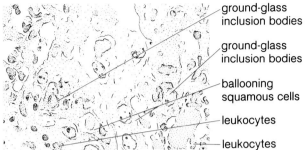

Fig. II.5.60 Same section as in Fig. II.5.58. Ballooning squamous cells with immature ground-glass intranuclear inclusions and leukocytic infiltrates.   HPS stain, ×1,000

ground-glass inclusion bodies

ground-glass inclusion bodies

ballooning squamous cells

leukocytes

leukocytes

Anal Cytomegalovirus Infection

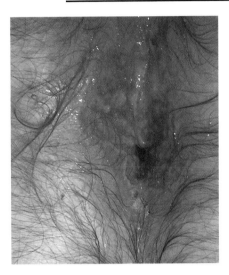

Fig. II.5.61 Anal CMV infection with large confluent clusters of vesicles.

Condyloma Acuminatum of Anus

Papillary, wartlike formation, 3.2 x 2.6 cm in size, in the anal area in a 31-year-old homosexual man.

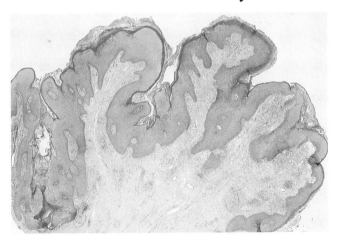

Fig. II.5.62 Broad papillae composed of fibroconnective cores with inflammatory lymphoplasmacytic infiltrates, covered by irregularly thickened stratified, keratinized squamous epithelium.   HPS stain, ×25

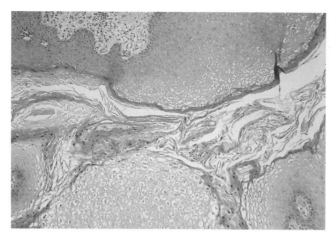

Fig. II.5.63 Papillae of condyloma acuminatum composed of fibroconnective cores with inflammatory infiltrates and thick, stratified, keratinized squamous epithelium with koilocytotic atypia.   HPS stain, ×100

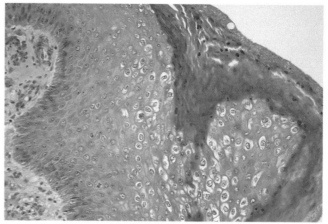

Fig. II.5.64 Tip of papilla in anal condyloma. Connective tissue core; stratified squamous epithelium; koilocytosis with vacuolated cells and large, atypical nuclei, deposition of keratin.   HPS stain, ×250

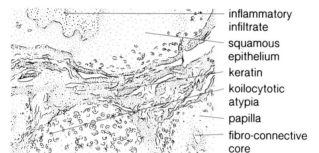

inflammatory infiltrate
squamous epithelium
keratin
koilocytotic atypia
papilla
fibro-connective core

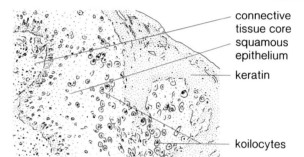

connective tissue core
squamous epithelium
keratin
koilocytes

Squamous Cell Carcinoma in Situ (Bowen's Disease) of Anus

A 33-year-old homosexual man presents with extensive pruritic, raised, plaquelike areas in the anal and perianal regions.

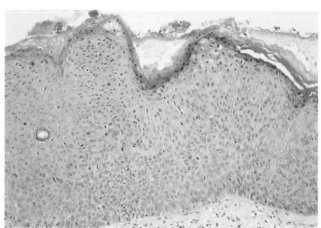

Fig. II.5.65 Anal biopsy specimen showing uniform thickening of squamous epithelium with cellular disorientation, incomplete maturation, and nuclear pleomorphism.
HPS stain, ×200

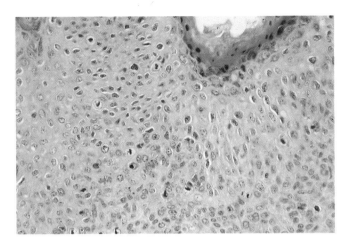

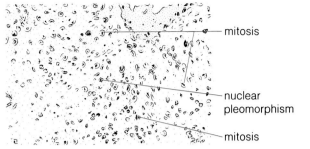

Fig. II.5.66 Same section as in Fig. II.5.65, showing parakeratosis, loss of cell orientation, and marked nuclear pleomorphism with frequent mitoses, involving the full thickness of squamous epithelium.   HPS stain, ×400

— mitosis

— nuclear pleomorphism

— mitosis

LIVER

Chronic Active Hepatitis

Hepatic needle biopsy in a 30-year-old HIV-positive drug addict

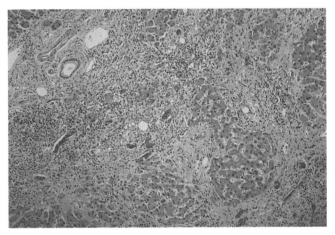

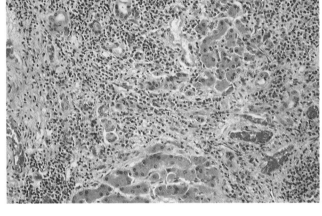

Fig. II.5.67 Massive fragmentation and replacement of hepatic lobules by inflammatory cells and fibrosis with progression to cirrhosis. Portal space with proliferating biliary ducts.   HPS stain, ×100

Fig. II.5.68 Same section as in Fig. II.5.67. Piecemeal necrosis of hepatocytes, abundant aggressive lymphocytic infiltrates, proliferation of bile ducts, and fibrosis.   HPS stain, ×200

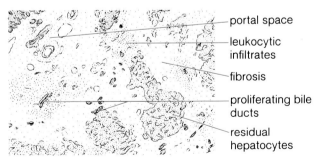

— portal space

— leukocytic infiltrates

— fibrosis

— proliferating bile ducts

— residual hepatocytes

Hepatic Tuberculosis

A 43-year-old Haitian man with HIV infection presents with low-grade fever and lymphadenopathy.

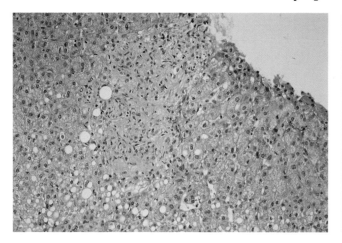

Fig. II.5.69 Hepatic needle biopsy specimen shows ill-defined granuloma and fatty change in adjacent hepatocytes.
HPS stain, ×200

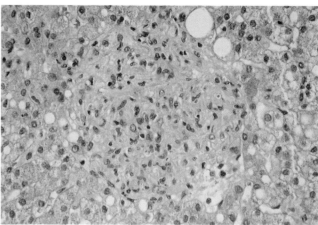

Fig. II.5.70 Granuloma composed of epithelioid cells and lymphocytes within hepatic parenchyma. Giant cells and caseation are not present. HPS stain, ×40

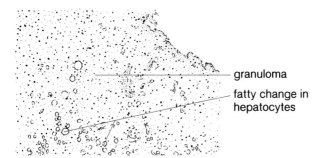

granuloma

fatty change in hepatocytes

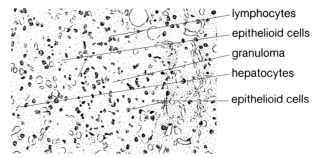

lymphocytes

epithelioid cells

granuloma

hepatocytes

epithelioid cells

Fig. II.5.71 Same section as in Fig. II.5.70. Scattered, clustered rod-shaped acid-fast bacilli between epithelioid cells in hepatic granuloma. Kinyoun's stain, ×100

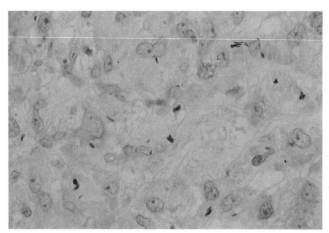

Hepatic Mycobacteriosis

Hepatic needle biopsy in 33-year-old man with fever and pancytopenia who tests positive for HIV-antibody.

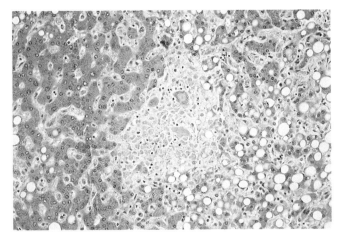

Fig. II.5.72 Nonnecrotizing granuloma composed of histiocytes and a giant cell in hepatic parenchyma, which shows marked fatty change.   HPS stain, ×200

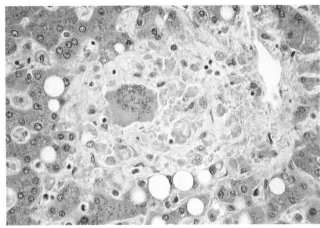

Fig. II.5.73 Same section as in Fig. II.5.72. Foamy histiocytes with multinucleated giant cell, forming hepatic granuloma. Hepatocytes with fatty change.   HPS stain, ×400

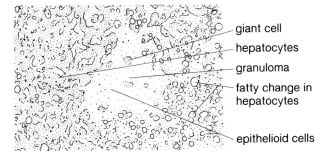

giant cell
hepatocytes
granuloma
fatty change in hepatocytes
epithelioid cells

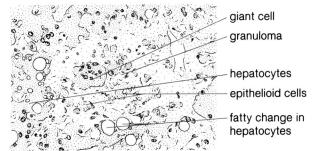

giant cell
granuloma
hepatocytes
epithelioid cells
fatty change in hepatocytes

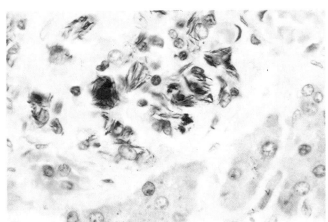

Fig. II.5.74 Foamy histiocytes in hepatic granuloma are filled with large amounts of acid-fast bacilli *(Mycobacterium avium-intracellulare).*   Kinyoun's stain, ×1,000

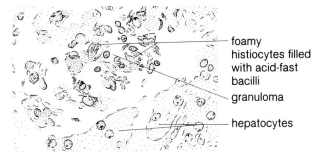

foamy histiocytes filled with acid-fast bacilli
granuloma
hepatocytes

Hepatic Histoplasmosis

Hepatic needle biopsy in a 31-year-old homosexual man with fever and bilateral small pulmonary infiltrates.

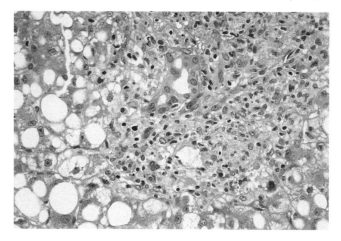

Fig. II.5.75 Nonnecrotizing granuloma in liver parenchyma composed of epithelioid cells, lymphocytes, and macrophages and containing faintly staining fine organisms. Fatty change of hepatocytes.
HPS stain, ×400

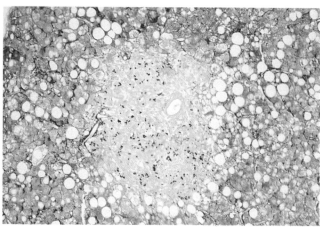

Fig. II.5.76 Same section as in Fig. II.5.75. Nonnecrotizing granuloma containing numerous organisms. Fatty change of hepatocytes.
GMS stain, ×400

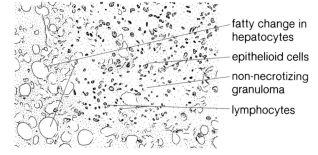

fatty change in hepatocytes

epithelioid cells

non-necrotizing granuloma

lymphocytes

Fig. II.5.77 Same section as in Fig. II.5.75. Numerous yeasts, single and in narrow-based budding forms. GMS stain, ×1,000

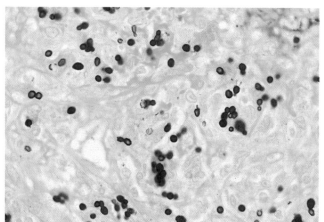

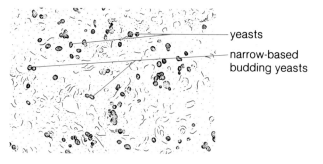

yeasts

narrow-based budding yeasts

Coccidioidomycosis in Liver

Systemic coccidioidomycosis in 52-year-old homosexual man.

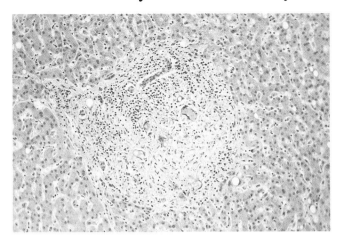

Fig. II.5.78 Nonnecrotizing granuloma in liver parenchyma. Accumulations of lymphocytes, epithelioid cells, and giant cells containing cysts, some with still distinguishable endospores. HPS stain, ×100

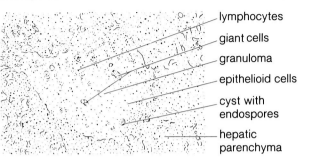

lymphocytes

giant cells

granuloma

epithelioid cells

cyst with endospores

hepatic parenchyma

Lymphoma in Liver

Disseminated non-Hodgkin's lymphoma (large noncleaved cell type) in 33-year-old homosexual man. At autopsy, most organs are involved.

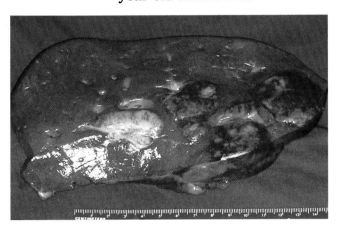

Fig. II.5.79 Large tumor nodules protruding on inferior aspect of liver.

GALLBLADDER

Cryptosporidiosis of Gallbladder

A 49-year-old homosexual man with noncalculous acute cholecystitis.

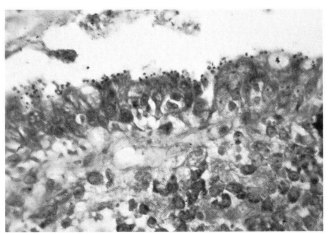

Fig. II.5.80 Gallbladder mucosa with small fine organisms attached to apical borders of lining columnar epithelial cells. Lymphocytes and plasma cells infiltrate the submucosa. Giemsa stain, ×400

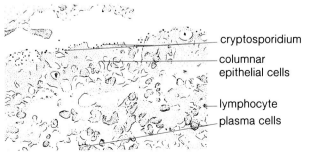

cryptosporidium

columnar epithelial cells

lymphocyte

plasma cells

PANCREAS

Tuberculosis of Pancreas

Miliary tuberculosis in a 44-year-old drug abuser.

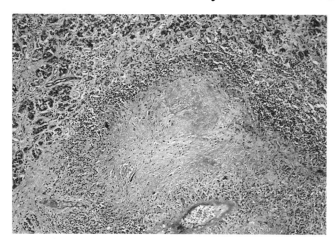

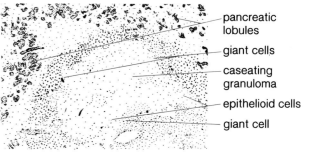

Fig. II.5.81 Granuloma with caseating center and peripheral rim of epithelioid cells, giant cells, and lymphocytes within pancreatic parenchyma. HPS stain, ×100

- pancreatic lobules
- giant cells
- caseating granuloma
- epithelioid cells
- giant cell

Cytomegalovirus Pancreatitis

Disseminated CMV infection in 43-year-old man.

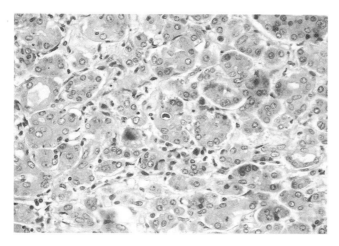

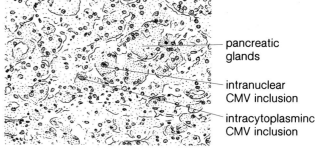

Fig. II.5.82 Intranuclear and intracytoplasmic CMV inclusions in pancreatic cells. HPS stain, ×400

- pancreatic glands
- intranuclear CMV inclusion
- intracytoplasminc CMV inclusion

OMENTUM

Coccidioidomycosis in Omentum

A 52-year-old homosexual man, with coccidioidomycosis meningitis who, after the placement of a ventriculoperitoneal shunt, developed an abscess in the peritoneal cavity.

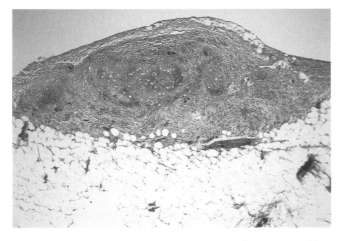

Fig. II.5.83 Granulomas in adipose tissues of omentum with focal areas of necrosis surrounded by cellular infiltrates with giant cells.   HPS stain, ×25

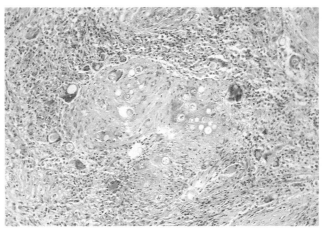

Fig. II.5.84 Granuloma with central area of necrosis containing multiple degenerated cysts surrounded by cyst-containing giant cells and lymphocytes.   HPS stain, ×100

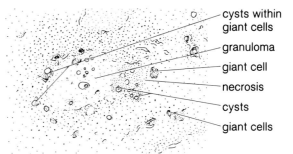

cysts within giant cells

granuloma

giant cell

necrosis

cysts

giant cells

Fig. II.5.85 Coccidiococcal cysts with degenerated endospores in area of necrosis. Giant cells, lymphocytes, and plasma cells.

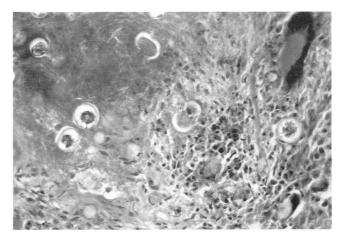

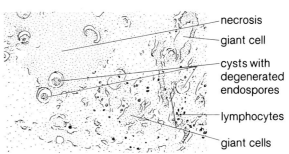

necrosis

giant cell

cysts with degenerated endospores

lymphocytes

giant cells

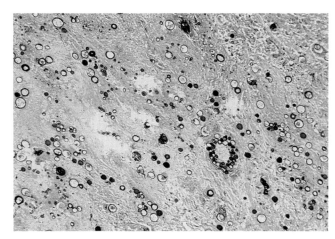

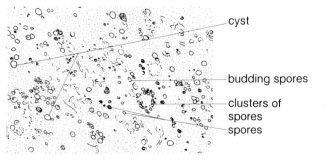

Fig. II.5.86 Silver-stained cysts and spores, single, budding, and in clusters in coccidiococcal granuloma of omentum.

GMS stain, ×250

cyst

budding spores

clusters of
spores

spores

RETROPERITONEUM

Non-Hodgkin's Lymphoma of Retroperitoneum

A massive tumor involving the retroperitoneal space, probably originating in the para-aortic lymph nodes, in a 33-year-old homosexual man.

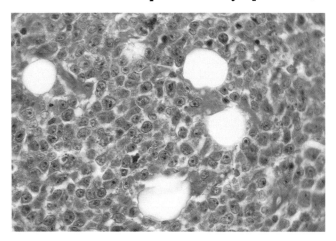

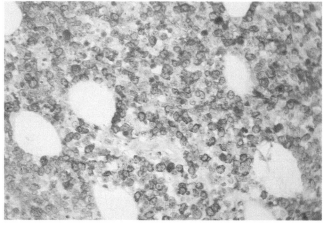

Fig. II.5.87 Sheets of lymphoma cells with large noncleaved nuclei including frequent mitoses infiltrate the lobules of adipose tissues.

HPS stain, ×250

Fig. II.5.88 Same case as Fig. 11.5.87. Sections show anti-κ monoclonal staining of lymphoma cells.

Perox-antiperox stain, ×250

Urinary Tract

KIDNEY

Focal, Segmental Glomerulosclerosis

A 54-year-old homosexual man who had hypergammaglobulinemia, hyponatremia, proteinuria, and gradually increasing uremia eventually died with diffuse cerebral dysfunction.

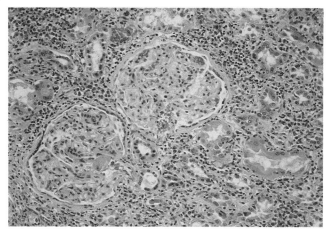

Fig. II.6.1 Renal cortex with focal interstitial inflammatory infiltrates, tubular degeneration, and segmental glomerulosclerosis. Glomeruli show lobulation, hypercellularity, and deposition of immunoglobulins with incipient sclerosis.
HPS stain, ×200

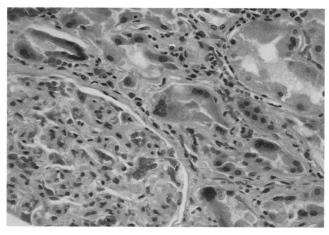

Fig. II.6.2 Glomerulus showing mesangial hypercellularity and deposition of immunoglobulins with segmental sclerosis. Marked tubular degeneration with nuclear fusion in the lining epithelial cells.
HPS stain, ×400

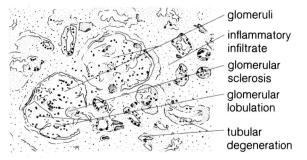

glomeruli

inflammatory infiltrate

glomerular sclerosis

glomerular lobulation

tubular degeneration

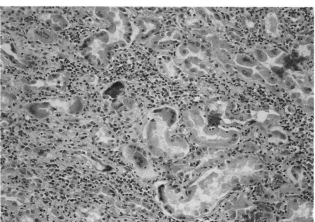

Fig. II.6.3 Intense diffuse interstitial inflammatory infiltrates made up of lymphocytes, granulocytes, and plasma cells in medulla. Tubular degeneration and atrophy, with nuclear fusion.
HPS stain, ×250

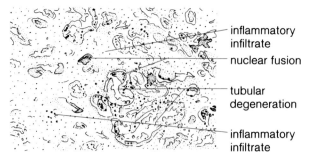

inflammatory infiltrate

nuclear fusion

tubular degeneration

inflammatory infiltrate

Cytomegalovirus Nephritis

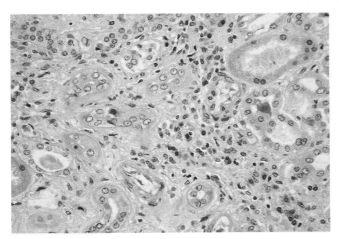

Fig. II.6.4 Inflammatory infiltrate in kidney parenchyma with tubular degeneration. Lymphocytes, plasma cells, and cytoplasmic and intranuclear CMV inclusion bodies in tubular epithelial cells.   HPS stain, ×400

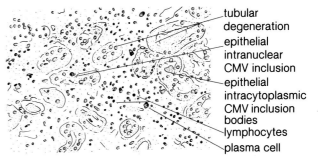

- tubular degeneration
- epithelial intranuclear CMV inclusion
- epithelial intracytoplasmic CMV inclusion bodies
- lymphocytes
- plasma cell

Candidiasis in Kidney

Disseminated candidiasis in 24-year-old homosexual man.

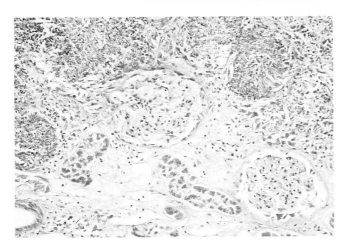

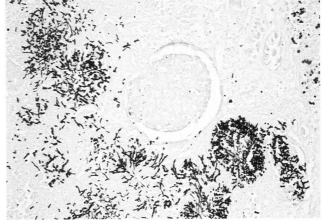

Fig. II.6.5 Massive invasion of glomeruli and renal tubules by large accumulations of pseudohyphae, resulting in areas of necrosis. Minimal inflammatory reaction.   GMS stain, ×200

Fig. II.6.6 Mycelial colonies in renal cortex surrounding glomerulus.   HPS stain, ×200

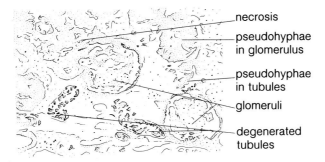

- necrosis
- pseudohyphae in glomerulus
- pseudohyphae in tubules
- glomeruli
- degenerated tubules

Coccidioidomycosis in Kidney

Systemic coccidioidomycosis in 52-year-old homosexual man.

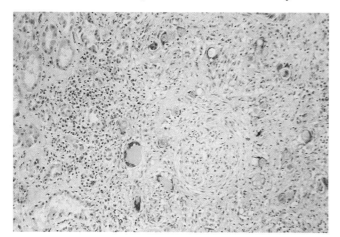

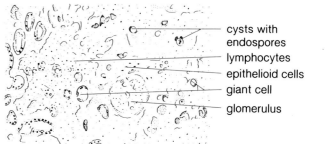

Fig. II.6.7 Nonnecrotizing, ill-formed granulomas surrounding fibrosed glomerulus. Accumulations of lymphocytes, epithelioid cells, and numerous giant cells containing degenerated cysts, some with visible endospores.

HPS stain, ×100

- cysts with endospores
- lymphocytes
- epithelioid cells
- giant cell
- glomerulus

Renal Toxoplasmosis

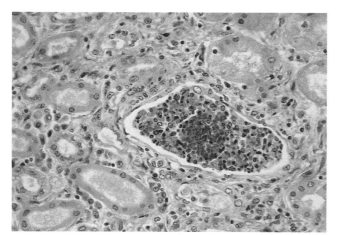

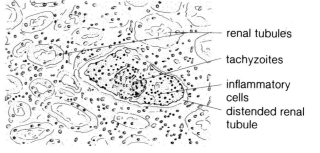

Fig. II.6.8 Distended renal tubule with large cluster of tachyzoites and inflammatory cells. HPS stain, ×400

- renal tubules
- tachyzoites
- inflammatory cells
- distended renal tubule

Non-Hodgkin's Lymphoma in Kidney

Disseminated non-Hodgkin's lymphoma (large noncleaved cell type) in 33-year-old homosexual man. Autopsy reveals that most organs are involved.

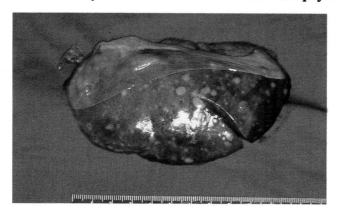

Fig. II.6.9 After the kidney capsule is stripped, numerous tumor nodules protrude from renal parenchyma.

BLADDER

Non-Hodgkin's Lymphoma in Urinary Bladder

A 46-year-old homosexual man has non-Hodgkin's lymphoma of the colon with extensive invasion of abdominal and pelvic organs.

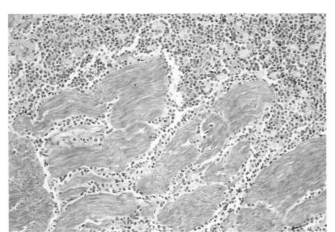

Fig. II.6.10 Massive infiltration and replacement of smooth muscle in urinary bladder wall by lymphoma (small-cell plasmacytic type). HPS stain, ×200

URETHRA

Condyloma Acuminatum of Urethra

A 45-year-old homosexual man manifests papillary growth in the meatus of the urethra.

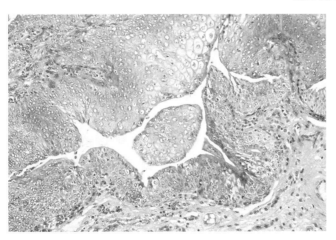

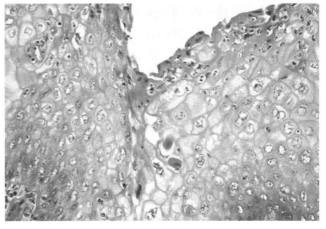

Fig. II.6.11 Urethral mucosa with broad, papillary protrusions into the lumen. Koilocytotic atypia in superficial layers. Chronic inflammation in stroma. HPS stain, ×200

Fig. II.6.12 Same section as in Fig. II.6.11. Koilocytotic atypia in upper third of squamous epithelium. Koilocytes are enlarged cells with clear cytoplasm and irregularly shaped, eccentric, hyperchromatic nuclei. HPS stain, ×400

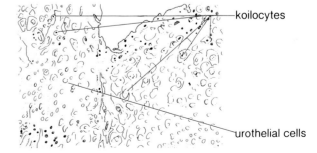

koilocytes

urothelial cells

Genital Tract

MALE GENITAL TRACT

Molluscum Contagiosum of Penis

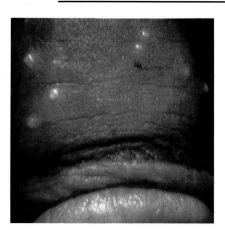

Fig. II.7.1 Multiple lesions on the penile shaft of a 30-year-old drug abuser.

Endophytic Condyloma of Penis

A 23-year-old homosexual man presents with a flat, raised, growth, 2 x 1 cm in size, on the penile shaft.

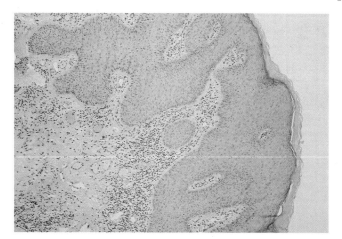

Fig. II.7.2 Broad, anastomosing tongues of squamous epithelium growing inward into the subjacent inflamed stroma. HPS stain, ×100

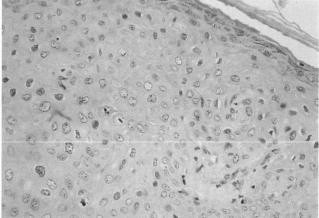

Fig. II.7.3 Same section as in Fig. II.7.2. Squamous epithelium showing acanthosis and koilocytosis. HPS stain, ×400

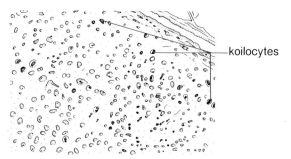

koilocytes

Penile Herpes

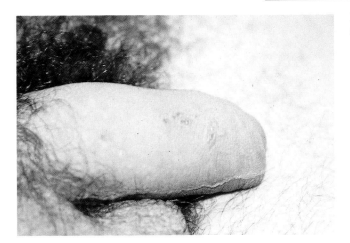

Fig. II.7.4 Cluster of ulcerated herpetic vesicles on penile shaft.

Kaposi's Sarcoma of Penis

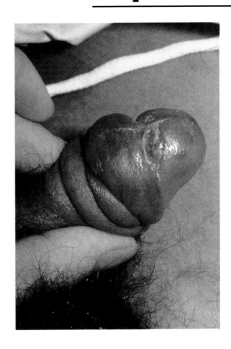

Fig. II.7.5 Ulcerated plaque of Kaposi's sarcoma on glans penis of 42-year-old homosexual man.

Cytomegalovirus Prostatitis

Autopsy reveals disseminated CMV infection in a 51-year-old homosexual man.

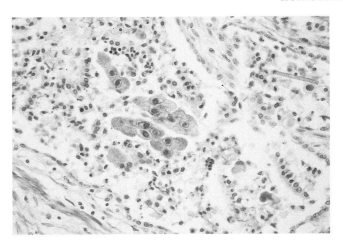

Fig. II.7.6 Largely distended prostatic gland with desquamated epithelial cells containing multiple intranuclear CMV inclusion bodies. Few lymphocytes are present.

HPS stain, ×400

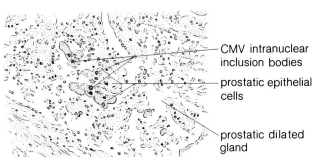

CMV intranuclear inclusion bodies

prostatic epithelial cells

prostatic dilated gland

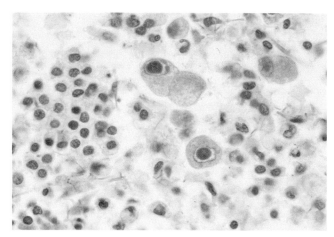

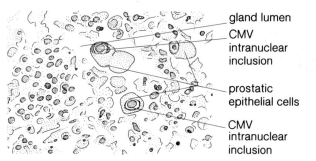

Fig. II.7.7 Same section as in Fig. II.7.6. Epithelial cells with intranuclear haloed CMV inclusion bodies within lumen of prostatic gland.   HPS stain, ×1,000

- gland lumen
- CMV intranuclear inclusion
- prostatic epithelial cells
- CMV intranuclear inclusion

Lymphoma in Seminal Vesicle

Retroperitoneal non-Hodgkin's lymphoma (large noncleaved cell type) in a 35-year-old homosexual man extends to the prostate and seminal vesicles.

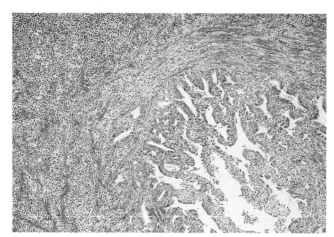

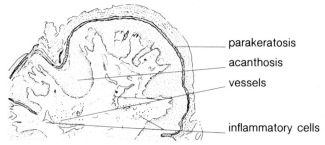

Fig. II.7.8 Masses of lymphoma cells infiltrate mucosal ridges, mucosa, and smooth muscle of seminal vesicle.

HPS stain, ×100

- smooth muscle
- lymphoma cells
- mucosa
- mucosal ridges
- lumen seminal vesicle

FEMALE GENITAL TRACT

Condyloma Acuminatum of Vulva

A verrucous, friable, soft lesion, 0.3 x 0.3 cm in size, on the labia minora of a 22-year-old woman.

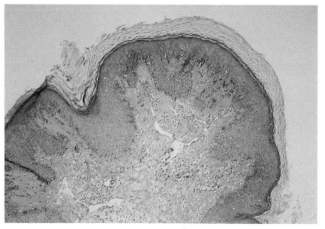

Fig. II.7.9 Warty raised area showing acanthosis, and broad, irregularly shaped rete pegs. Subjacent stroma with chronic inflammation and vascularization.   HPS stain, ×100

- parakeratosis
- acanthosis
- vessels
- inflammatory cells

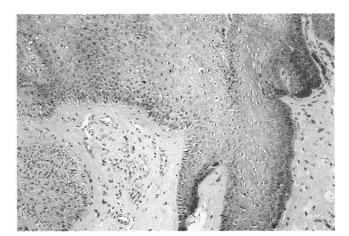

Fig. II.7.10 Acanthotic surface squamous epithelium with thickened rete pegs, showing marked koilocytosis.

HPS stain, ×200

Herpes of Vulva and Anus

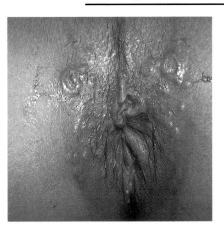

Fig. II.7.11 Numerous perivulvar and perianal herpes vesicles and confluent ulcers.

Endocrine System

THYROID

Candidiasis of Thyroid

Disseminated candidiasis in a 24-year-old homosexual man.

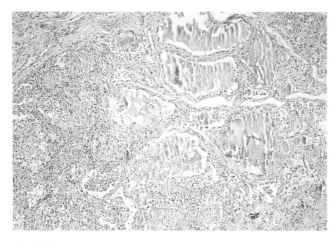

Fig. II.8.1 Thyroid follicles invaded and replaced by colonies of mycelia. HPS stain, ×200

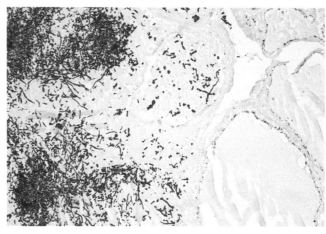

Fig. II.8.2 Colloid-filled thyroid follicles surrounded, infiltrated, and replaced by large colonies of mycelia. GMS stain, ×200

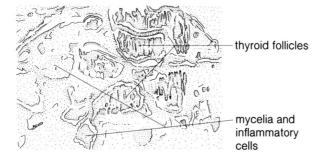

— thyroid follicles

— mycelia and inflammatory cells

ADRENAL GLANDS

Cytomegalovirus Adrenalitis

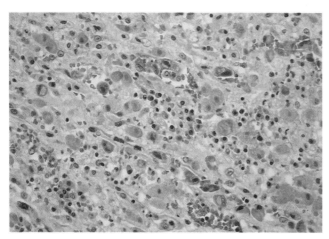

Fig. II.8.3 Extensive inflammation and necrosis of both adrenals at autopsy in a 43-year-old man. Cells of adrenal cortex either showing intranuclear CMV inclusion bodies or necrosis. Focal hemorrhages and infiltrates made up of lymphocytes and plasma cells. HPS stain, ×400

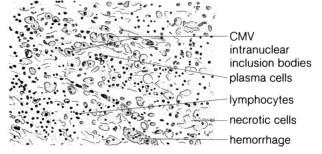

— CMV intranuclear inclusion bodies
— plasma cells
— lymphocytes
— necrotic cells
— hemorrhage

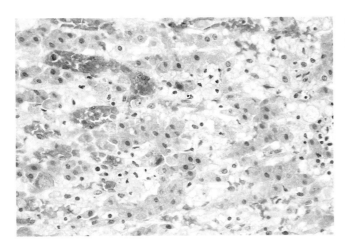

Fig. II.8.4 Extensive necrosis, focal hemorrhages, and inflammation in adrenal cortex. Numerous intranuclear CMV inclusion bodies.   HPS stain, ×400

Central Nervous System

BRAIN

Subacute Encephalitis

A 30-year-old woman who is a long-term IV drug abuser exhibits neurologic motor symptoms and progressive dementia.

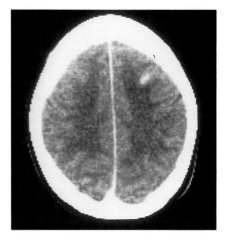

Figure II.9.1 Small, well-defined area of contrast enhancement with minimal surrounding edema at corticomedullary junction of left frontal lobe. Contrast-enhanced CT scan.

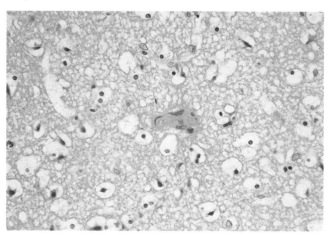

Fig. II.9.2 Extensive area of demyelination with multinucleated giant cell in cerebral cortex.   HPS stain, ×400

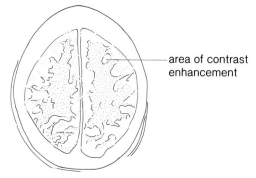

area of contrast enhancement

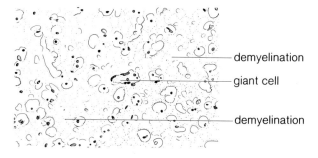

demyelination

giant cell

demyelination

Fig. II.9.3 Demyelination, scattered lymphocytes, glial cells, and a multinucleated giant cell with overlapping nuclei.
HPS stain, ×400

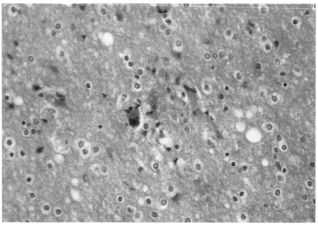

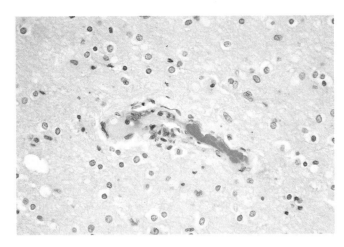

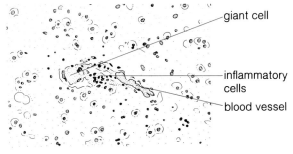

Fig. II.9.4 Focus of perivascular small inflammatory cells with multinucleated giant cell.   HPS stain, ×400

giant cell

inflammatory cells

blood vessel

A 49-year-old homosexual man shows progressive signs of encephalitis. Marked cerebral atrophy is found at autopsy.

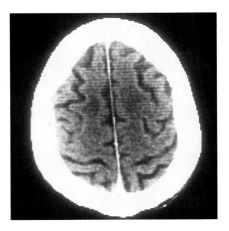

Fig. II.9.5 Bilateral enlargement of sulci, indicating cerebral atrophy. Contrast-enhanced CT scan.

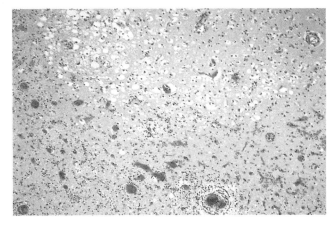

Fig. II.9.6 Extensive area of demyelination surrounded by congested vessels, with perivascular accumulations of inflammatory cells.   HPS stain, ×100

Fig. II.9.7 Cerebral cortex with two arterioles. Abundant mineralization (siderocalcinosis) of arteriolar walls.
HPS stain, ×200

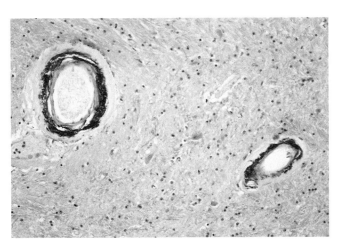

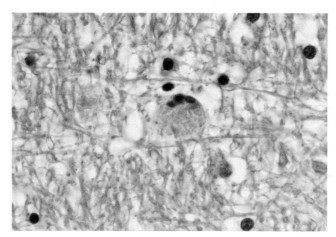

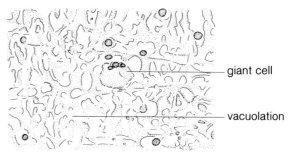

Fig. II.9.8 Demyelination and extreme vacuolation of cerebral white matter. A giant cell with fine, pale cytoplasm and small overlapping nuclei.   HPS stain, ×100

giant cell

vacuolation

Herpes Simplex Encephalitis

A 36-year-old heroin addict male with herpes simplex encephalitis.

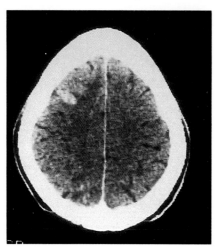

Fig. II.9.9 Oval-shaped area of contrast enhancement with minimal surrounding edema in right frontal lobe. Contrast-enhanced CT scan.

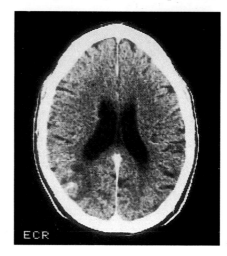

Fig. II.9.10 Irregular area of contrast enhancement with surrounding edema in the periphery of right parietal lobe. Contrast-enhanced CT scan.

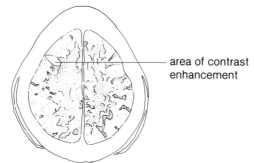

area of contrast enhancement

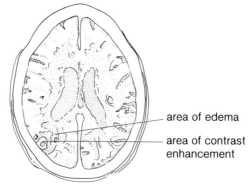

area of edema

area of contrast enhancement

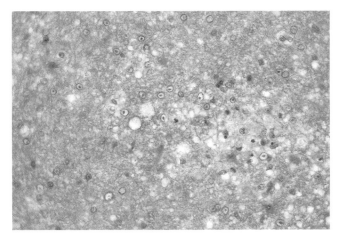

Fig. II.9.11 Parietal region with palely staining area of disorganization produced by demyelination. Numerous glial cells with a prominent centrally located intranuclear viral inclusion body. No inflammatory reaction is present.

HPS stain, ×250

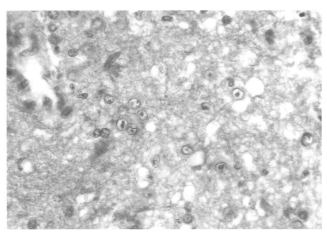

Fig. II.9.12 Viral inclusion bodies in center of glial cell nuclei. Characteristic halo is formed by peripheral margination of chromatin. Area of demyelination and neuronal degeneration.

HPS stain, ×400

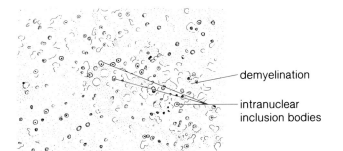

demyelination

intranuclear inclusion bodies

Brain biopsy in a 47-year-old homosexual man.

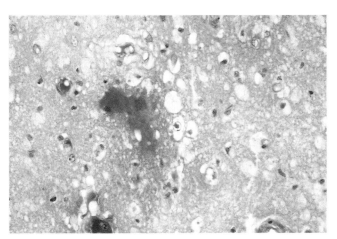

Fig. II.9.13 Brain biopsy specimen shows focal hemorrhage, edema, a zone of demyelination, and a haloed intranuclear inclusion body.

HPS stain, ×400

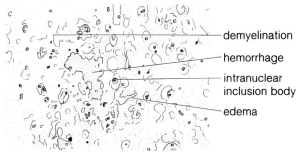

demyelination

hemorrhage

intranuclear inclusion body

edema

Progressive Multifocal Leukoencephalopathy (PML)

A 42-year-old homosexual man exhibits progressive motor and sensory nerve deficits.

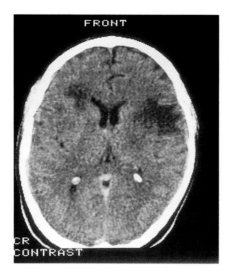

Fig. II.9.14 Two areas of decreased attenuation in white matter of cerebral hemisphere: a large area within right frontal lobe and a smaller area adjacent to frontal horn of left frontal lobe. Nonenhanced CT scan.

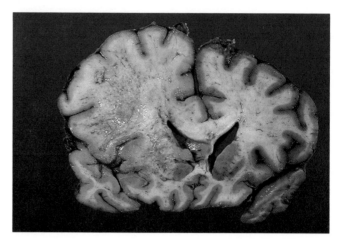

Fig. II.9.15 Multiple confluent areas of discoloration representing degeneration of white matter in left frontal, parietal, and temporal lobes. HPS stain, ×200

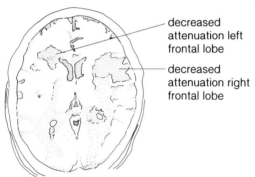

decreased attenuation left frontal lobe

decreased attenuation right frontal lobe

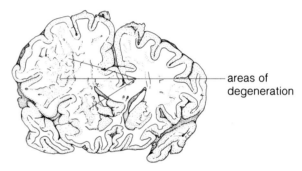

areas of degeneration

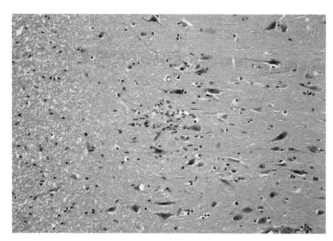

Fig. II.9.16 Microglial nodule at periphery of area of demyelination.

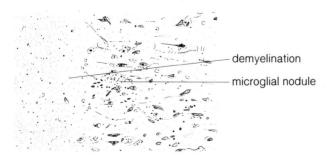

demyelination

microglial nodule

Fig. II.9.17 Accumulation of macrophages filled with lipid material from demyelinated white matter. HPS stain, ×400

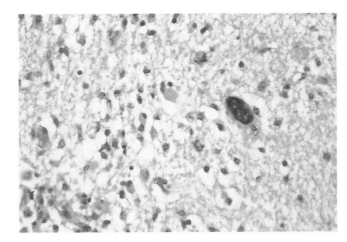

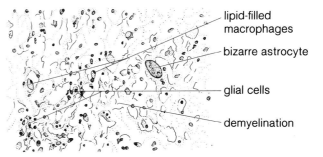

Fig. II.9.18 Large, bizarre, hyperchromatic astrocyte (gemistocyte), lipid-filled macrophages, and glial cells accumulating in area of demyelination.　　HPS stain, ×400

lipid-filled macrophages

bizarre astrocyte

glial cells

demyelination

PML in 32-year-old man with progressive ataxia and dementia.

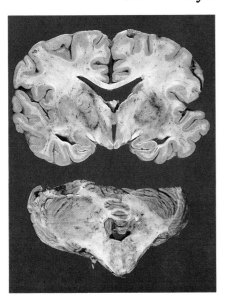

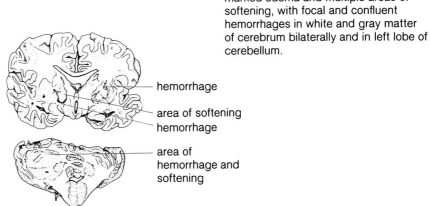

Fig. II.9.19 At autopsy, brain shows marked edema and multiple areas of softening, with focal and confluent hemorrhages in white and gray matter of cerebrum bilaterally and in left lobe of cerebellum.

hemorrhage

area of softening
hemorrhage

area of hemorrhage and softening

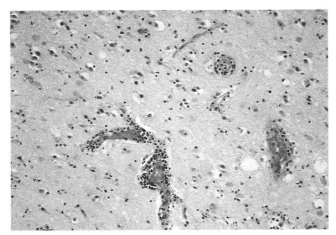

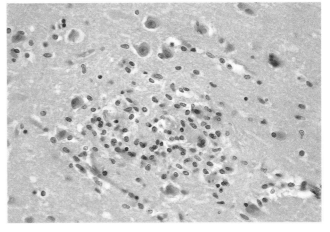

Fig. II.9.20 Accumulations of inflammatory cells, lymphocytes, and oligodendrocytes around blood vessels at the periphery of demyelinating area.　　HPS stain, ×250

Fig. II.9.21 Microglial nodule composed of lymphocytes, oligodendrocytes, and hyperplastic, hyperchromatic astrocytes.　　HPS stain, ×400

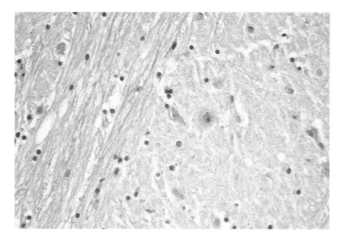

Fig. II.9.22 Intranuclear haloed inclusion body in white matter of parietal lobe. HPS stain, ×400

A 59-year-old homosexual man with florid PML.

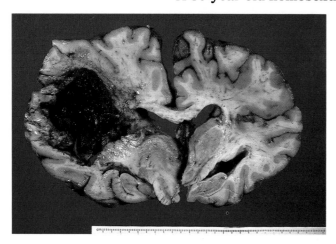

Fig. II.9.23 Large area of hemorrhagic necrosis in left cerebral hemisphere and herniation with hemorrhagic necrosis of brain stem were found at autopsy.

Tuberculous Meningoencephalitis

A 54-year-old homosexual man with an extensive history of smoking and chronic obstructive pulmonary disease has tuberculous meningitis with noncharacteristic radiographic changes and only moderate alterations of cerebrospinal fluid. Diagnosis was made at autopsy.

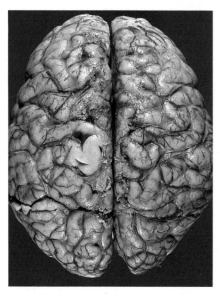

Fig. II.9.24 Congestion of meningeal vessels and patches of white exudate in leptomeninges of cerebral hemispheres.

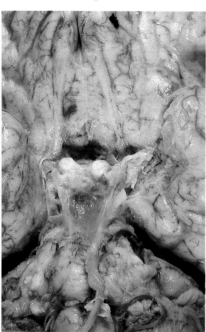

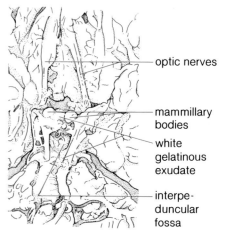

Fig. II.9.25 Leptomeninges at base of brain, thick and opaque, covered by white, gelatinous exudate that partially obscures optic nerves, mammillary bodies, and interpeduncular fossa.

optic nerves

mammillary bodies

white gelatinous exudate

interpeduncular fossa

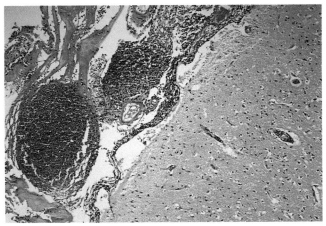

Fig. II.9.26 Leptomeninges markedly thickened by congestion of vessels, edema, and inflammatory exudate, including formation of 1 to 3 mm nodules of caseation necrosis and fibrin. Cerebral cortex with congested vessels.

HPS stain, ×100

- leptominges
- nodules of caseous necrosis
- congested vessel
- cerebral cortex

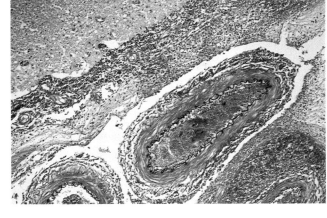

Fig. II.9.27 Leptomeninges with abundant inflammatory exudate and congested vessels at base of cerebrum.

EVG stain, ×100

- cerebral cortex
- inflammatory exudate
- arteriole
- inflammatory exudate
- arteriole

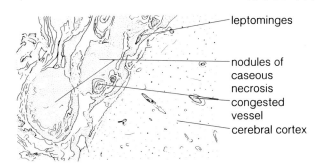

Fig. II.9.28 Massive meningitis with abundant fibrinous, partially necrotic exudate extending along fissures into cerebral matter. HPS stain, ×100

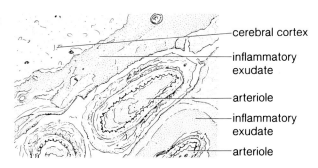

Fig. II.9.29 Infiltrate composed of lymphocytes and monocytes around meningeal artery, with numerous acid-fast *Mycobacterium tuberculosis* bacilli. Granulomas, epithelioid cells, and giant cells are not present. Kinyoun's stain, ×1,000

Fig. II.9.30 Large necrotic area with abundant infiltration of mononuclear cells in cerebral parietal cortex. HPS stain, ×250

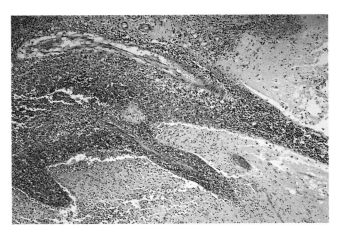

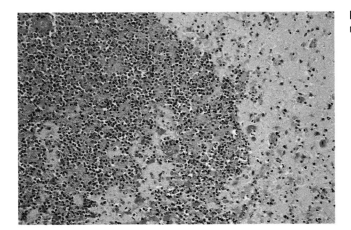

Cerebellar Nocardiosis

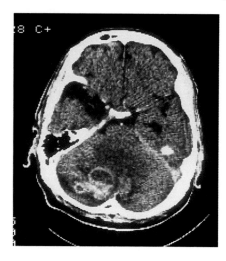

Fig. II.9.31 *Nocardia* asteroides abscess in cerebellum. Multiple irregular, ring-shaped areas of contrast enhancement with surrounding edema involving left cerebellar hemisphere. There is compression of fourth ventricle. Contrast-enhanced CT scan.

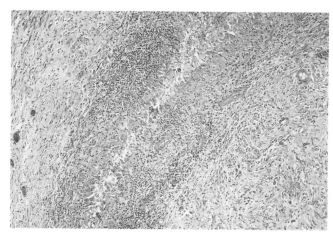

Fig. II.9.32 *Nocardia* asteroides abscess in cerebellum. Large accumulations of inflammatory cells, mostly granulocytes, with central area of necrosis and peripheral fibrosis.

HPS stain, ×100

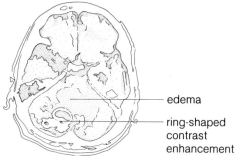

edema

ring-shaped contrast enhancement

Cryptococcal Meningoencephalitis

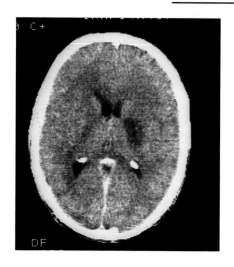

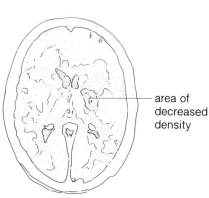

Fig. II.9.33 Oval-shaped area of decreased density within right basal ganglia. Contrast-enhanced CT scan.

area of decreased density

A 40-year-old homosexual man has meningoencephalitis with no other manifestations.

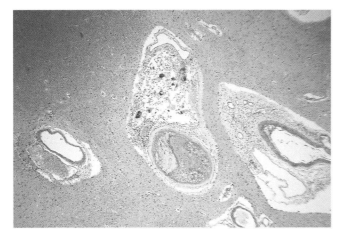

Fig. II.9.34 Leptomeninges around blood vessels in cerebral sulci with edema and inflammatory infiltrates.   HPS stain, ×25

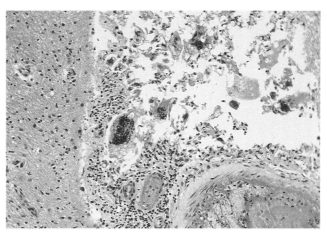

Fig. II.9.35 Cerebral tissue of parietal lobe, and meninges infiltrated by lymphocytes and giant cells containing yeasts.
HPS stain, ×100

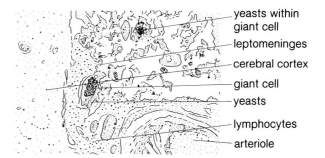

yeasts within giant cell
leptomeninges
cerebral cortex
giant cell
yeasts
lymphocytes
arteriole

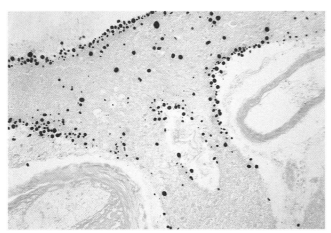

Fig. II.9.36 Silver-stained *Cryptococcus* yeasts of varying size in inflamed meninges.   GMS stain, ×100

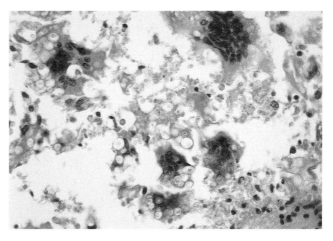

Fig. II.9.37 Multinucleated giant cells in leptomeninges, containing numerous *Cryptococcus* yeasts within intracytoplasmic vacuoles.   HPS stain, ×250

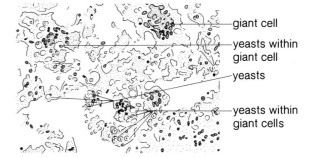

giant cell
yeasts within giant cell
yeasts
yeasts within giant cells

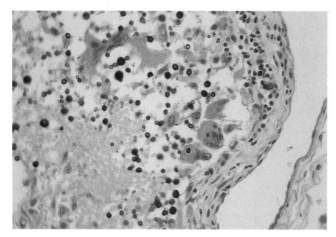

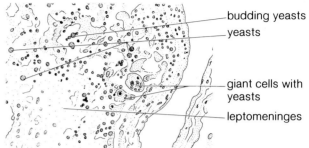

Fig. II.9.38 Mucicarmine-positive *Cryptococcus* yeasts, single or budding, scattered or engulfed in giant cells within inflamed leptomeninges.　　　　Mucicarmine stain, ×250

budding yeasts
yeasts
giant cells with yeasts
leptomeninges

Coccidioidomycosis Meningoencephalitis

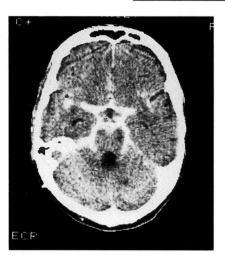

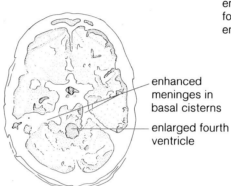

Fig. II.9.39 Intense meningeal enhancement of the basal cisterns. The fourth ventricle is enlarged. Contrast-enhanced CT scan.

enhanced meninges in basal cisterns

enlarged fourth ventricle

Cerebral Toxoplasmosis

Six months after admission for *Pneumocystis carinii* pneumonia, a 33-year-old homosexual man began to manifest neurologic symptoms; he died two months later. At autopsy, multiple large hemorrhagic foci of necrosis are present bilaterally in the cerebral cortex, right midbrain, and basal ganglia.

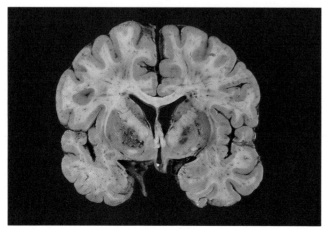

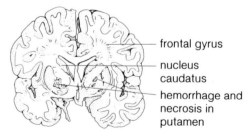

Fig. II.9.40 Coronal brain section. Foci of hemorrhage and necrosis in white matter of frontal gyrus, nucleus caudatus, and putamen.

frontal gyrus
nucleus caudatus
hemorrhage and necrosis in putamen

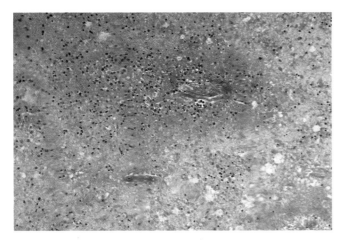

Fig. II.9.41 Cerebral cortex with perivascular area of hemorrhage, necrosis, and accumulation of mononuclear inflammatory cells. H&E stain, ×200

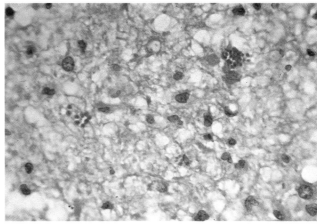

Fig. II.9.42 Cerebral cortex with marked edema, demyelination and two clusters of free tachyzoites. H&E stain, ×400

Fig. II.9.43 Free tachyzoites in midbrain tissues. Congested blood vessel and a few scattered mononuclear inflammatory cells. H&E stain, ×400

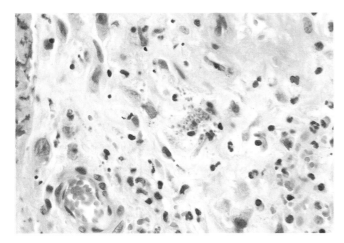

A 40-year-old heroin addict with cerebral toxoplasmosis.

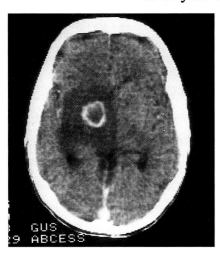

Fig. II.9.44 Irregular ring-shaped area of contrast enhancement within left basal ganglion region, with extensive surrounding zone of edema. Contrast-enhanced CT scan.

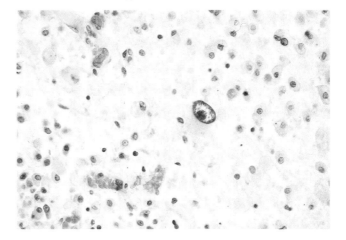

Fig. II.9.45 Pseudocyst with bradyzoites in occipital lobe. No reactive inflammatory cells are present. HPS stain, ×400

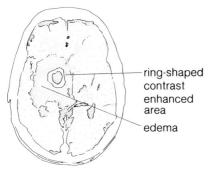

ring-shaped contrast enhanced area

edema

Non-Hodgkin's Lymphoma of Brain

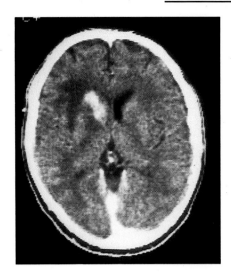

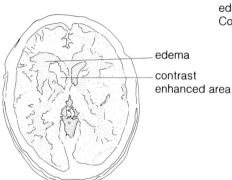

Fig. II.9.46 Amorphous area of contrast enhancement with surrounding edema involving left head of cordate. Contrast-enhanced CT scan.

edema

contrast
enhanced area

**Primary non-Hodgkin's lymphoma of the brain diagnosed in a 40-year-old man
with HIV infection.**

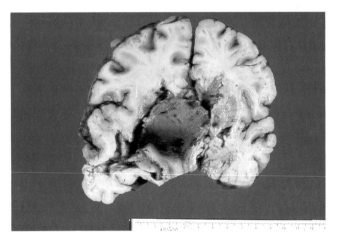

Fig. II.9.47 Firm, focally necrotic, and hemorrhagic 6 x 6 x 10 cm tumor mass, extending from anterior putamen to posterior portion of thalamus, occupying third ventricle and protruding laterally into left parietal and temporal lobes.

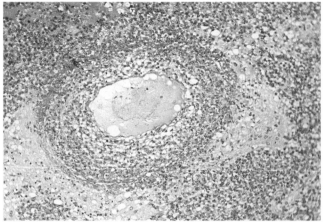

Fig. II.9.48 Dense infiltration of lymphoma cells surrounding a blood vessel and replacing cerebral tissues in temporal lobe.
HPS stain, ×100

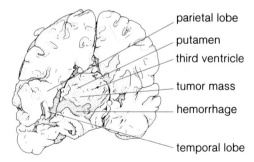

parietal lobe

putamen

third ventricle

tumor mass

hemorrhage

temporal lobe

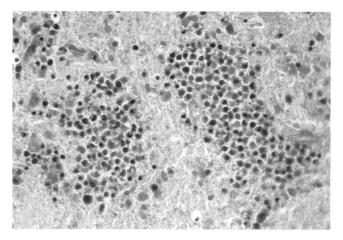

Fig. II.9.49 Large area of necrosis in thalamic region involving both cerebral tissues and lymphoma cells.
HPS stain, ×250

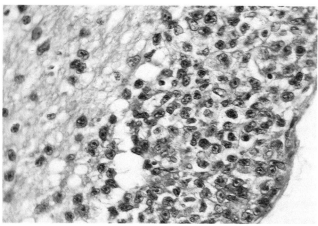

Fig. II.9.50 Lymphoma cells with round nuclei and conspicuous nucleoli accumulating next to third ventricle.
HPS stain, ×400

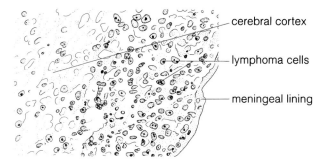

cerebral cortex

lymphoma cells

meningeal lining

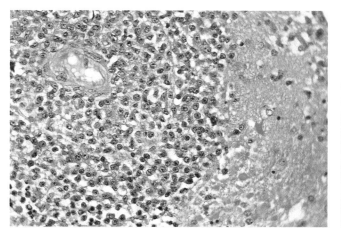

Fig. II.9.51 Uniform population of undifferentiated lymphoma cells with round nuclei, conspicuous nucleoli, and occasional mitoses replacing gray matter of basal nuclei around blood vessel.
HPS stain, ×250

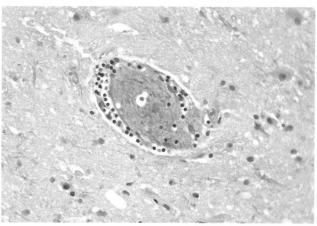

Fig. II.9.52 Lymphoma cells in perivascular space of Virchow-Robin. Vascular lumen is thrombosed; cerebral gray matter is not involved.
HPS stain, ×250

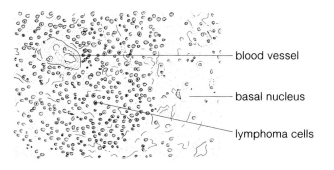

blood vessel

basal nucleus

lymphoma cells

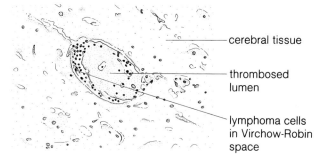

cerebral tissue

thrombosed lumen

lymphoma cells in Virchow-Robin space

A 46-year-old bisexual man is diagnosed as having primary non-Hodgkin's lymphoma (large cleaved cell type).

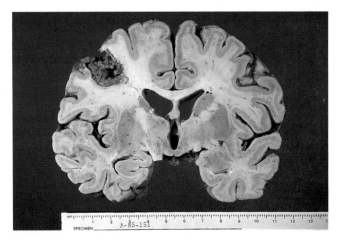

Fig. II.9.53 Coronal brain section. Cavitary, necrotic 2 x 2 cm tumor in cortex of left frontal lobe.

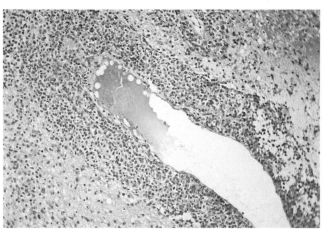

Fig. II.9.54 Large infiltration of lymphoma cells, more dense around vascular space in white matter of frontal lobe.
HPS stain, ×100

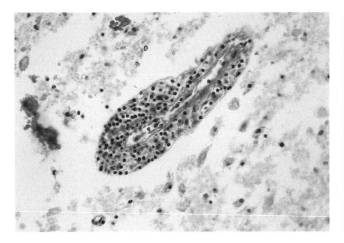

Fig. II.9.55 Lymphoma cells in Virchow-Robin space of cerebral arteriole. Isolated lymphoma cells in cerebral tissue.
HPS stain, ×250

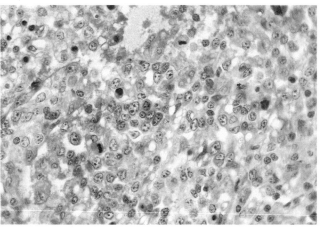

Fig. II.9.56 Non-Hodgkin's lymphoma (undifferentiated Burkitt's-cell type) of cerebrum. Uniform population of lymphoma cells with round nuclei containing several conspicuous nucleoli and frequent mitoses.   HPS stain, ×400

Fig. II.9.57 Undifferentiated lymphoma cells (Burkitt's cell type) with moderate amount of cytoplasm, containing few mitochondria and few cisternae of endoplasmic reticulum. Round nuclei with peripheral chromatin and several nucleoli.
(×10,600)

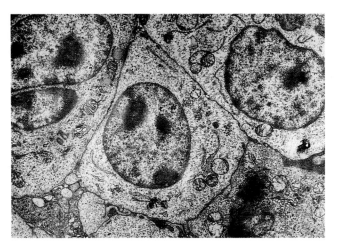

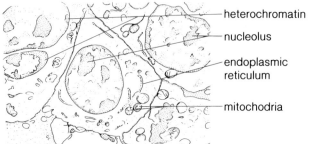

heterochromatin

nucleolus

endoplasmic reticulum

mitochodria

Non-Hodgkin's Lymphoma Cells in CSF

Cytospin of CSF in a 31-year-old homosexual man with non-Hodgkin's lymphoma (large cleaved cell type) of the brain.

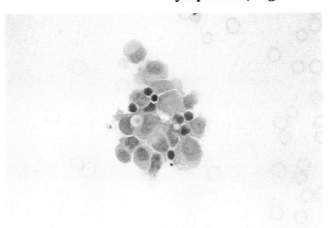

Fig. II.9.58 Cell cluster of lymphoma cells and small mature lymphocytes shows size, proportion, and nuclear shape of the two cell types.   Papanicolaou stain, ×400

Cytospin of CSF in a 37-year-old homosexual man with non-Hodgkin's lymphoma (undifferentiated Burkitt's-cell type) of the brain.

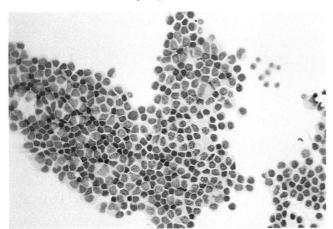

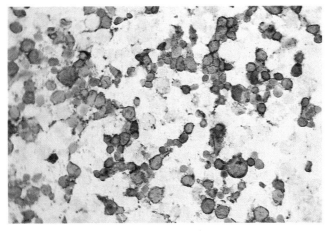

Fig. II.9.59 Homogeneous population of lymphoma cells with large, rounded, pale nuclei, some appearing darkly stained and pyknotic. Few monocytes are included.

Giemsa stain, ×250

Fig. II.9.60 Same section as in Fig. II 9.59. Positive membrane staining of lymphoma cells for κ light-chain immunoglobulin. Staining for λ immunoglobulin was negative.

Perox-antiperox immunostaining with anti-κ antibody, ×250

SPINAL CORD

Vacuolar Myelopathy

Vacuolation of the spinal cord is observed in a man with AIDS.

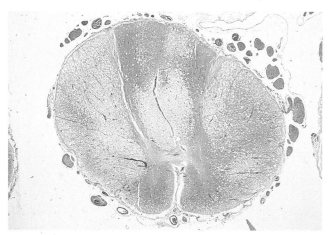

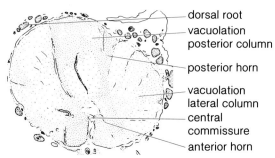

Fig. II.9.61 Lower thoracic spinal cord with marked confluent vacuolation in posterior and lateral columns and mild to moderate vacuolation in anterior columns. (Courtesy of CK Petito)
H&E stain, ×7.92

dorsal root
vacuolation
posterior column
posterior horn
vacuolation
lateral column
central
commissure
anterior horn

Vacuolar myelopathy in a man with AIDS.

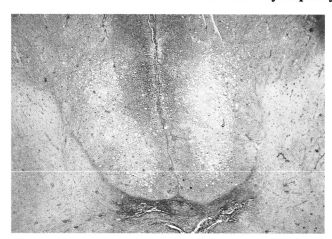

Fig. II.9.62 Cervical spinal cord showing vacuolization of the dorsal columns, most prominently in the cuneate fasciculi. (Courtesy of HV Vinters)
Holzer stain, ×10.5

PERIPHERAL NERVES

Peripheral Neuropathy

An AIDS patient with disseminated Kaposi's sarcoma and polyneuropathy.

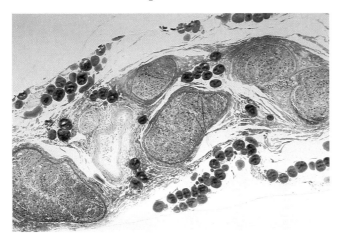

Fig. II.9.63 In a cross section of sural nerve note severe loss of small and large myelinated fibers. The loss is disproportionately greater for the large fibers. (Courtesy of HV Vinters)   Toluidine stain, ×16

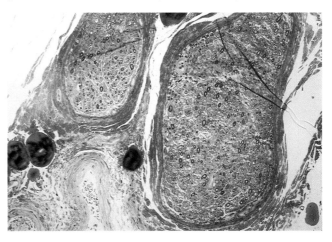

Fig. II.9.64 Higher power view of same section as in Fig. II.9.63 shows marked loss of myelinated fibers. Inflammatory reaction is minimal. (Courtesy of HV Vinters)
Toluidine stain, ×40

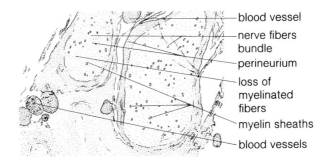

- blood vessel
- nerve fibers bundle
- perineurium
- loss of myelinated fibers
- myelin sheaths
- blood vessels

Eyes

chapter

ten

Kaposi's Sarcoma of Eyelid

A 26-year-old man presents with a raised red-purple nodule, 0.6 x 0.3 cm, on
the medial third of the lower eyelid.

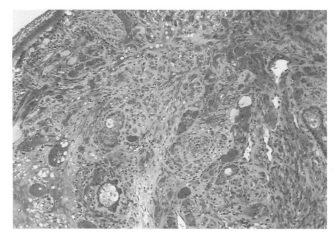

Fig. II.10.1 Eyelid, with hair shafts, gland ducts, and
meibomian glands infiltrated by bundles of spindle-shaped
neoplastic cells and numerous blood vessels.

HPS stain, ×100

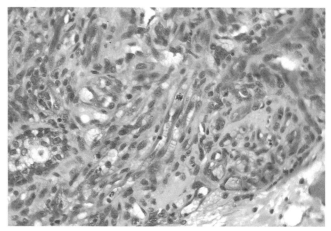

Fig. II.10.2 Neoplastic cells with spindle-shaped nuclei lining
newly formed vascular clefts with red blood cells, having
replaced subcutaneous tissues of eyelid. Residual meibomian
gland.

HPS stain, ×250

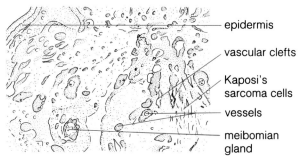

- epidermis
- vascular clefts
- Kaposi's sarcoma cells
- vessels
- meibomian gland

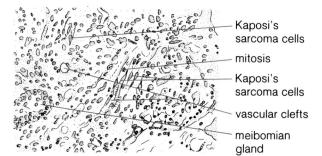

- Kaposi's sarcoma cells
- mitosis
- Kaposi's sarcoma cells
- vascular clefts
- meibomian gland

Fig. II.10.3 Kaposi's sarcoma cells aggregated in bundles or
lining vascular clefts. Nuclei with conspicuous nucleoli and
mitoses.

HPS stain, ×400

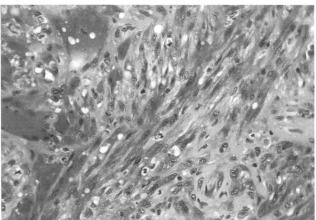

EYE

Cotton Wool Spots

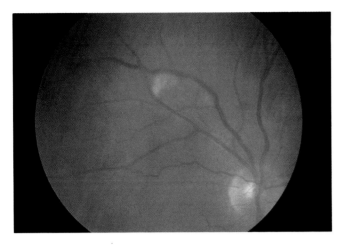

Fig. II.10.4 Retina of right eye, with cotton wool spot lying between superior temporal vein and artery.

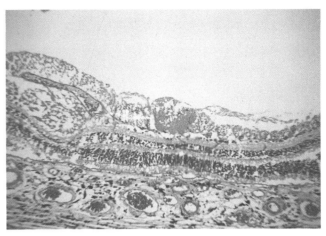

Fig. II.10.5 Cytoid body located in the retina.
H&E stain, ×100

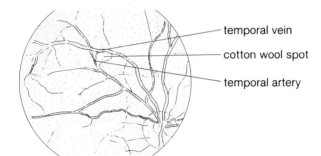

temporal vein

cotton wool spot

temporal artery

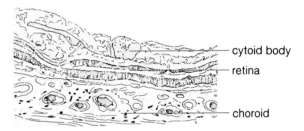

cytoid body

retina

choroid

Fig. II.10.6 Cytoid body in retina, showing markedly swollen axons.
H&E stain, ×600

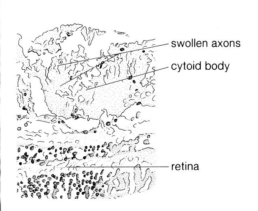

swollen axons

cytoid body

retina

Cytomegalovirus Retinitis

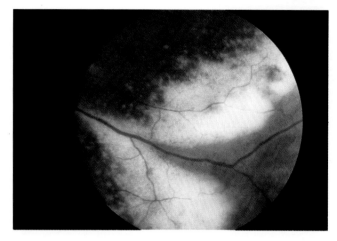

Fig. II.10.7 Areas of retinal necrosis adjacent to retinal vessels with associated intraretinal hemorrhages.

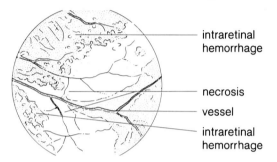

- intraretinal hemorrhage
- necrosis
- vessel
- intraretinal hemorrhage

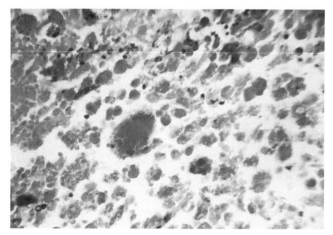

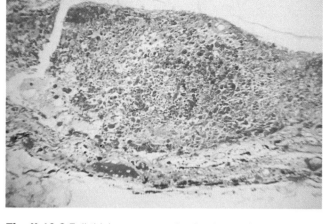

Fig. II.10.8 Full-thickness necrosis of retina and retinal pigment epithelium. Retinal architecture is totally destroyed.
H&E stain, ×150

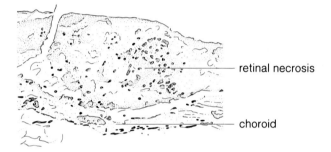

- retinal necrosis
- choroid

Fig. II.10.9 Retinal necrosis with CMV inclusions within retinal cells.
H&E stain, ×600

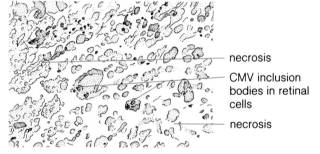

- necrosis
- CMV inclusion bodies in retinal cells
- necrosis

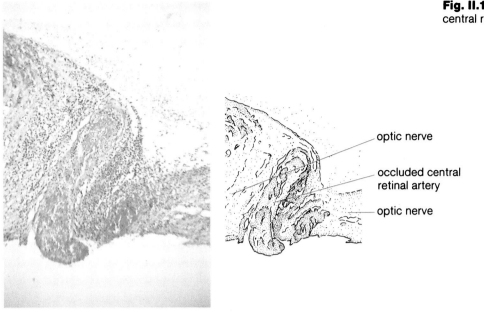

Fig. II.10.10 Optic nerve with occluded central retinal artery.   H&E stain, ×150

optic nerve

occluded central retinal artery

optic nerve

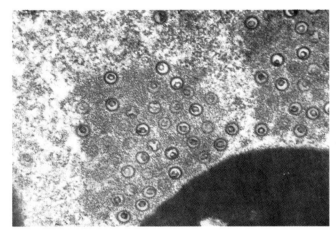

Fig. II.10.11 CMV particles within nucleus of infected retinal cell.   (×60,000)

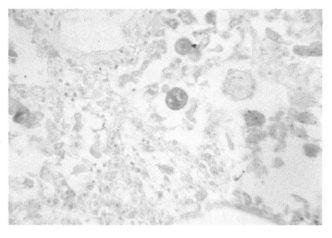

Fig. II.10.12 CMV particles stained with anti-CMV antibody, and indirect immunoperoxidase.   ×625

Fig. II.10.13 Retina with abundant leukocytic infiltrate in AIDS patient with CMV retinitis treated with Gancyclovir.
H&E stain, ×300

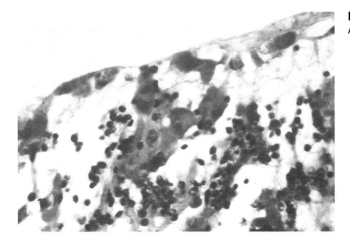

Herpes Simplex Virus Retinitis

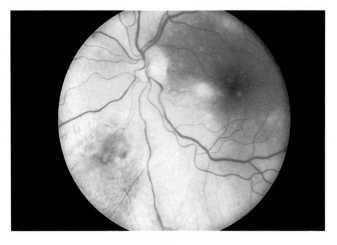

Fig. II.10.14 Areas of retinal necrosis found in AIDS patient with HSV retinitis around the optic nerve.

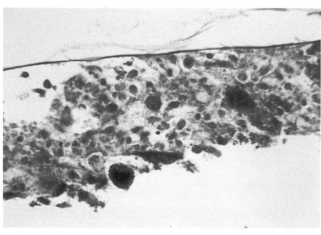

Fig. II.10.15 Necrotic retina with total destruction of retinal structures.

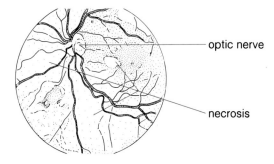

optic nerve

necrosis

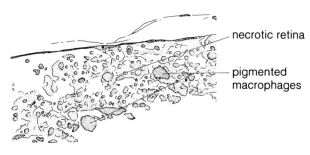

necrotic retina

pigmented macrophages

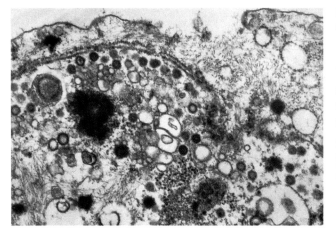

Fig. II.10.16 Occluded retinal vessel.

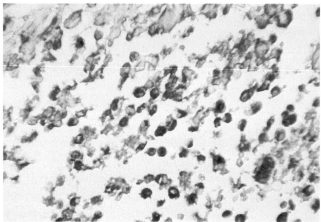

Fig. II.10.17 HSV-1 particles in necrotic retina. Immunoperoxidase stain wtih anti-HSV-1 antibody, ×625

Fig. II.10.18 Multiple HSV-1 particles within nucleus of retinal cell.   (×40,000)

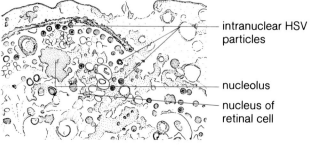

intranuclear HSV particles

nucleolus

nucleus of retinal cell

Ophthalmic Infections with Herpes Zoster Virus

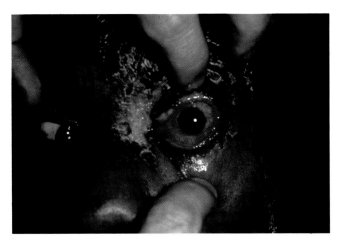

Fig. II.10.19 HZV vesicular lesions with severe epidermal necrosis on distribution area of first division of trigeminal nerve. Patient also has ophthalmoplegia and is unable to abduct the left eye.

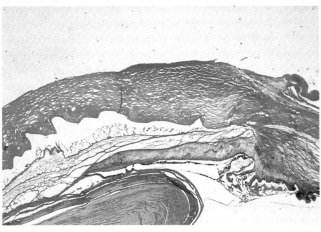

Fig. II.10.20 Necrotic cornea. Fibrinous exudate in anterior chamber. Necrotic iris.

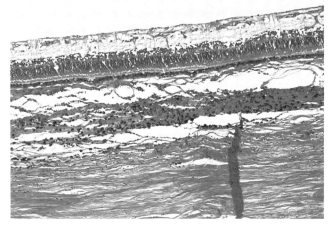

Fig. II.10.21 Atrophic retina. Ganglion cell layer and internal nuclear layer are absent. Long ciliary nerve is degenerated.

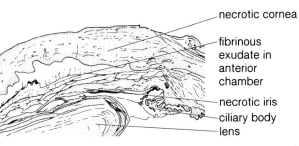

necrotic cornea

fibrinous exudate in anterior chamber

necrotic iris
ciliary body
lens

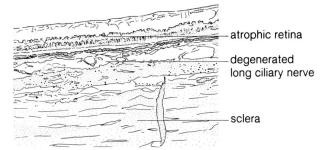

atrophic retina

degenerated long ciliary nerve

sclera

Fig. II.10.22 Demyelinated long ciliary nerve.

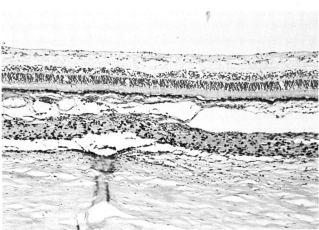

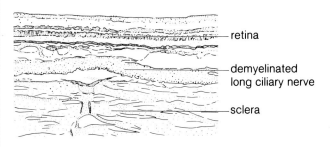

retina

demyelinated long ciliary nerve

sclera

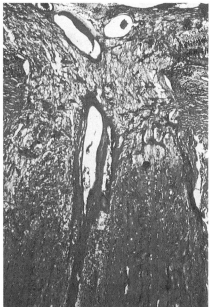

Fig. II.10.23
Necrosis of anterior portion of optic nerve.

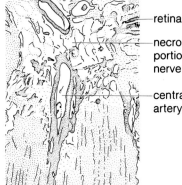

retina

necrotic anterior portion of optic nerve

central retinal artery

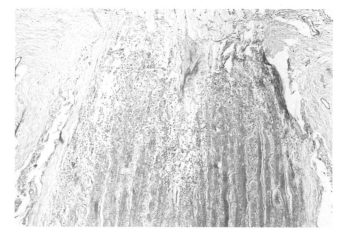

Fig. II.10.24 Demyelination of optic nerve shown by luxol-fast-blue stain. One area of nerve is less affected.

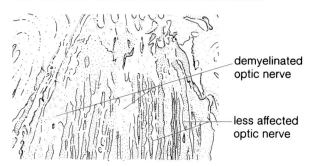

demyelinated optic nerve

less affected optic nerve

Ophthalmic Infections with *Toxoplasma gondii*

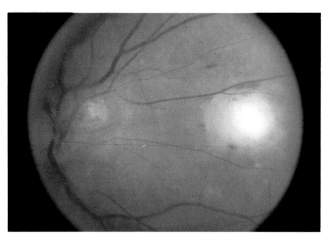

Fig. II.10.25 Involvement of the retina in an AIDS patient with cerebral toxoplasmosis. Circumscribed white lesions in the fundus.

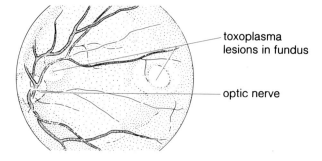

toxoplasma lesions in fundus

optic nerve

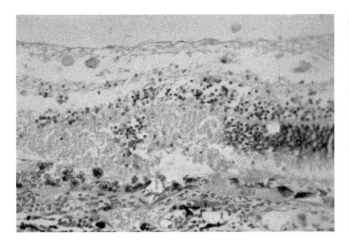

Fig. II.10.26 Focal area of necrosis in the retina with disruption of retinal pigment epithelium. Choroid with diffuse inflammation.   H&E stain, ×150

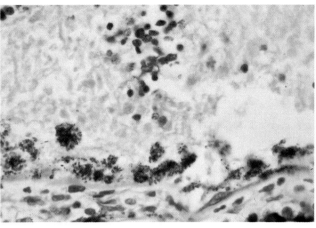

Fig. II.10.27 Same section as in Fig. II.10.26, showing the presence of *Toxoplasma gondii* tachyzoites in necrotic retina.
                              H&E stain, ×450

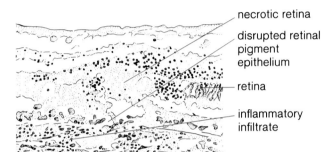

necrotic retina

disrupted retinal pigment epithelium

retina

inflammatory infiltrate

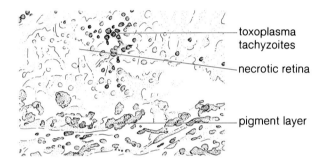

toxoplasma tachyzoites

necrotic retina

pigment layer

Candida albicans Retinitis

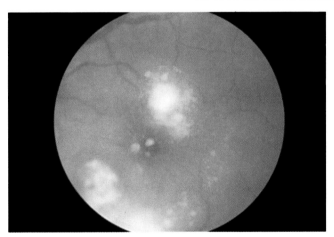

Fig. II.10.28 Multiple lesions, isolated and confluent, in retina of male IV drug addict.

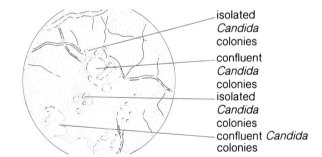

isolated *Candida* colonies

confluent *Candida* colonies

isolated *Candida* colonies

confluent *Candida* colonies

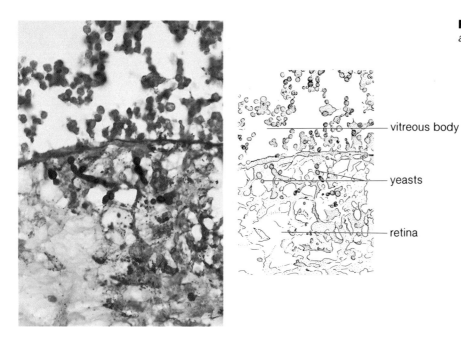

Fig. II.10.29 Yeasts of *Candida albicans* in retina.

vitreous body

yeasts

retina

Endophthalmitis with *Hemophilus influenzae*

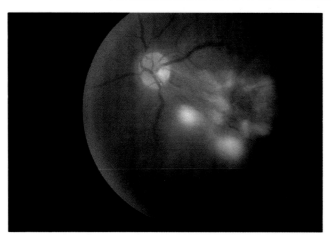

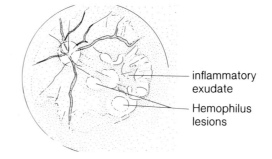

Fig. II.10.30 Left eye with two lesions and exudative inflammation on macular area that progressed to full-blown endophthalmitis.

inflammatory exudate

Hemophilus lesions

Non-Hodgkin's Lymphoma of Eye

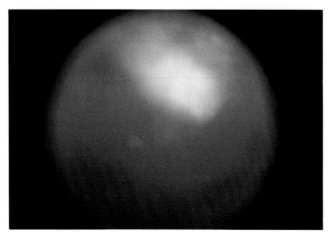

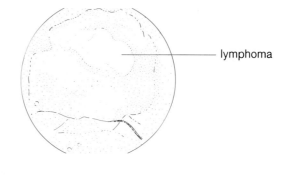

Fig. II.10.31 Large lesion with indistinct borders in fundus of eye.

lymphoma

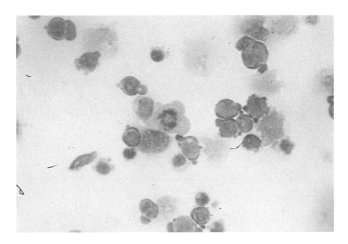

Fig. II.10.32 Non-Hodgkin's lymphoma cells (large-cell type) in aspirate of vitreous body. Lymphoma cell in mitosis at center.   Giemsa stain, ×400

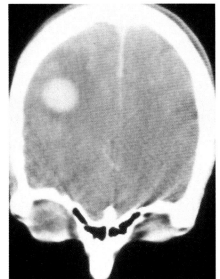
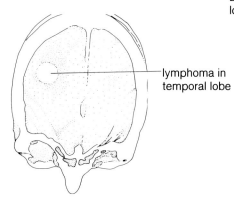

Fig. II.10.33 Same patient as in Fig. II.10.32, also had cerebral lymphoma. Large round tumor apparent in temporal lobe on CT scan.

lymphoma in temporal lobe

INDEX

Note: The numbers in **boldface** type refer to Figure numbers

Esophagitis
  in candidiasis, 51, 174–175, **II.5.23–24**
  cytomegalovirus, 175, **II.5.24–25**
  herpetic, 31, 175, **II.5.26**
Esophagus, Kaposi's sarcoma of, 176, **II.5.27**
Eye disorders, 94–95
  Candida albicans retinitis, 51, 241–242, **II.10.28–29**
  cotton wool spots in, 95, 235, **II.10.4–6**
  cytomegalovirus retinitis, 26, 28, 94, 236–237, **II.10.7–13**
  endophthalmitis with *Hemophilus influenzae*, 242, **II.10.30**
  herpes simplex retinitis, 94, 238, **II.10.14–18**
  herpes zoster infections, 239–240, **II.10.19–24**
  Kaposi's sarcoma of lid, 83, 95, 234, **II.10.1–3**
  lymphoma, 89, 95, 242–243, **II.10.31–33**
  in toxoplasmosis, 72, 95, 240–241, **II.10.25–27**

F

Foreign-body granulomas, pulmonary, 161, **II.4.56**
Fungal diseases, secondary, 50–65
  aspergillosis, 52–54, **I.5.2,** 150–151, **II.4.21–25**
  blastomycosis, 62–63, **I.5.6,** 156–157, **II.4.39–41**
  candidiasis, 50–51. *See also* Candidiasis
  coccidioidomycosis, 60–61, **I.5.5.** *See also* Coccidioidomycosis
  cryptococcosis, 58–59, **I.5.4.** *See also* Cryptococcosis
  histoplasmosis, 56–57, **I.5.3,** 154, **II.4.32–34,** 192, **II.5.75–77**
  mucormycosis, 64–65, **I.5.7,** 157–158, **II.4.42–45**
  nocardiosis, 54–55, 222, **II.9.31–32**

G

Gallbladder, cryptosporidiosis of, 74, 193, **II.5.80**
Gastrointestinal tract. *See specific gastrointestinal organs*
Gemistocytic astrocytes in progressive multifocal
  leukoencephalopathy, 38, **I.3.8,** 219, **II.9.18, 21**
Genital tract
  carcinomas of, 91–92
  condylomata of, 33–34, 204, **II.7.2–3,** 206–207, **II.7.9–10**
  cytomegalovirus prostatitis, 28, **I.3.3,** 205–206, **II.7.6–7**
  herpesvirus infections, 30, 205, **II.7.6,** 207, **II.7.11**
Giant cells, multinucleated
  in progressive encephalopathy of childhood, 105
  in subacute encephalitis, 9, **I.1.6,** 214–215, **II.9.2–4,** 216,
    II.9.8
Glomerulosclerosis, focal and segmental, 21–22, 198, **II.6.1–3**
Granulomas
  in blastomycosis, 62, 156, **II.4.39–40**
  in bone-marrow, 14–15, 121, **II.2.4–5**
  in coccidioidomycosis, 61
  in cryptococcosis, 59, 152, **II.4.27–28**
  in histoplasmosis, 56
  in mycobacteriosis, 46
  pulmonary, foreign-body, 161, **II.4.56**
Gums, lymphoma of, 171, **II.5.12–13**

H

Hassall's corpuscles in thymic dysplasia, 13
Heart
  in aspergillosis, 53
  in candidiasis, 51
  cardiomyopathy of, 140, **II.3.1–3**
  lymphoma of, 88, 141–142, **II.3.4–7**
  in toxoplasmosis, 72
Hemophilus influenzae, endophthalmitis with, 242, **II.10.30**
Hepatitis, chronic active, 189, **II.5.67–68**
Herpes simplex infection
  anal, 31, 186–187, **II.5.58–60,** 207, **II.7.11**
  and carcinomas of genital tract, 91
  cutaneous, 30–31, **I.3.4–5,** 112–114, **II.1.2–9**
  encephalitis, 31–32, 216–217, **II.9.9–13**
  esophagitis, 31, 175, **II.5.26**
  gastric, 30, 176–177, **II.5.28–29**

tuberculosis of, 45, 190, **II.5.69–71**
Lung conditions. *See* Respiratory tract
Lymph nodes, 123–135
   coccidioidomycosis of, 132, **II.2.46**
   cryptococcal lymphadenitis of, 130–132, **II.2.38–45**
   Hodgkin's lymphoma of, 134–135, **II.2.52–53**
   isosporiasis of, 76
   Kaposi's sarcoma of, 84, 133–134, **II.2.48–51**
   lymphoma of, 88, **I.7.4C,** 89, 135, **II.2.54–55**
   mycobacteriosis of, 128–130, **II.2.32–37**
   persistent generalized lymphadenopathy of, 2–5, 123–128
      type I or type A, 2, 123–125, **II.2.12–20**
      type II or type B, 5, 127, **II.2.26–27**
      type III or type C, 3, 127–128, **II.2.28–31**
      Langerhans cells stained with anti-S-100 antibody in, 3,
        I.1.1, 126, **II.2.23**
      morphologic features of viral particles in, 4, **I.1.3,** 126,
        II.2.24
      tubuloreticular structures and vesicular bodies in, 4–5, **I.1.4–**
        5, 125–126, **II.2.21–21**
      virus antigen deposits in, 3, **I.1.2,** 126, **II.2.25**
   salivary gland lymphadenopathy of, 23–24, 171–173, **II.5.14–**
      19
   toxoplasmosis of, 71, 133, **II.2.47**
Lymphoma, 80, 87–90, **I.7.4–6**
   of bladder, 201, **II.6.10**
   of bone marrow, 15, 122, **II.2.8–9**
   of brain, 88, 226–229, **II.9.46–60**
   of cervical lymph nodes, 89, 135, **II.2.54–55**
   of colon, 183–184, **II.5.50–51**
   of eye, 89, 95, 242–243, **II.10.31–33**
   of gums, 171, **II.5.12–13**
   of heart, 88, 141–142, **II.3.4–7**
   Hodgkin's. *See* Hodgkin's lymphoma
   of ileum, 180–181, **II.5.39–41**
   of kidney, 89, 200, **II.6.9**
   of liver, 193, **II.5.79**
   of lung, 163–165, **II.4.61–67**
   of lymph nodes, 88, **I.7.4C,** 89, 135, **II.2.54–55**
   of rectum and anus, 185–186, **II.5.54–57**
   of retroperitoneum, 89, **I.7.6,** 196, **II.5.87–88**
   of salivary glands, 23, 173–174, **II.5.20–22**
   of seminal vesicle, 206, **II.7.8**
   of skin, 89, 118, **II.1.22–23**
   of stomach, 177, **II.5.31**

Macrophages
   in histoplasmosis, 56
   in mycobacteriosis, 46–47, **I.4.2**
Meningoencephalitis, tuberculous, 45, 220–221, **II.9.24–30**
Mineralization of blood vessels in subacute encephalitis, 9, **I.1.7,**
   215, **II.9.7**
Molluscum contagiosum, 100–101, **I.9.1,** 114–115, **II.1.11–13**
   of penis, 204, **II.7.1**
Mouth
   candidiasis of tongue, 50–51, **I.5.1,** 169, **II.5.7**
   hairy leukoplakia of tongue, 35–36, **I.3.6,** 168–169, **II.5.1–6**
   Kaposi's sarcoma of, 83, 169, **II.5.6,** 170, **II.5.8–11**
   lymphoma of gum, 171, **II.5.12–13**
Mucormycosis, 64–65, **I.5.7,** 157–158, **I.4.42–45**
Multinucleated cells
   in blastomycosis, 63, **I.5.6,** 156, **II.4.40**
   giant cells
      in progressive encephalopathy of childhood, 105
      in subacute encephalitis, 9, **I.1.6,** 214–215, **II.9.2–4,** 216,
      II.9.8

Respiratory tract
  aspergillosis, pulmonary, 52–54, **I.5.2**, 150–151, **II.4.21–25**
  blastomycosis, pulmonary, 62, I.5.6, 156–157, II.4.39–41
  candidiasis, pulmonary, 51, 149–150, **II.4.16–20**
  coccidioidomycosis, pulmonary, 60, 155–156, II.4.35–38
  cryptococcosis, pulmonary, 59, 152–153, **II.4.26–31**
  cytomegalovirus pneumonitis, 26–27, 31, **I.3.1–2**, 147,
    II.4.10–11
  foreign-body granuloma, pulmonary, 161, **II.4.56**
  histoplasmosis, pulmonary, 56, **I.5.3**, 154, **II.4.32–34**
  Kaposi's sarcoma, pulmonary, 84, 161–162, **II.4.57–60**
  Legionella pneumonia, 42–43, **I.4.1**, 147–148, **II.4.12–14**
  lymphocytic interstitial pneumonitis, 7, 144, **II.4.1–3**
    in children, 104, 145–146, **II.4.4–9**
  lymphoma of lung, 163–165, **II.4.61–67**
  mucormycosis, pulmonary, 64, **I.5.7**, 157–158, **II.4.42–45**
  mycobacteriosis, pulmonary, 46, 148, **II.4.15**
  pneumocystosis, 68–70, **I.6.1**, 158–160, **II.4.46–55**
  toxoplasmosis, pulmonary, 71, I.6.2, 72
Retina, cotton wool spots in, 95, 235, **II.10.4–6**
Retinitis
  Candida albicans, 51, 241–242, **II.10.28–29**
  cytomegalovirus, 26, 28, 94, 236–237, **II.10.7–13**
  herpes simplex, 94, 238, **II.10.14–18**
  in toxoplasmosis, 72, 240–241, **II.10.25–27**
Retroperitoneum, lymphoma of, 89, **I.7.6**, 196, **II.5.87–88**
Rhinocerebral lesions in mucormycosis, 64

Salivary glands
  lymphadenopathy of, 23–24, 172–173, **II.5.14–19**
  lymphomas of, 23, 173–174, **II.5.20–22**
Sarcoma, Kaposi. *See* Kaposi's sarcoma
Seborrheic dermatitis, 99, 112, **II.1.1**
Secondary diseases
  bacterial, 42–47
  fungal, 50–65
  neoplastic, 80–92
  protozoal, 68–76
  viral, 26–38
Seminal vesicles, lymphoma of, 206, **II.7.8**
Siderocalcinosis of blood vessels in subacute encephalitis, 9,
  I.1.7, 215, **II.9.7**
Skin conditions, 98–101
  cryptococcosis, 59
  herpes simplex infection, 30–31, **I.3.4–5**, 112–114, **II.1.2–9**
  herpes zoster infection, 30, 114, **II.1.10**
  Kaposi's sarcoma, 83, 115–117, **II.1.14–21**
  lymphoma, 89, 118, **II.1.22–23**
  molluscum contagiosum, 100–101, **I.9.1**, 114–115, **II.1.11–13**
  mucormycosis, 64
  seborrheic dermatitis, 99, 112, **II.1.1**
Spinal cord, vacuolar myelopathy of, 11, 230, **II.9.61–62**
Spleen
  candidiasis of, 51
  coccidioidomycosis of, 138, **II.2.63**
  in immune thrombocytopenic purpura, 17, 136–137, **II.2.56–
    59**
  mycobacteriosis of, 46, 137–138, **II.2.61–62**
  tuberculosis of, 137, **II.2.60**
Sporangia in coccidioidomycosis, 60, 61, **I.5.5**, 155, **II.4.36–37**
Sporozoites in isosporiasis, 76, **I.6.5**
Stomach
  herpesvirus infection of, 30, 176–177, **II.5.28–29**
  Kaposi's sarcoma of, 177, **II.5.30**
  lymphoma of, 177, **II.5.31**
  mucormycosis of, 64